Suspension Fitness

The Easy Way to Improve Strength, Endurance, and Overall Health

Tracy Christenson, M.S.

Suspended Fitness

ACKNOWLEDGMENTS

This has been a three-year endeavor that has consumed thousands of hours. I've been through several editors and revisions as we fought the clock to bring this book to fruition.

I need to thank the following people:

My husband, Coach Richard Wharton, and my parents, Mark and Alison Christenson, for their support and belief in me on so many levels. You helped me overcome the many setbacks I encountered along the way and reach the finish line.

Dean Markham for the time and work he has provided with the photography and videography over the last several years.

My friends and clients Melissa, Travis, and CJ, and Michele for being outstanding models.

Richard "Ro" O'Conner, who came along just in time to help me get this project back on track. Unfortunately, he passed away before the completion. I am extremely grateful for his expertise and guidance.

My two dogs, Petey and Jake, for putting up with many missed walks and broken promises of playtime that got pushed aside for work.

All those who have been willing to share their knowledge by providing opportunities for continuing education, seminars, conferences, and certification courses that I have been fortunate enough to attend through the years. You gave me the knowledge and confidence to put this manual together and get it out in the public eye.

CONTENTS

Preface

Health-related problems due to obesity, stress, and inactivity are a huge concern for both individuals and society. Furthermore, people are busier than ever. I see the struggles people have trying to balance the immediate demands of everyday life, with a desire to be fit and healthy. Most often, people understand and truly want to be more active, fit, and healthy. However, there is always something competing for time and opportunities, and the immediate need usually takes precedent over a long-term plan for better health and fitness.

I see these struggles in the lives of my friends and clients. I have also experienced these struggles myself through the demands of running a small business, managing advanced education, handling a fixer-upper house full of dogs, and needing to generate income through additional means while building the business (and putting together this book). Even in my case, when I had all the tools and knowledge, it was still tough.

It was tough, but it was doable.

I wanted to bring those tools and knowledge to the people I saw around me who were struggling to bring better health and fitness into their lives. Individuals who truly wanted change but didn't have the resources. Those who didn't have the time available to attend exercise classes or make the trip to the gym several times a week. People who didn't have the resources to hire a personal trainer. People who didn't know where to start.

I also wanted to show people something different. When I go into traditional fitness centers, I still see people walking around through rows of machines, each machine isolating one area of the body. Sometimes they are following a workout routine that they have been doing for months or years. They look bored, they are rarely sweating or breathing even moderately hard, and often they are poorly fitted to the machine. Although training with suspension is not new, I feel it is vastly underused, and most people don't realize the incredible benefits.

When I have introduced a suspension and body-weight training approach to clients or friends, they have been exceptionally receptive.

The following comments really stood out:

"This is fun…like water-skiing!"

"The machines at the gym make my wrist hurt, but this feels OK."

"I can really feel this in my core!"

In addition to working with the general population through personal training, working with a community of cyclists, runners, and triathletes through our cycling studio gave me a whole different perspective. A lot of them actually did have time (although it was often limited) or made time for their training, but it usually wasn't easy. There was also less time left for strength work after their endurance workouts. Because they loved to run or ride, that's what they wanted to do with the time they had, and strength workouts often got pushed off the cliff. Those who did go to the gym often performed programs too reliant on traditional machine work that was less unique to the demands of their endurance activity. Machine work didn't always transfer over in the most efficient way to support their training goals. I wanted to do something for them as well.

Coming Up with a Solution

Training with suspension and your own body weight is a method that works. It's not a gimmick, and it can benefit a wide range of abilities and goals. It's also fun, and it can be done anywhere! I can't think of a better approach for achieving greater strength and fitness, especially for busy professionals, or those looking for better performance, emphasizing moving their body weight, versus moving plates and dumbbells. You achieve more in less time. You improve the ability of your muscles to function together and work as one unit, which transfers most efficiently to real-world physical demands. You can also tailor any workout to your level and goals.

What I love is that this is so useful for so many different fitness populations. Beginners, advanced exercisers, seniors, athletes, stay-at-home moms, working professionals, and post-rehab clients are all people with whom I have used suspension training, and we've experienced successful outcomes. However, until the writing of this book, the information out there was still sparse and inconsistent and not always of the greatest quality. My goal is to display what I use and have been able to share with my clients, to a wider audience, at a lower cost than I could ever offer through group or individual training. I want this book to achieve the following:

- Introduce people to a method of achieving better health and fitness to which they have never been exposed.

- Provide a higher confidence level to those who want to try it at a fitness center or at home.

- Provide motivation to start or continue with a fitness approach by providing information on the substantial benefits to health and performance.

- Provide direction on how to get started and how to design your own workouts and programs based on your goals and other active endeavors in perpetuity.

I hope I have been successful in that, and I hope I am able to provide at least some enhancement to your personal fitness program.

Introduction

I began my career as a personal trainer at a large fitness center in Dallas, Texas. Early in my time there, I remember seeing one of the more innovative instructors—who was also a cycling and triathlon coach—experiment with a suspension trainer during off-peak hours. This took place in the corner of the fitness center's free-weight area. It was like nothing I had seen before. As a young and relatively new trainer, educated in the traditional approach, combining machines, free weights, and some cardio, I filed this new method away in my mind.

A couple of years later, a little more confident as a strength and conditioning professional and looking to expand my skill set, I purchased my own suspension training kit and started to experiment. A TRX® Suspension Training Certification course came soon after, and I started a gradual but complete shift in my training style for my clients, as well as myself. This change wasn't a conscious move, but the suspension method felt so much better than what I'd been teaching. I gravitated toward it, made it a focus of my fitness program, and it was well received by my clients.

I shifted away from machines and isolation exercises toward a more functional approach to supporting and strengthening whole-body movement patterns we all use in everyday life as well as in our chosen sports. This method requires the body to work as a unit, and I learned ways to develop and improve techniques to achieve this, and then tailor them in unique ways for individuals. Suspension training fits very well into my evolving philosophy of what an outstanding training program should be.

TRX® is the pioneer equipment brand and is the most widely recognized name among many high-quality suspended products available. The equipment is easy to obtain, and with basic setup prices relatively low, suspension training has, not surprisingly, become widely known and practiced across the world in recent years. A significant population of professional and amateur athletes and fitness enthusiasts have heard of it and tried it, and many now even own a suspended trainer. But because it requires a little more technique and body awareness, suspension training has a learning curve and can be a little intimidating to novices.

People with more experience in physical conditioning are often more comfortable self-starting with suspension training, but when those individuals come to me for some fine-tuning or to learn about working very specific movement patterns, I sometimes see fundamental positional errors that have been ingrained through repetition and have become bad habits.

My goal with this book is to provide all the basic information on how to get the most out of this type of training, whether it be as supplemental resistance training for endurance athletes; as a means of achieving general fitness to assist with overall well-being and daily life; or a short, do-anywhere workout for business travelers for whom something is a lot better than nothing. Resources in this book will guide you in learning to use suspension training in the gym, at home, or on the road.

I hope this book helps you discover the rewards of suspension training and that you achieve the same success with it as my clients and I have.

How to Use This Book

This book is divided into three main sections. I recommend you read all of section 1, dip into section 2 as relevant to your needs and interests, and use section 3 as a referenced instructional resource.

Section 1: Chapters 1–4

This section covers essential information about the basics, including equipment setup, the progression in adjusting resistance levels, technique, external loading, and how to be comfortable training with suspension anywhere, at any level, and for any objective.

Section 2: Chapters 5–12

Here you'll find specific applications of suspension training and programs designed for building a solid foundation of strength and stability. I'll guide you through designing a program for specific goals, such as cardiovascular fitness, strength, and flexibility. There are also sections on strength training for cycling, running, and improved bone health. Each of these applications has its own chapter for quick reference, with guidance for readers at distinct levels of skill and experience. For several of the chapters, there are corresponding sample workouts at the end of the book with precise instructions on performing each exercise.

Section 3: Exercise Libraries and Toolbox Section

I've included comprehensive exercise libraries divided into upper, lower, core, and full body. These include exercises performed with suspension, as well as body-weight movements that require no additional equipment. Each movement contains detailed written and photographic instructions, with progressions and modifications for readers as their requirements develop. The toolbox chapter offers some ideas for workout sets and approaches to prevent things from getting stagnant and keep your program fun and interesting. The sample workouts give you programs to get started and a template to use going forward when designing your own workouts.

Section 1

Setup and Technique

.

Chapter 1

What It Is, and Who It's For

Origins and Development

Training with suspension using your own body weight is at the heart of everything in this book. Training with suspension is not new, but it has evolved and is being more widely recognized as a valuable and useful tool. Evidence of rope training dates back to the mid-1800s for many athletes, while gymnasts and trapeze artists have long performed aspects of their sports using suspension. If you have ever watched the "rings" competition in gymnastics, you have seen a form of suspension training.

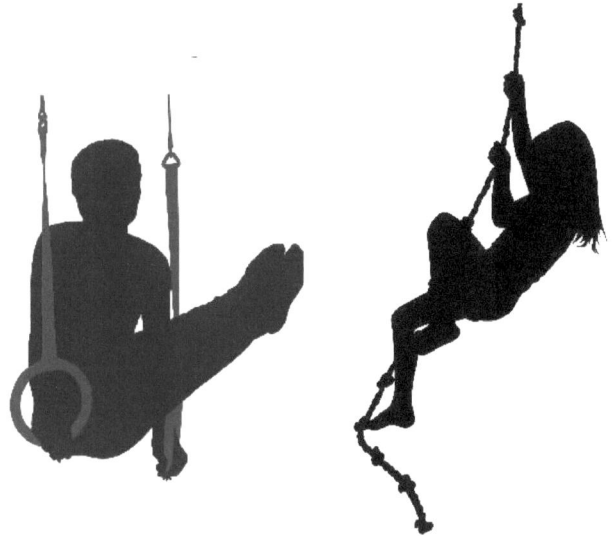

Since the mid-1990s, a variety of suspended training systems have been commercially available to professional trainers, home users, and the like. The most popular and widely recognized system is the TRX® Suspension Trainer.

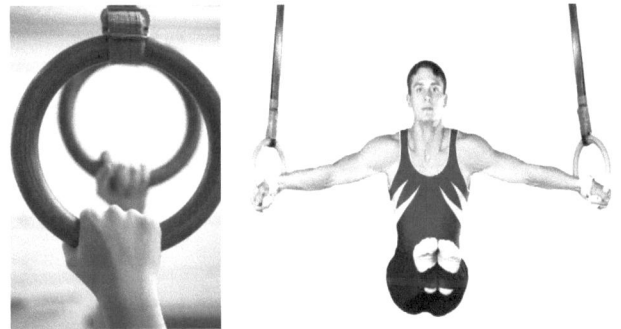

Randy Hetrick, a former US Navy SEAL and Stanford MBA graduate, developed the Total Resistance eXercise (TRX®) equipment and the associated suspended training body-weight exercises in the 1990s. As a SEAL out in the field, he developed what would later become the popular TRX® Suspension Trainer with an old Jiu-Jitsu belt and some surplus parachute webbing.

The suspension exercises and concepts discussed in this book are not limited to the TRX® Suspension Trainer, but can be practiced with a variety of suspension training brands available at a range of price points.

What It Is

Suspension training uses your own body weight as resistance. It is portable, extremely versatile, and can be used for building functional strength, balance, core stability, and flexibility. Most movements in suspension training can be easily modified to suit a variety of fitness and ability levels.

By using suspension training as a tool, new exercisers, as well as experienced fitness enthusiasts and athletes, can create workouts to suit a variety of objectives and ability levels. Novice exercisers will appreciate the joint-friendly and easily adjustable resistances offered by the movements. Athletes at advanced fitness levels will appreciate the progressions and easy transitions between movements. Athletes using suspension training notice significant gains in the performance of everyday activities as well as when cycling, running, and swimming. If done correctly, suspension training can be one of the most functional and efficient ways to train the body in both solo and group settings.

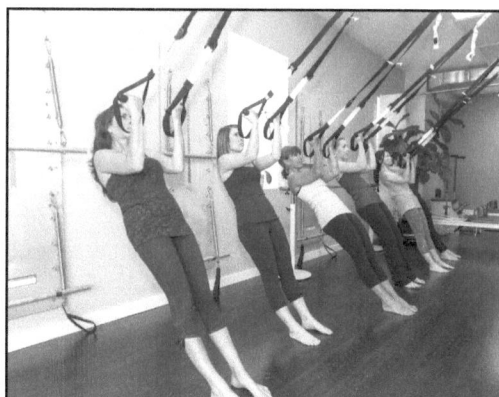

Suspended Training Alone or Combined

Scientific studies evaluating suspended-type training, point to the value of its use as a stand-alone tool, or as a combined component of your workout program. One study of trunk muscle activation looked at the "plank" movement, performed on a stable surface, such as a floor, and compared it to performing the same movement with the feet and arms suspended. The highest level of abdominal muscle activation was shown to occur when the arms and/or the feet were suspended.[1] as is practiced in suspended training. A study by Behm and Kible demonstrated that instability resistance training is effective, and suggested that it be incorporated in conjunction with traditional, stable training, to provide a greater variety of training experiences.[2]

In a resistance training program for strength or rehabilitation, including both stable and unstable exercises is an effective way to make sure you are training your capacity for both strength as well as balance, by challenging the neuromuscular system through a range of movements.[3]

Suspended Training Is Appropriate for All Ability Levels

Suspended training makes body-weight training accessible to a broad spectrum of abilities. This is because the resistance levels are so easy to adjust. When you are hanging on the straps, whatever percent of your body weight is being supported by the straps is the weight with which you will ultimately be working. This could range from a small percent, resulting in a very light load, or the weight of your entire body. Your body position relative to the straps and the ground will determine how much weight with which you will be working. I will talk more about that in the upcoming chapters. You can also adjust on the fly if you didn't get the most appropriate resistance at the start of the set or want to work with increasing or decreasing amounts of resistance during your set. This makes it a versatile tool for people at many different ability levels.

Suspended Training Is Ergonomic

Performance coach Mike Gillette talked about the ergonomics of suspension training in his book *Rings of Power*, and he described how this aspect had benefited him.[4] As his age advanced, he began to experience painful shoulder, elbow, and wrist problems in his training. After transitioning to suspension training through rings, he was gradually able to perform pain-free workouts. Training with rings, he wrote, reshaped his approach to strength training and allowed him to once again train hard without pain.

> *A suspended trainer gives the hands, wrists, and arms greater scope to rotate and adjust as needed throughout the movement.*

A suspended trainer works in a very comparable manner to the rings with which Mike Gillette had such success. It appears to be joint friendly, because it does not lock you into any set position as you move. The ability to constantly adjust your position during the movement, allows for the optimal amount of flexibility, and freedom of movement. When using a bar or machine, you are usually locked into a fixed position throughout that movement. This focused positioning can overly stress joints as you pass through the range of motion. A suspended system provides the freedom to rotate your wrist and hands around more as needed. This results in less stress transferred through the joints, and often less pain for those with joint discomfort.

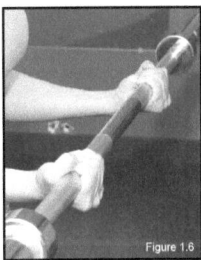
Figure 1.6

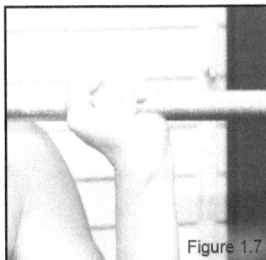
Figure 1.7

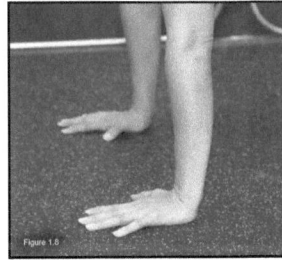
Figure 1.8

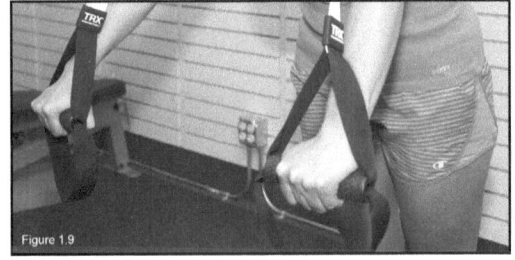
Figure 1.9

A Note for Those Suffering Joint Pain

Mike Gillette's book is a compelling anecdotal account. If you experience joint pain, there are no guarantees a suspended trainer will eliminate discomfort. But I do believe that it will increase the chances of being able to perform movements with less pain. In addition, several of my own clients, who struggle with joint pain, can successfully perform movements on a suspended trainer, that they are unable to perform without pain using other variations, machines, or tools.

Suspended Training Is Functional

The strength gained from suspension training helps in everyday activities, as well as your chosen sport. The key is that almost every movement in suspension training requires the use of core muscles to stabilize or move the body. In addition, it works the body as a unit. Too often, when you go into a fitness center, you'll see a line of machines… all designed to exercise distinct parts of the body. For example, you may go through a bicep curl, triceps contraction, chest press, and leg extension as part of your circuit. For most of these, you might be seated with a backrest so you can focus on just the targeted muscle.

This is not how the body moves during everyday tasks, and it's not how I would recommend training. You are missing out on the development of critical motor patterns that go along with the acquired strength. In addition, you are not learning stability or how to use your core to create a solid center of mass that your extremities can rely on, to both transfer force and hold proper alignment when required to lift or move objects. This is especially true when handling asymmetrical loads (such as picking up a heavy bag of groceries, a suitcase, or a small, wiggling dog). It doesn't matter how many plates you can chest press, if you throw out your back when moving a piece of furniture or picking up your child. You may suffer injury if your core doesn't know how to properly activate and stabilize the load you're trying to support with your arms and shoulders. Training your body in suspension will better prepare you to handle the demands of your chosen current fitness endeavors, and the physical demands of everyday living activities.

Suspended Training Is Time Effective

There's no traveling between machines with suspended training. It's all right in front of you. Those who are pressed for time will appreciate the quick transition from one movement to the next without lag time.

For those whose objective is burning calories, this time efficiency gives you a lot of bang for your buck. You can plan a workout that elevates your heart rate, burns more calories per unit of time, and replaces some of the more traditional cardio activities. In addition, it can be much more dynamic and fun. Because the equipment is lightweight and packs up easily, you can also take it with you on the road when traveling.

Chapter 2

Getting Set Up and Getting Started

Suspended trainer users can set up their equipment in a variety of ways, both indoors and out. In this chapter I talk a little about each venue and give you some examples. I'm using a TRX Suspension Trainer as an example. If you're using another brand, there may be some slight differences in the features, but the general principles should be the same.

Home Setup

The simplest way to set up a suspended trainer inside your home is to use a door anchor. Some trainers will come with one, but if not, they are readily available online. If you're buying a door anchor separately, or even making your own, make sure it's solid enough to sufficiently support your body weight. I say this because some door anchors are made for anchoring bands, and I would not recommend using one of those for a suspended trainer. A standard door anchor will have a hard, square-shaped block attached to a nylon loop, as in figure 2.1.

Some people opt for more permanent anchoring solutions (figure 2.2), which bolt onto a wall or beam and are available ready-made as kits. Others prefer to fashion their own using an I-bolt from the local hardware store. If making your own, be sure it's long enough to be inserted to a depth sufficient to hold the anticipated weight load. Also, make sure the material you are inserting it into it is solid and sturdy enough to hold the anchor.

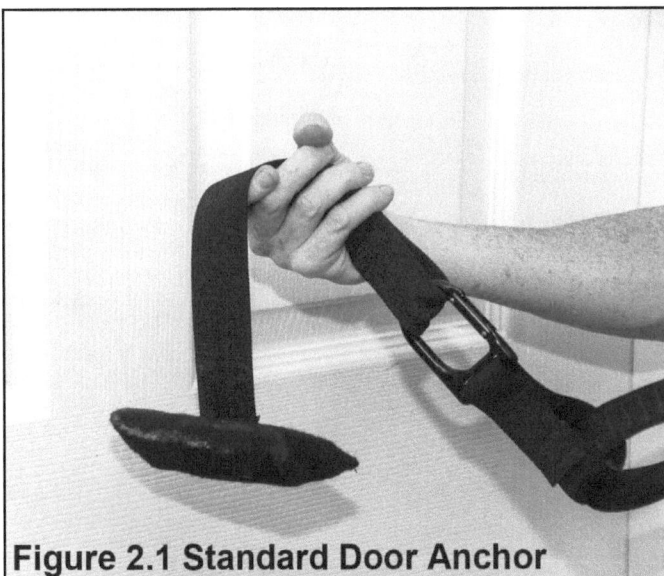

Figure 2.1 Standard Door Anchor

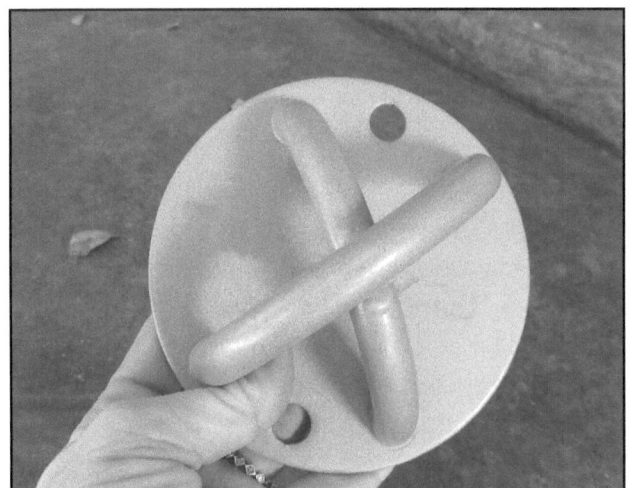

Figure 2.2 Suspension Training Mount

Door Anchor Setups

I strongly advise you to set up your workout space with the door closing toward you. This gives a much stronger support for your equipment and prevents the scenario of the door not being completely secured and possibly opening toward you when you're working out on the suspended trainer.

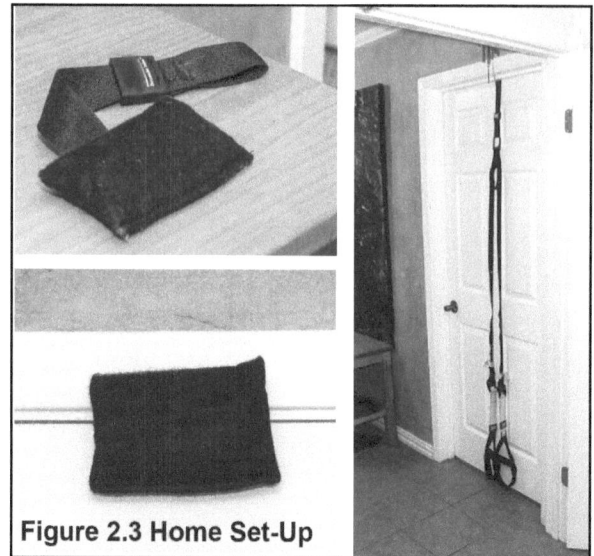

Figure 2.3 Home Set-Up

1. Choose a suitable door with enough space for your workout. You will need a good eight to ten feet of clear space in front   the door.

2. Place the hard square on the back side of the door, midway along the top edge, with the nylon strap feeding through the crack, to the side facing you (figure 2.3). Close the door.

3. Attach the suspended trainer to the nylon loop. Tug on it once or twice to make sure it's secure before beginning your workout!

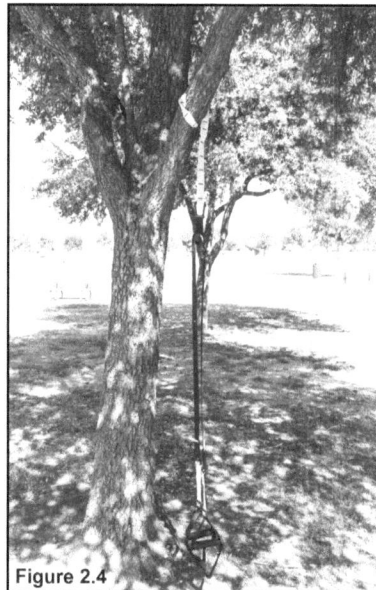

Figure 2.4

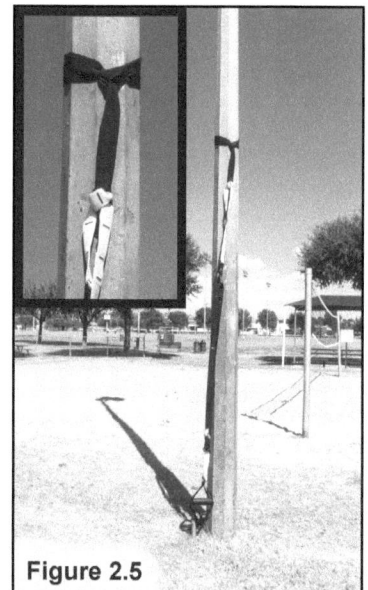

Figure 2.5

Outdoor Setups

Outdoor venues offer a variety of options. Trees, fences, poles, beams, and playground equipment can provide good anchoring points for your equipment (figures 2.4 and 2.5). Just make sure whatever you fasten it to won't flex, is securely bolted down, and is strong enough to support the load you'll place on it. Always err on the side of caution. There are times you may need an extender if you are anchoring high up, or if you need to wrap around something thick such as a beam or thick pole (figure 2.5). Special extender straps for suspended trainers are commercially available, but webbing made for rock climbers works equally well and will provide multiple small loops to clip onto. Figure 2.6 shows three pieces included as part of one training kit: the straps, the anchoring extender, and an extra extender like what is used in figure 2.5. If possible, try to set

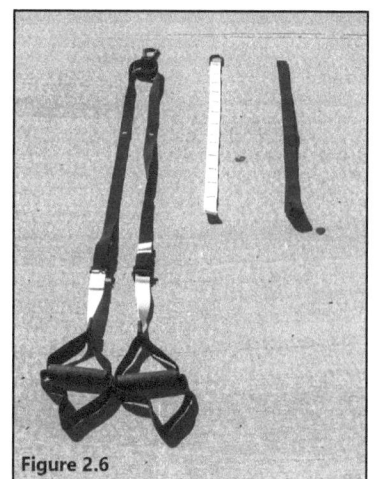

Figure 2.6

up your suspended training equipment, so the handles hang about six inches off the ground when the straps are fully extended. If that's not possible, just try and get it as close to six inches as you can.

Lengthening and Shortening Your Suspended Trainer

Most suspended trainers will have a buckle enabling you to adjust the strap length. For the purpose of my examples, I'm using the TRX brand, so if you are using a different brand, just be aware there may be some slight differences in the type of buckles used.

Shorten the strap by pushing the buckle down and pulling the yellow adjustment tab up to the desired height (figures 2.7 and 2.8).

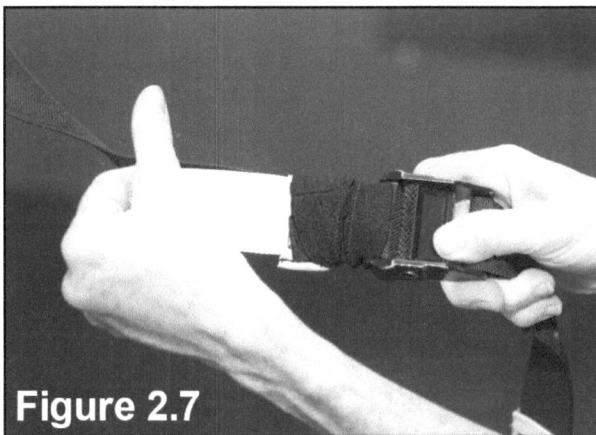

Figure 2.7

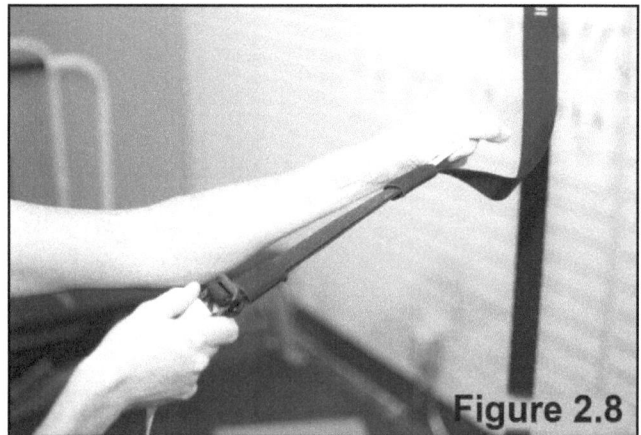

Figure 2.8

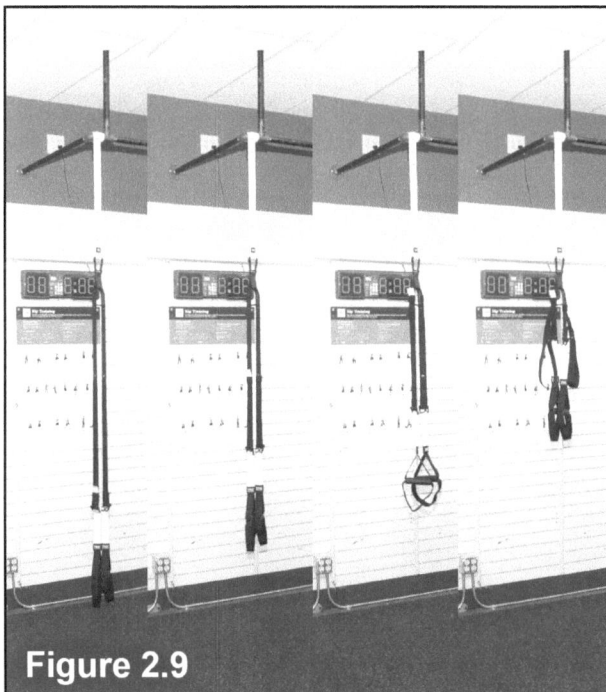

Figure 2.9

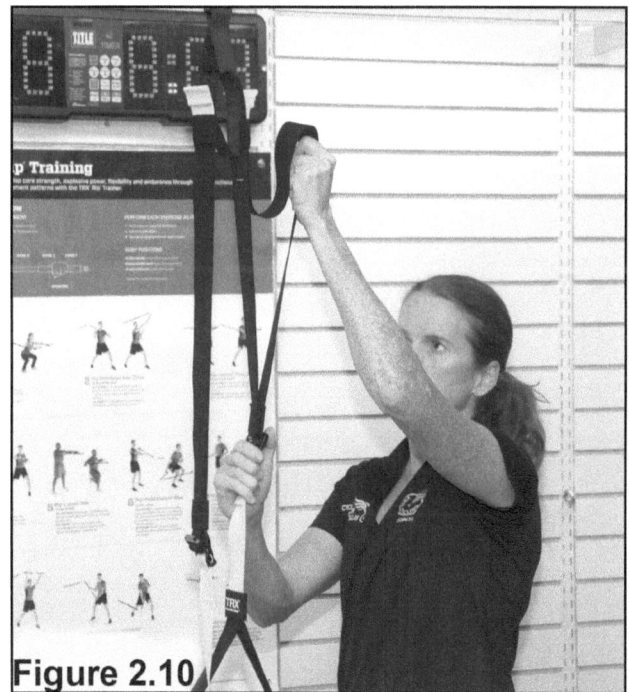

Figure 2.10

Figure 2.9. Four primary strap lengths: fully extended, mid-length, short, and super-short.

Figure 2.10. To adjust to the super-short length, pull up on the outside strap and then allow it to remain loose, hanging down on the sides like dog ears.

Using a Single Handle Only

Some exercises require you to use only one of the handles, such as the single-arm row.

Depending on your suspended training equipment, you might need to tie the handles together to create a single handle. One way to find out is by checking the top of your suspended trainer. If you have a nylon loop at the very top that prevents you from pulling one strap down more than a couple of inches past the other, you probably won't have to adapt your straps to single-handle mode. However, if your equipment doesn't have this loop, you will pull one side all the way through if you pull on just the single opposite handle. You can prevent this by using the single-handle mode when you're putting your weight on only one side. Either way, make sure and test the load before doing the exercise.

Currently, all of my own suspended trainers have anchoring loops. I still prefer to use single-handle mode, however, because it keeps the strap not being used from swinging around during the movement I am performing, which can be annoying.

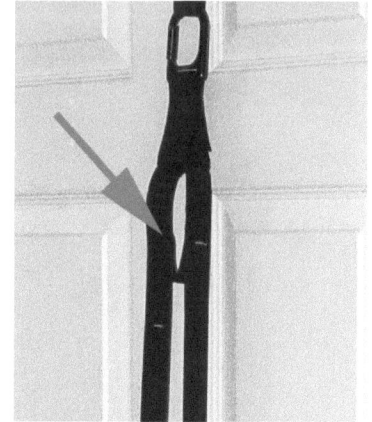

Figure 2.12 Anchoring loop

Single-Handle Mode

To tie the handles together:

1. Hold one handle in each hand. The one in your right hand is handle one; the one in your left hand is handle two.

2. Put handle one through the triangle of handle two, and then switch hands. Handle two is now in your right hand (figure 2.11).

3. Repeat this action by putting handle two through handle one.

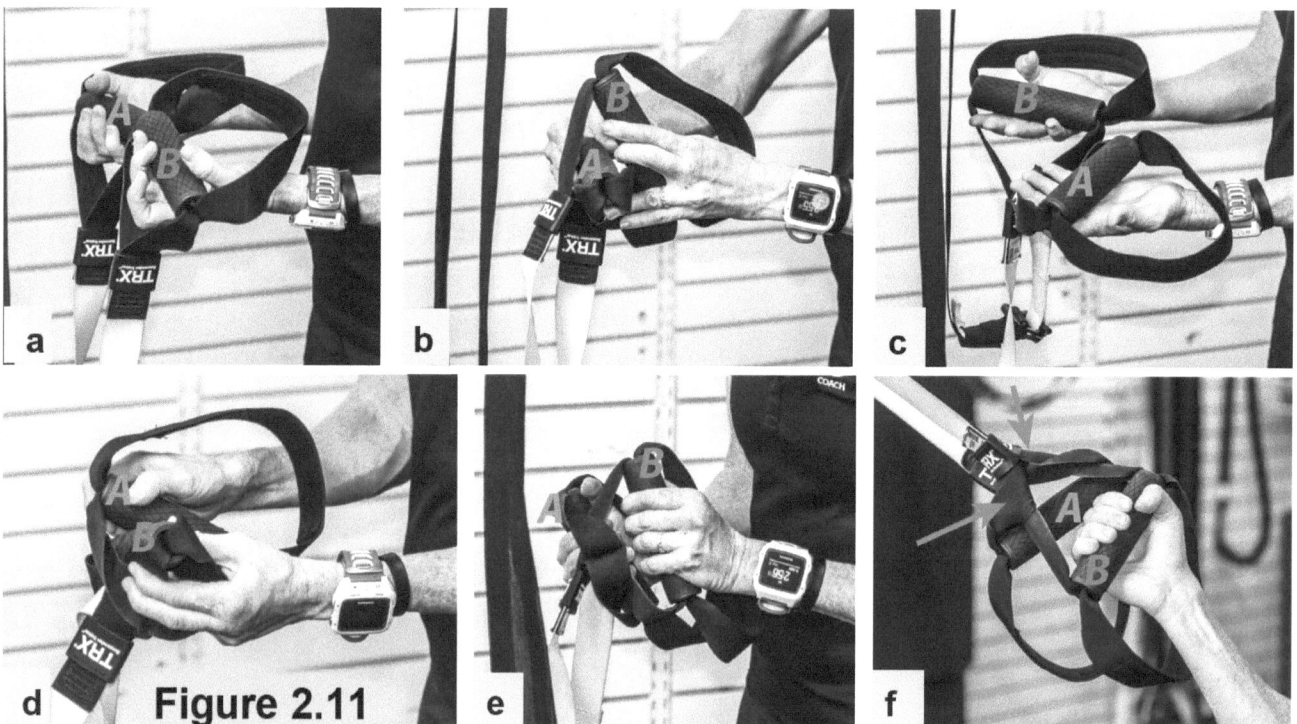

Figure 2.11

Safety Note

If you are working with a suspended trainer without an anchoring loop, it's critical that you hold the correct handle when in single-handle mode. The webbing attached to the handles should look like a mustache, right above the handle you are holding (figure 2.11). Grabbing the incorrect handle could result in one handle slipping through the other during the exercises, which would cause the tie to come undone, possibly resulting in a fall during the movement. Models of suspended trainers with an anchoring loop at the top avoid this, by preventing the straps from being pulled all the way down on one side (figure 2.12).

Using the Foot Cradles

Foot cradles enable you to perform many of the movements in the lying position, either face down or up. For movements where you start on your back, you will place your heels in the cradles. When lying on your stomach, you will place your toes in the cradles. The easiest way I have found to get in each of those positions is shown below.

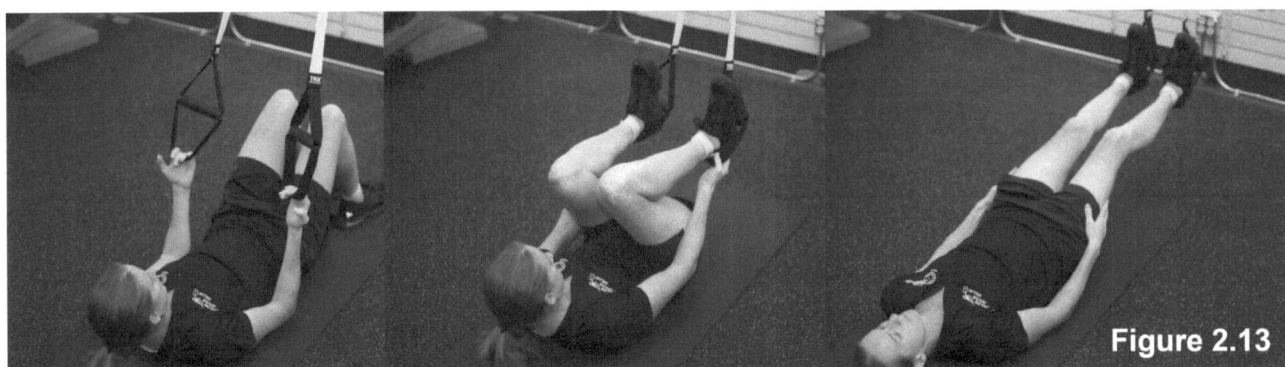

Figure 2.13 Putting your heels in the cradles

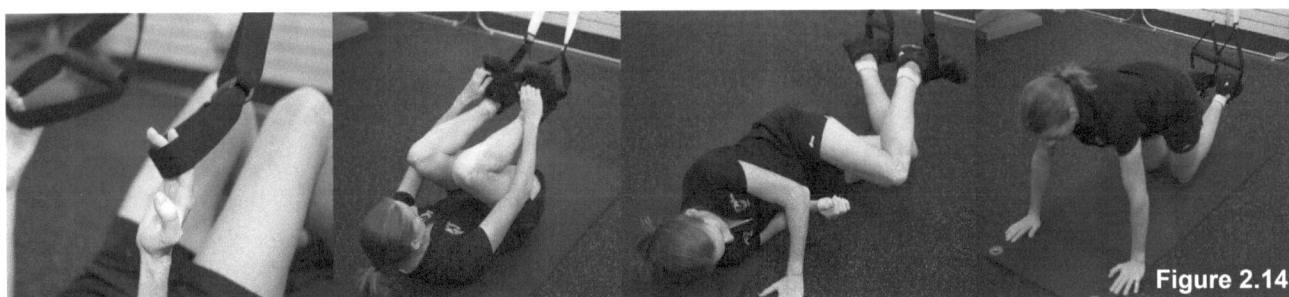

Figure 2.14 Putting your toes in the cradles

Conclusion

In this chapter, I covered the basics of setting up your suspended training equipment, the single-handle mode, and use of the foot cradles. These are the basics of your equipment setup and should give you the tools to be able to set up your trainer anywhere. You can adjust the length, and make use of the foot cradles for floor-based movements. With this information, you will be able to prepare for any of the movements you find in this book.

Chapter 3

Adjusting Resistance Levels

In this chapter, you will learn how to use your body position to modify exercises that match your fitness level and challenge you appropriately. I will show you how to do this by increasing and decreasing both the resistance and the stability of the movements you perform standing up. Finally, I will talk about how to modify the difficulty level of movements you perform from the ground position.

Changing the Resistance Level from the Standing Position

Most movements will have you starting in a standing position. From this position, you can use the angles of your body position to load varying percentages of your body weight onto the straps. This allows a beginner to safely and easily make adjustments to find his or her starting point. It also allows a more experienced user to increase the resistance, as well as perform sets of varying resistance, without interruption. Finally, it allows several users of various abilities to do the same workout together, yet perform the movements at their individual levels of resistance. I find this pretty cool! There is no need to take off or put on weight plates, mess with machines, or trade in dumbbells. You can make these changes quickly and even mid-set if needed.

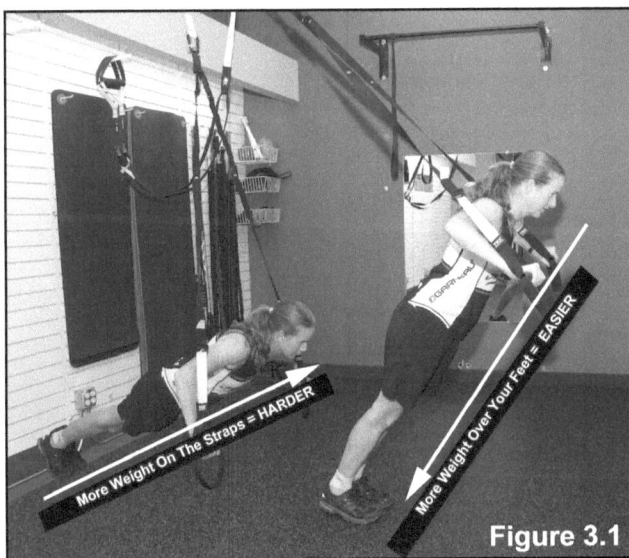

Figure 3.1. Above is an example of two levels of resistance during a suspended push-up. The more upright you are, the more body weight you're supporting with your legs and not having to push with your arms. If you want more resistance, simply step back farther to load more weight onto the straps. All the angles between the hardest (most horizontal) and the easiest (most upright) can be used to load any desired amount of weight onto the straps.

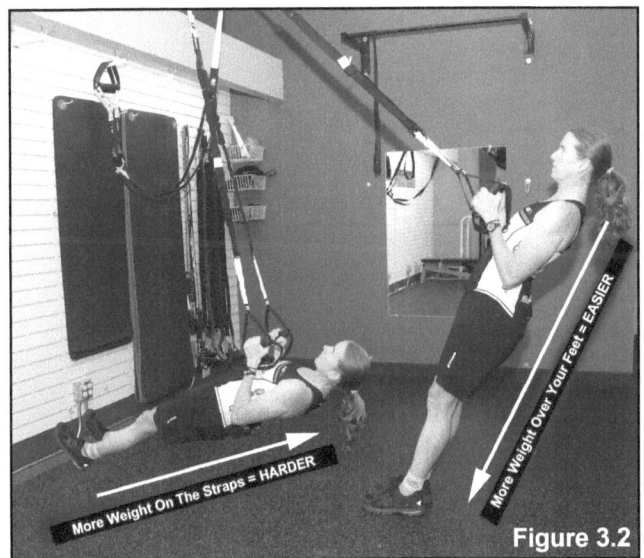

Figure 3.2. demonstrates the same concepts during a rowing (pulling) exercise. The farther you step underneath the straps, the more weight is hanging on the straps that you will have to pull up during the movement.

Changing the Resistance Level from the Ground Position

You can adjust the resistance to some degree, from the ground-based position, by changing where you are in relation to the point directly underneath the anchor.

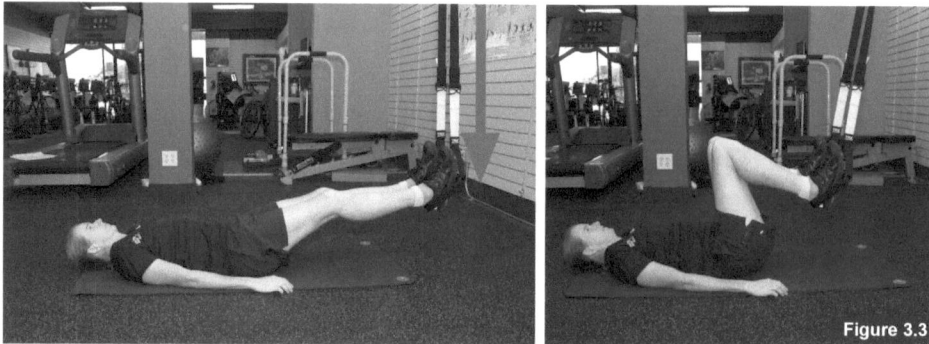

Figure 3.3

When you're doing movements with your feet in the cradles, you can use your position relative to the center spot, right under the anchor and gravity, to add or reduce resistance.

Neutral is right under the anchor point (see figure 3.3 above).

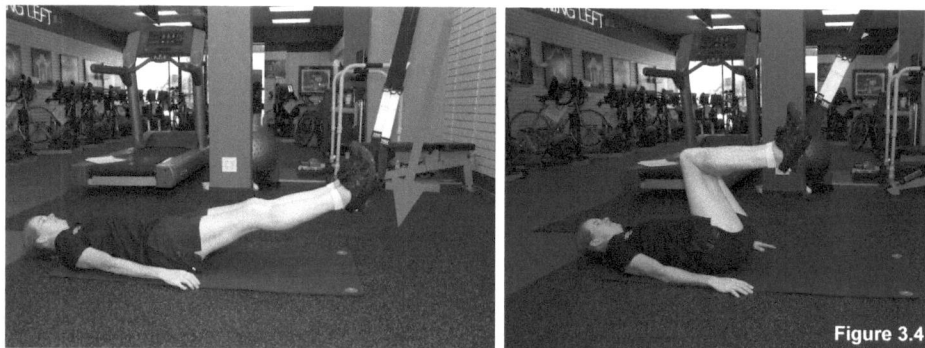

Figure 3.4

Moving out, so that your starting position is in front of the anchor point, will start the movement at a higher level of resistance. You will be pulling against gravity during the movement, making it harder (see figure 3.4).

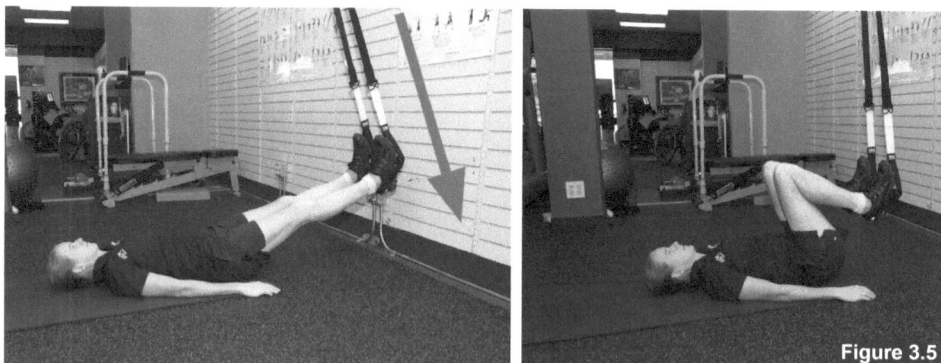

Figure 3.5

Moving further underneath the anchor point will have the opposite effect. You will be pulling with gravity until the point where you cross neutral (see figure 3.5).

Adjusting the Level of Stability

The instability of suspended training is much of what makes it so highly functional and relevant, to both everyday movements, and to the movement demands of cyclists and runners. Stability can be added or taken away, depending on where your feet are during your standing position. If you are a novice at suspension training, start with the most stable foot position until you feel comfortable with the movement.

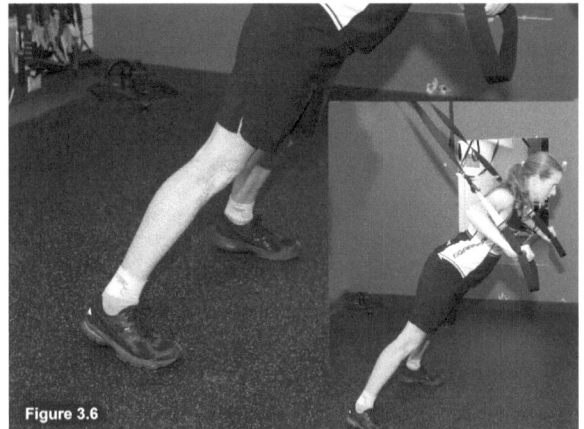

Figure 3.6

- **Wide base of support:** Stability is maximized with a broad base of support and your center of gravity in the middle of that base. If you are performing a push-up and have a wide stance, you will be more stable during that exercise, and it will be easier to balance than if you have a narrow stance.

- **Narrow your support base when using a suspended trainer:** If you would like to challenge your ability to stabilize yourself, bring your feet closer together to create a narrow stance, or do the exercise on just one foot. Decreasing the distance between your feet, decreases the width of the base upon which you are standing. This will be more challenging to your stability, because you are performing the movement on a narrower base of support.

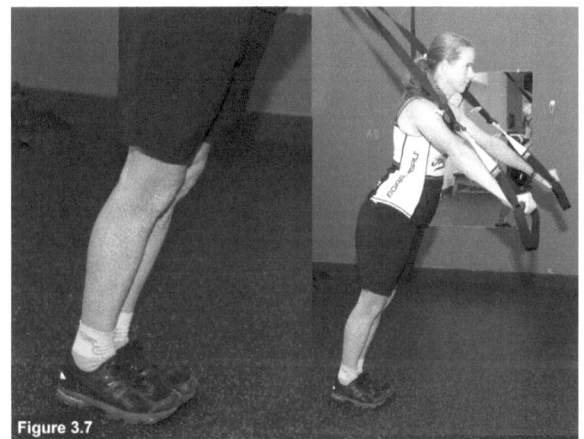

Figure 3.7

- **Offset stance:** Place one foot in front of the other. An offset stance gives you more stability going from front to back and allows you to shift weight forward and back during the movement. It's a convenient way to self-spot when performing movements with tougher angles. A longer offset position will provide more stability than a shorter one. As with the narrow and wide foot positions shown in figure 3.8, you can adjust your foot placement as needed before or during the movement.

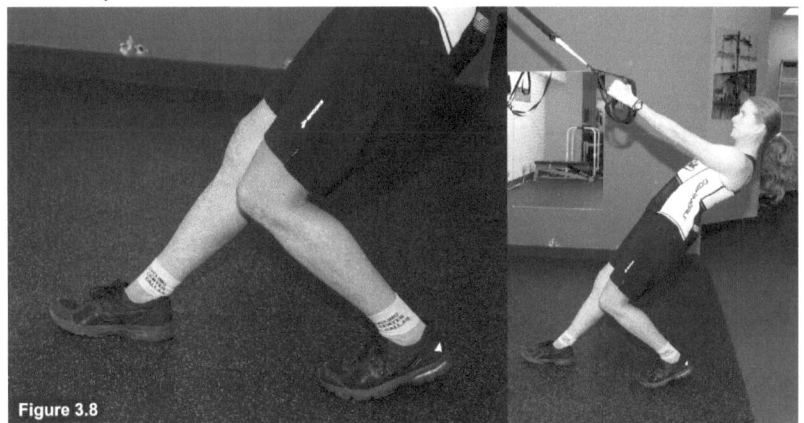

Figure 3.8

If you are using suspension training for the first time: It's OK to be conservative until you feel comfortable with it. If you're doing an exercise for the first time, start with a position in which you can do about 15 repetitions. It's OK to adjust your position as many times as you need until you feel you're fatiguing your muscles within your goal repetition range while still being able to execute the movement with good form.

If you have a specific workout goal: Choose a resistance level that fits your goal. If you're training for strength, go with a high amount of resistance. If you are looking for more of a cardio, calorie-burning workout, get in a position that loads a lower amount of resistance on your suspended trainer so you can perform the exercise for longer or perform several exercises consecutively.

> *Tip*: To increase the intensity within one movement, perform a drop set. Start with a resistance where you can only do 4 to 5 reps with good form. At that point, adjust your position to make it just easier enough to do another 4 to 5 reps. Adjust your position again, and finish with one last block of 5 reps. Ouch. Your muscles will thank you later.

Now that you know how to adjust the resistance levels, account for this when you are planning a workout or doing a workout from this book. For example, if you are working on muscle endurance and a set calls for 20 repetitions, adjust the resistance from the start to find a level where you feel you can complete 20 repetitions without having to adjust mid-set. If you're working more on strength, you will want to start with a harder resistance, knowing that you will only be doing 6 to 8 repetitions. Always try to find the level that will challenge you and fatigue you at the desired number of repetitions while still allowing you to maintain good form and technique throughout the set.

Chapter 4

Proper Technique

Perfecting Your Form

The term "form" in suspended training is so important that it's worth defining. "Form" is the exact shape and position of the entire body, from head to toe, and includes specific parts of the body when performing suspended training moves.

Having correct form during suspended training movements is extremely important. To help demonstrate some fundamentals of correct form, I will use a traditional isometric (static) exercise popularly called the "plank." Many people have heard of the "plank" and have experience using it in a training program.

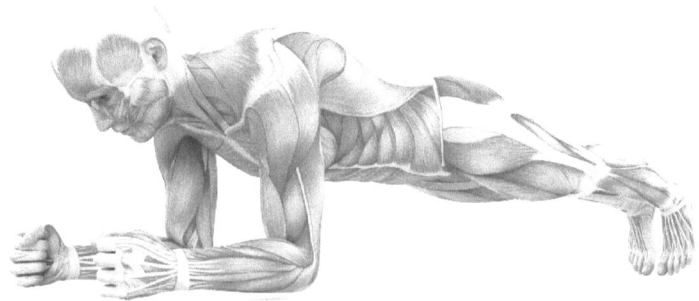

How to Properly Perform a Plank:

1. Start in a ground position facing down.

2. Consciously contract all the muscles you can feel, from your toes to your shoulders.

3. Raise your body up as one unit, so you are contacting the ground with only your forearms and toes.

4. Make sure your body forms a straight line from your shoulders to your ankles.

5. Engage your core by sucking your belly button into your spine.

6. Hold with good form until you get tired.

Plank form tip: Before going into the plank position, preload the muscles with tension by pulling your toes toward your knees, and squeezing all the muscles of your legs, glutes, abdomen, and back before raising your body off the ground. This may feel different from previous plank positions, if you have never performed the plank without preloaded muscle tension.

If you have never done the plank, practice it several times over three to four workout sessions before starting a suspended training program. Suspended training requires that you have a good feeling for engaging the core muscles as demanded by correct performance of the plank. If you have done the plank in the past but not recently, a little refresher would be good to reinforce the muscle memory. Time yourself, and focus on increasing the number of seconds you can hold this position. You should aim for at least thirty to sixty seconds before progressing to a more advanced variation such as the suspended plank.

Just Starting Out?

If you are new to strength training, or if it has been a while since you've done it, go ahead and start with a modified version of the plank until your body develops the strength and ability to hold the harder version. To do the modified version, simply hold the position from your knees instead of your toes as shown in figure 4.1. When you can properly hold this position for a full minute, progress to your toes. Initially, reduce the amount of time you attempt to hold the plank when you move up to the more challenging position. Make it a goal to increase your time by five seconds each week until you reach one minute. At this point, you may move to the suspended trainer. Don't rush the progressions, and give your body time to increase its strength and stability during each one.

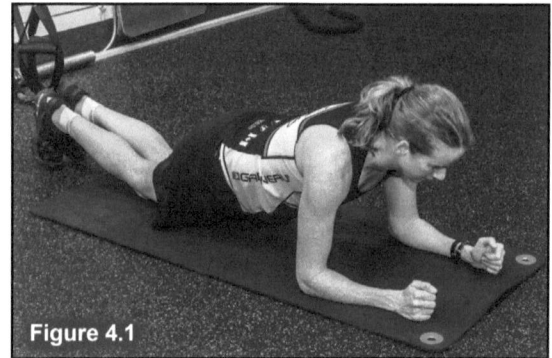

Figure 4.1

Why Does the Plank Matter If We Are Doing Suspension Training?

Performing a plank correctly, gives your body the foundation of muscle control needed for most movements that you will perform on a suspended trainer. You need to stabilize your core, while your arms and legs have the job of moving the weight of your body. Your body will need to know how to properly engage the right muscles in the correct order, and have the strength to hold the position throughout the movement. Losing your plank during a movement on the suspended trainer will result in losing your form.

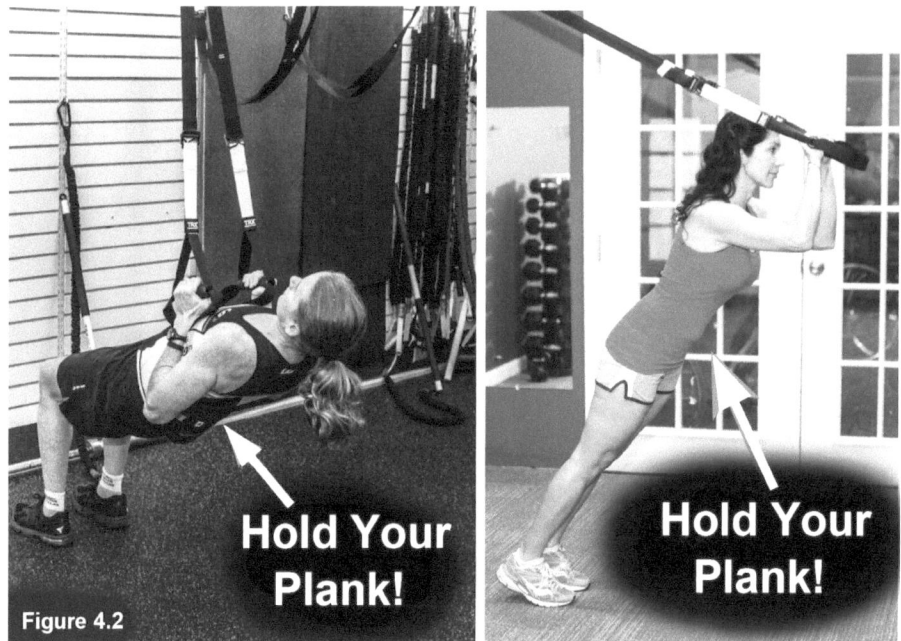

Hold Your Plank!

Figure 4.2

Hold Your Plank!

Suspended Training Technique and Common Form Errors

Many beginners make the same mistakes at first with their technique. I will point these errors out here, so you'll know not to make them! Incorrect starting position is often where problems begin, so get this right, and you'll be on a good track. Lack of concentration during the movement is another common error. When it comes to form, the mantra is "Start strong and stay strong." If you cannot maintain your form throughout your set, it's likely you're trying to achieve too much, so adjust your resistance angle until you can maintain your form.

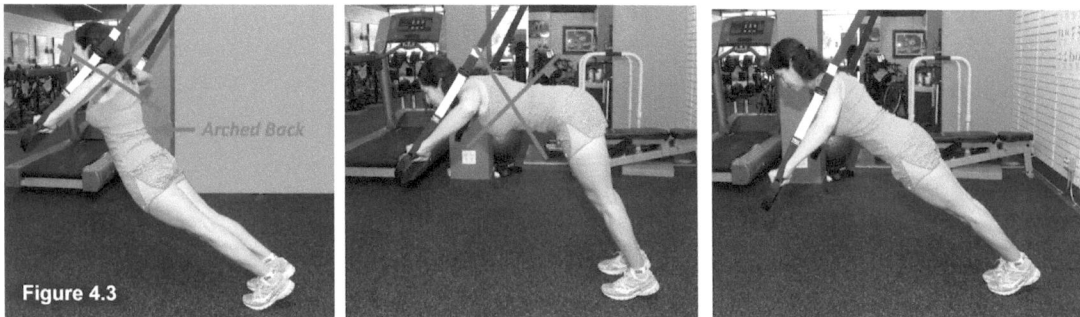
Figure 4.3

Hips: Both poor form and good form of the hips are shown above in figure 4.3. Keep a straight body, like a board. Avoid sagging or having slack in the midsection. Avoid allowing your hips to be up in the air.

Shoulders: Avoid shrugging during the movement, like in figure 4.4. Keep the shoulders down. To help with this, think about maintaining space between your ears and shoulders, and pulling your shoulder blades down toward your butt. Also, lift your chest and maintain good posture in a stand-up-straight type of way.

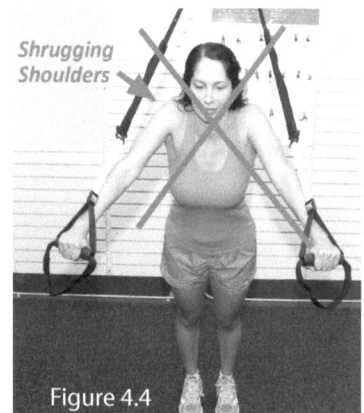
Figure 4.4

Core: Keep a tight core, beginning before you even start the movement, until you are finished. Contract and preload the muscles in your abdomen as if someone is going to punch you in the stomach. Pulling your belly button to your spine is also an analogy I use with people. Also, envision making your body as straight as a surfboard or table.

Head and Neck: Keep alignment of the head with the spine. A common error is to look down or up, which often causes other poor posture habits, such as a rounded back and shoulders. See figure 4.5 for examples of poor form and good form of the head and neck.

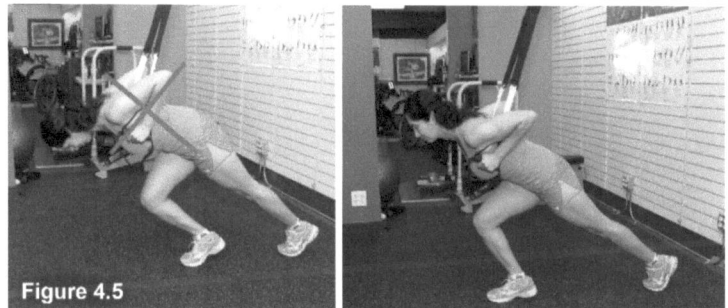
Figure 4.5

Wrists: Keep your wrists straight. Avoid a soft wrist, where you allow your wrist to bend back during the movement. See figure 4.6 for examples of poor wrist form and good wrist form.

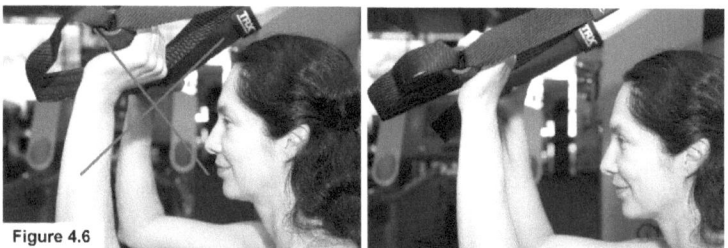
Figure 4.6

Knees: For the most part, your knees will maintain alignment with your hips and feet. They should not cave inward or bow outward during squatting or lunging movements, and they should stay centered over your feet during most of those movements. Figure 4.7 shows a common error of form, allowing the hips to drop back on a split-squat movement, resulting in the knee being misaligned with the foot.

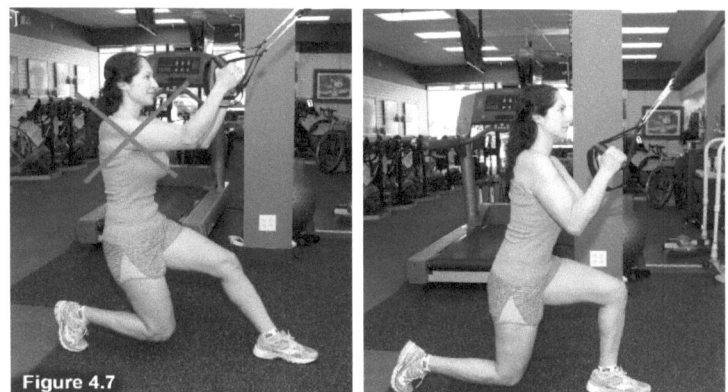
Figure 4.7

Loose Straps: When using a suspended trainer, the straps should always have tension throughout any movement. A common mistake is to allow the straps to lose tension at the top or the bottom of your movement. If you find the straps are loose at any point during the movement, adjust your position to put tension back on them.

Sawing: Keep the straps even at all times. Sawing happens when one arm or leg pulls harder than the other and the strap moves back and forth through the support strap at the top. Most suspended trainers are not made to perform as a pulley. Sawing is not only poor form; it will also wear out your suspended trainer faster.

Now, some suspended trainers, such as the CrossCore®, are made with a pulley rotation device at the top. These are designed for rotation movements with very specific purposes that are beyond the scope of this book. If your suspended trainer includes a pulley system, it should have a locking device that enables it to be used as you would any of the suspended trainers you see in this book.

Conclusion

If you become familiar with what is considered good form, you will go into your movements ready to execute them with the highest quality, get the most from them, and reduce chances of strains or injuries resulting from poor form. Once you know what good form feels like, be sure to check in with yourself as you fatigue when performing sets of any movement. It's during this time that errors in technique tend to be made. It's also the time when you're giving your body the stimulus it needs to get stronger and fitter. You must teach your muscles to maintain the highest quality of movement execution during this time as well.

Section 2

Specific Applications

Chapter 5

Developing a Strong Foundation

This is the most important chapter of the book when it comes to developing fitness, strength, and stamina through suspension training. This chapter will give you the tools to help you put together a training program and improve overall strength at your level. It will also give you a foundation of fitness that will set you up for success when progressing your program to more specific goals.

I will go over why it's important to consider your long-term goals and what you want to get out of your training program. This will prevent you from making the mistake of jumping into a random collage of workouts, repeating the same workout for too long, or running out of ideas to keep you engaged and progressing, which can cause you to gradually lose interest. A suspended trainer is the only tool required for designing workouts using this book, with any fitness objective in mind. However, it's not mandatory that you use suspension training for all exercises, and it's not necessary that you limit yourself to only suspension training if you have the resources to include other types of training.

Designing a medium-term or long-term program is not necessary to start training. However, it can give you direction and help you progress properly toward your medium and long-term goals. It can also help you stay on track and hold yourself accountable. With that said, the structured approach may work better for some than for others. If your style is more on the unstructured side, this is still the best place to start out, and you may still find yourself returning to this section as your fitness level advances.

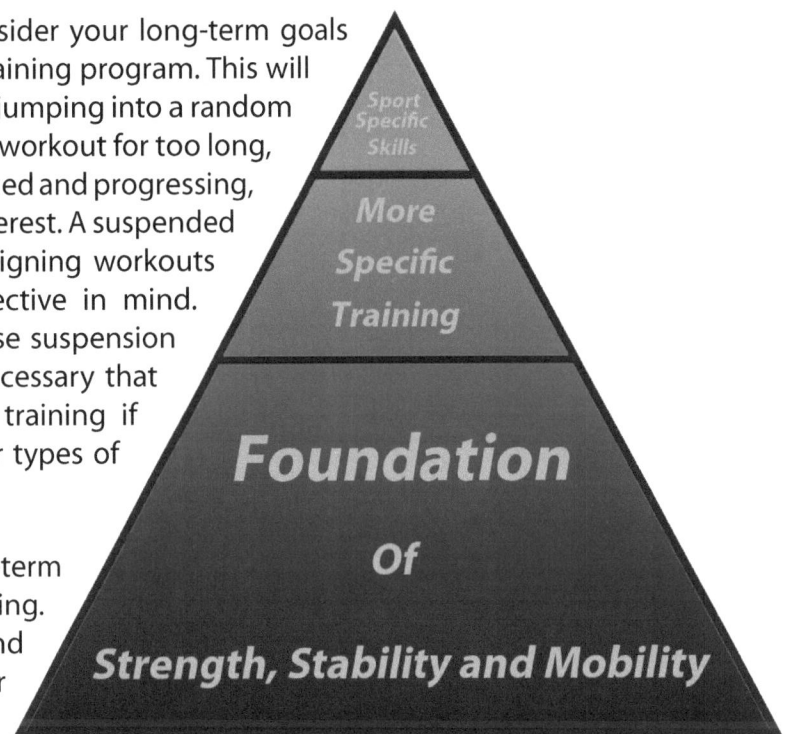

What Is Periodization?

Having spent time in the personal training world, I have too often come across people who exercise consistently but have reached a permanent plateau. The most common scenario is that they have been stuck on the same program for months or even years—the same exercises, same repetition ranges, and same amounts of resistance. Their bodies have already adapted to the program and are not getting any overload or demands that require any more change. Whether you are a performance-oriented endurance athlete or someone who wants to lose weight and obtain better general fitness, the way to do that is to continually challenge your body with new demands. In a variety of studies, periodization has been shown to result in more fitness gains.[1]

Periodizing your training into phases or blocks that will keep your body working harder and adapting to new demands, while getting adequate rest to recover and rebuild, is the route to continuing improvement. Generally, each phase has certain objectives, and you work on targeting things during your workouts that will best result in you meeting those objectives. The following chapters go into further detail on a variety of aspects, such as cardio, strength, performance for running, or bone density, that you may want to focus on during a training phase. These phases may build on one another, focusing on just one aspect at a time, or they may shift in focus to completely distinct aspects.

Periodization can be done within a block of training. The simplest approach would be to focus on increasing the amount of resistance you can move at a targeted repetition range. You could also reverse this and aim to increase the repetitions you can perform at a given resistance. Another approach might be to increase the number of sets or duration of work intervals over the course of a block of training.

Periodization can be done over the span of several blocks of training. A traditional approach would be shifting from using sets of lower resistance and higher repetitions in one training phase, to sets of higher resistance and lower repetitions in the next training phase. Another example would be a recreational cyclist, or general fitness enthusiast, designing a six-week training plan to focus on general strength, followed by a six-week training program to focus on cardio and weight loss. Finally, a competitive cyclist might transition from a general strength program, to a strength maintenance program, to coincide with an on-the-bike training program.

> **Periodization:** Conditioning programs can use periodization to break up the program into phases or training blocks. Each block has specific aspects and goals on which it will focus. A phase can be built on the work achieved during the phase preceding it, or it can shift focus to a different objective.

After you have obtained a general ability and comfort level performing movements on a suspended trainer, you should start thinking about your goals for the next training block. You may want to plan your upcoming phases by choosing to alter any number of variables, depending on your goals or preferences, with the goal being to improve on those aspects and keep your program dynamic and effective.

For instance, if you are interested in targeting more cardiovascular benefits or are pressed for time, it would be beneficial to plan a four-to-six-week block of workouts that include movements which use multiple muscle groups and/or have short, or no, rest periods between sets. If you are concerned about osteoporosis and want to improve bone density, you could choose exercises that work large muscle groups with high resistance, or exercises that involve some impact. If you are combining suspension training with other methods, you have limitless options when it comes to program design.

Things you can change within a workout:

- movements performed

- the number of sets performed

- the number of repetitions performed

- doing sets of repetitions versus time-based sets

- the level of resistance

- the rest between sets
- the number of exercises
- the speed at which you perform the exercises

Things you can target within a training phase:

- building a solid foundation
- building strength
- gaining muscle
- improving cardiovascular health
- targeting weight loss
- improving balance and stability
- improving flexibility
- improving bone density
- sport-specific strength

Start Your Program Off Right

A solid foundation to your fitness program is not unlike a solid foundation to your house. It may not always be the sexiest part of the program, but it's the most important building block. If you want to be able to perform advanced progressions or intensity, a solid foundation will provide necessary support, and you will be more likely to handle the higher intensities and complex movement demands. However, adding intense training on top of a weak or cracked foundation may result in bad technique, less efficient workouts, or even breakdown and injury.

To build your foundation, start with a general all-around workout that targets multiple movements and challenges strength, endurance, and stability. Maintain balance in your exercise selections by including movements that counter each other. For example, employ a pushing movement and a pulling movement that work opposing muscle groups, like push vs pull. A movement that targets the anterior chain of muscles in the front of your body counters a movement that focuses on the posterior chain of muscles on the backside of your body. Select basic movements and perform them at a comfortably challenging resistance level. I recommend a repetition range of about 15 reps per set during this phase. This will give you a moderate degree of resistance and enough reps to develop muscle memory and coordination of the movement.

The unstable platform of the straps is something your body may not be used to, and this will allow it time to learn the most efficient muscle-firing patterns, as well as stabilizer recruitment of the muscles involved. I also suggest an initial block of at least four to six weeks to develop this. If you are new to strength training, make that six to eight weeks, and consider doing more than one training block of foundation work. Everyone will have his or her own level of experience, ability, and comfort. If you don't have much experience strength training, a longer block of time or multiple training blocks of foundation work will allow for your strength, balance, coordination, flexibility, and overall kinesthetic awareness to further develop.

You may experience improvements during this time, as you become comfortable with the movements. Many of these initial gains will be neuromuscular as the body becomes more efficient and figures out which muscles to turn off and which ones to activate. The neuromuscular system is a quick learner. The structural components of your muscle fibers, tendons, and ligaments take a little longer to catch up and adapt to the new demands being placed them. Be patient, and give them the chance to do so.

You may still periodize within this phase, over multiple foundation blocks, by progressing the movements. Your ultimate goal should be improving all-around strength and stability. As you get stronger, you should be able to advance in movement progressions or in the resistance utilized for each given movement selected.

Getting Started with Your Program

A good start would be to choose one or two movements from the beginner/intermediate section of the exercise library with each focusing on a different movement pattern.

- pushing
- pulling
- legs and hips
- core

> ***Earn your progression!*** Don't move to the more advanced movements until you have mastered the movement or progression on which you are focused.

Once you've completed this phase, and have achieved an adequate comfort and ability level with a program of basic movements, you may want to change things up. This may involve simply continuing to build on that foundation with a modification of the exercises you select. Changing or progressing the movements performed, while keeping the repetitions, sets, and rest periods the same will accomplish that. You may also want to shift the focus to strength, cardio, or a sport-specific strength program.

Sample Workouts to Get You Started

Reference the level 1 and level 2 foundation workouts at the back of the book to begin. Both are well-rounded programs that include a variety of general movements. Level 1 consists of exercises selected from the beginner-level category. Level 2 consists of more movements from the intermediate level.

Which Workout Should I Start With?

Start with the level 1 (page 212) workout if you are a novice exerciser, are coming back from a break from working out, or are coming back from an injury or health issue. If you are unsure about which program would be best to start with, begin here. You can always move up to level 2 if you decide you need more of a challenge.

Start with the <u>level 2</u> (page 215) workout if you are already performing resistance training or have a strong fitness/athletic background. Each movement is adjustable, so find the most appropriate level of resistance and stability for you. You want to be challenged, but you also should be able to complete 15 reps of each set with good form. You may advance the progression of any given exercise selection as needed.

Conclusion

Start your training off right with the recommendations in this chapter.

You will achieve a balanced program with movements that complement each other. You will also develop a strong foundation of strength and stability that you can build on, or transition to focus on other aspects of your fitness. Some of these additional aspects include cardiovascular training, improving bone density, increasing maximal strength, improving flexibility, or sport-specific training. These are all covered in the following chapters.

Progress at your own pace. Don't worry about what exercises others may be doing. Find the exercise, progression, and resistance level that are right for you and your goals within that workout. It should be challenging to finish each set while performing the targeted number of repetitions. You should also be able to complete the targeted number of repetitions without changes to form or a reduction in the range of motion. Don't move to the next progression or more advanced movement until you have mastered the current one.

Consider all the variables you can manipulate within each workout and each training phase. You may change any of these variables to target your fitness goals, or simply to keep things interesting and prevent plateaus in your fitness. Periodization to your program can be done over weeks, months, or even years.

Consistency is key. Stick with it.

Chapter 6

Improving Cardiovascular Health

You Don't Need a Treadmill or Stationary Bike to Get Benefits to Your Cardiovascular System

When you think of traditional aerobic or cardio workouts, you may envision the stationary bike or elliptical machine. What if I told you that you could get the same or even greater benefits to your cardiovascular system through a body-weight and suspension training program? This method might be more fun and interesting than counting down the minutes on the stationary bike or treadmill.

Cycling, jogging/walking, or any type of traditional aerobic workout continues to be a significant activity, and it can produce a lot of health and fitness benefits. However, in this chapter, I present an approach centered around using a suspended trainer that can produce those same benefits (and possibly even more). It's also an option that is much more versatile and convenient for frequent travelers who don't want to worry about finding a fitness center in every new destination.

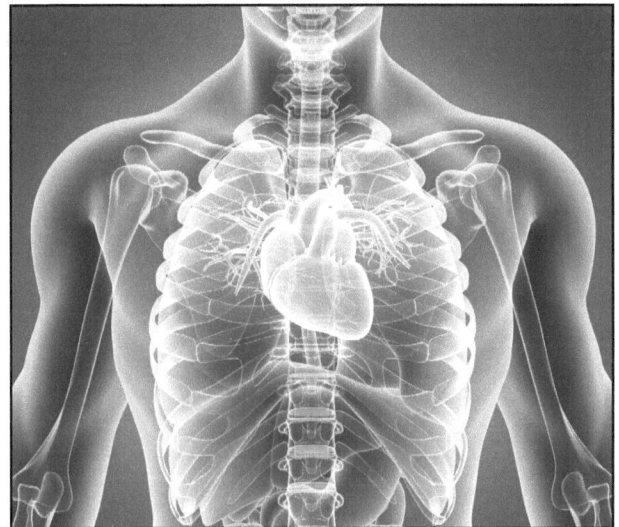

Your Body Generates Energy Using Two Primary Systems

Aerobic: Most of the energy for work comes from oxygen. This is what you are doing most of the day, whether you are sitting at a desk at work, or walking around the grocery store. This is also what happens during lower-intensity, sustained exercise efforts.

Anaerobic: This is when the demand for oxygen surpasses either the supply or the amount that can be processed, and other forms of energy must kick in to provide the muscles what they need to continue to work. This happens during hard and usually short efforts. Examples would be sprinting across a parking lot, or daily living activities such as carrying a heavy load up a flight of stairs.

Your fitness training can target one or both systems depending on what you do in your workouts. Most strength training tends to focus on the anaerobic systems because they consist of shorter efforts followed by recovery.

The cardio-focused workouts here can be considered "combination training".[1] These are workouts that target both the aerobic and anaerobic systems. The workouts presented within this chapter fall under this category and will develop the abilities of both systems. The strength sets are longer and less intense. The recovery between hard sets is even less intense but keeps you moving and primarily targets the aerobic system. These recovery periods from the harder efforts still involve keeping an effort level that is benefiting the aerobic system.

You can recover from the hard effort while still getting the training benefits of the less intense but aerobic effort. During the recovery periods, you are still training your aerobic system, but you are also allowing your body to clear lactic acid out of the blood and recover from the oxygen debt that your last effort created.

An article in the *Strength and Conditioning Journal*[2] described the benefits of "High-Intensity Interval Training" (HIIT). This training involves alternating high-intensity and low-intensity work during your workout session.

When compared to traditional aerobic training, the benefits of this approach include a greater reduction in body fat, improvements in blood pressure and strength of the contractions of the heart, and greater VO2 max improvements (Volume of Oxygen that you can utilize under max strain). Improvements in these areas will result in greater cardiovascular health. They will also prevent, or even reverse to some extent, cardiovascular diseases.

> Increasing *anaerobic abilities* means your body is able to perform more work during your hard efforts or sustain harder efforts longer at the same intensities.
>
> Increasing *aerobic abilities* means you can do more repeated or longer workouts without getting fatigued and having to stop.

The higher intensity that targets the anaerobic system can improve endurance at the lower exercise intensities as well. This means you can last longer until you fatigue on your walks, while hiking, or when you ride a bike. The reason for this is that the higher-intensity demands you are putting on your lungs, heart, and muscles force them to get stronger and adapt to meet this intensity. This is a good thing because it's giving your body the stimulus to say, *"Hey, we need to meet this new demand. Let's adapt to get stronger and more efficient so we can do just that."*

Interval Training

You've probably heard of this term. It essentially refers to those hard, short efforts that fall under the anaerobic category. Most people refer to interval training when they talk about cycling, running, or a program on a StairMaster® or elliptical machine. However, that's not the only context in which interval training can be used. We are going to use the same concept when building our workouts around a suspended trainer.

The ability to perform more work for longer periods of time equals more calories burned. It also increases your ability to do daily living activities or any of the active endeavors you might enjoy. You may notice you're a lot less winded after total body movements, such as going up the stairs to your office or bedroom, carrying your child, or lifting and moving a heavy object.

Designing a Program to Improve Cardiovascular Health, Stamina, and Weight Loss

Interval and anaerobic training are tough. Some of the workouts in this category will be among the hardest you will attempt. They will leave you winded and may require some suffering to get through the sets or intervals.

When designing these workouts, choose movements that target multiple muscle groups at the same time. Also, include movements that target large muscle groups. The plyometric exercises are an excellent choice for a routine of this type. You may use either repetitions or time for your sets. Keep the resistance moderate to light to allow for quick transition between movements, with very short recovery times between consecutive movements of zero to fifteen seconds. Alternate circuits of consecutive movements with sets of easier, more steady efforts of walking or easy jogging, a side-to-side shuffle, easy jumping jacks, stairs, step-ups, or a cardio machine, or combine with a step or free-standing aerobics routine.

For Beginners or Those Not Currently Exercising Regularly

It's important that you are cleared by your doctor before starting an intense exercise program. This is especially true if you've had any cardiovascular issues in the past. It also helps to have a base of several weeks of steady-state traditional aerobic work. Be conservative when choosing the intensity of your intervals. It's better to err on the side of it being too easy. You can always increase the intensity as you get more comfortable with the program. If you're unable to keep the rest intervals at or below fifteen seconds, the difficulty level of the movements may be too high for this program, and you should lower it. The work-to-rest ratio for recovering between sets of circuits should be around 1:2. This means if it took you two minutes to complete your exercise circuit, you should do your lower intensity cardio activity for four minutes. For those who are less fit, increasing the rest to 1:3 or 1:4 is perfectly acceptable until your body gets used to the new demands. Choose activities such as walking or lower intensities on a cardio machine.

For Those at an Intermediate or Advanced Fitness Level

Choose movements and intensities that challenge you but still allow you to complete the sets or circuits without having to take extra rest. Shoot for a timed work-to-rest interval of 1:2. You may want to choose more intense cardio activities such as running, stair climbing, or jumping rope. However, remember that you also want to keep the intensities low enough that you are ready to tackle the next circuit or set at a high intensity.

The sample workouts located at the end of this chapter are examples of how you can build a workout around suspension training to target improving cardiovascular endurance. Feel free to use them in their entirety, or use parts of them to help build your own daily program. You may also change them up, simply by choosing different but comparable exercise selections to drop into the same sets.

Conclusion

When building and performing your workouts, remember that long-term adherence to exercise is the key to fitness, weight loss, and maintenance of that weight loss. You want results, but you also want a program you enjoy. Select the exercises and intensities based on your goals, but also keep things at an intensity that keeps it fun. Even the best-designed programs only work if they are implemented. If you ultimately design a program that is intense and effective but you dread doing it because it's so hard, it's time to change that program. There is no shame in backing off on the intensities or extending rest periods if it keeps you doing the work and helps you stay consistent.

Chapter 7

Building Muscle and Strength

Why Do We Get Stronger?

Strength and muscle gains are a result of both improved neural activation and increased diameter of the muscle fibers.[1] Basically, your body learns how to turn on more fibers, and those fibers get bigger. The improved neural activation is especially prevalent in those just starting a program. This is the focus from which most of your strength improvements will initially come. This is also part of why doing a foundation block is so beneficial to your long-term training. Your body and your brain are learning to selectively activate the fibers needed to meet the demands you are expecting. The muscle growth will follow.

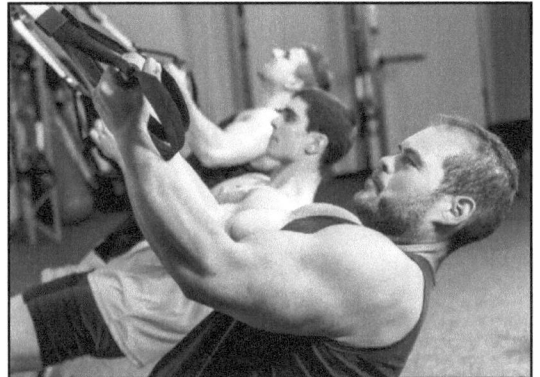

Training specifically to improve strength or gain muscle requires different approaches at the intermediate and advanced levels. The person with the most muscle mass is not always the strongest, and the strongest person is not always the biggest. If your training goals are more aesthetic in nature and you want a killer physique that turns heads at the beach, you should follow the training approach below for muscle gains, along with a nutrition plan that supports minimal fat storage while maximizing muscle gain. If your goals are more performance oriented, lean your approach more toward the strength section.

Rest and Recovery Matters

<u>Within a workout:</u> Rest is needed between sets to allow the body to recover from the intense demand you've placed on it, and then get ready for the next round. The amount of rest time taken between sets is often an afterthought for most people. The next set is usually started whenever you may feel you're ready or there is a break in the conversation between people working out together. There is nothing wrong with this approach if you are working out for general fitness, enjoyment, and camaraderie. However, if you have specific goals and want to get the most out of each workout and accomplish these goals, you need to structure your rest into your workout the same way you would your work intervals. The amount of rest required between sets is both determined by what was previously performed, and the goal of the next set. Training for strength requires a different approach than training to gain muscle. The following sections will talk more about this.

<u>Between workouts:</u> Muscles do not get stronger or bigger during your exercise sets or during any given workout. They are subjected to demands that actually break them down, and they may even experience some minor damage. This is OK because it's a needed stimulus. This is also why you might feel sore the next day after a hard workout or after performing a new exercise movement. Your body then knows to rebuild these muscle fibers stronger, so they can better withstand the demand being placed on them. Rest is needed in the day or two after hard workouts to allow the body to do this.

Training to Gain Muscle

If your primary goal is more muscle, make it a goal to get more volume in during your workouts. This means more sets, more repetitions, and more movements. Muscle growth is produced by repeated bouts of high-intensity muscle contractions, and is an adaptation to the work the muscles do. Resistance training increases muscle protein synthesis, which builds more muscle.

Doing multiple sets versus single sets has been shown to result in increased muscle gains. When initially starting a program, three sets per movement, alternated with recovery days, has been recommended by professional research.[3] You want to give your muscles enough stimulus to respond, without giving them too much. Remember that they need to recover and rebuild as they adapt to your new strength training program. If you already have sufficient training time under your belt, you may want to consider adding volume through even more sets, up to as many as 4 - 6, as that was also shown in research to result in even greater gains.

Increasing the number of movements themselves in your program will also add to the volume, in those who have already been doing some training. Also keep in mind that increases in muscle mass are smaller and come after strength increases. So be patient, and make sure you have developed a solid foundation to support long-term success before you add more sets and exercises to increase the volume of your program.

A gain in muscle mass results from increased diameter of your existing muscle fibers. It takes more time for the muscle fibers to increase in their size or thickness, than it does to make the neuromuscular gains that result in strength gains more quickly. However, the increased ability of the neuromuscular system to activate more muscle fibers is an important part of stimulating the muscles, and triggering the body's response to support growing the size and thickness of the muscle fibers.

How to Build Muscle Mass
• **Higher volume**
• **Multiple sets**
• **More exercises**
• **Moderate load**
• **More rest time between sets**

Because the number of exercises and sets are higher in a program designed for muscle growth, it's often appropriate to divide up movements into different days. For example, designate a day for pushing movements, followed by a day for pulling movements, followed by a rest day or day for light cardio. You could also do an upper-body day followed by a lower- body day. This will allow you to get the volume you need and strength train multiple days in a row, while still giving each group of muscles a chance to recover after being stressed. Consider combining suspension training with dumbbell, bar, or machine work as well. This will have the added benefit of providing more options for exercise variations.

Nutrition is a significant component of muscle gain as well. You need to give your body the fuel and building blocks through high-quality calorie intake, both before and after workouts, as well as throughout the day, to be able to respond to the stimulus you're placing on it, to build muscle. Getting nutrient-rich food and adequate amounts of protein, carbs, and healthy fats are crucial to recovering from workouts and providing your body with the building blocks to build muscle.

What to Do *during* Sets to Gain Muscle

How much weight should I use? Using moderate loads allow for more repetitions to be performed and have been shown to result in greater amounts of growth hormone produced. The research supports using 70 to 85 percent of the maximum amount of weight you can do for one repetition.[1] A less technical approach would be to use a resistance level that fatigues you between 8 and 12 repetitions, while still being able to complete the last rep without failing. If you're not sure about what weight to use or how much load to put on the suspended trainer through the angle of your body, just make a conservative guess. If you can complete more than 15 repetitions, increase the load. If you can't do 8 reps without breaking your form or failing on a rep, decrease the load.

How long should each repetition be? Aim for three to four seconds per repetition, resulting in a work period of about forty seconds per set.[2] I don't recommend going to failure during your sets if your goal is to gain muscle. This approach results in higher than moderate loads and may have a detrimental effect on following sets. Focus on the volume and number of exercises, quality of movement, and post- and pre-workout nutrition.

Movements using larger and multiple muscle groups should be a priority. Presses, squats, lunges, pull-ups, and rows are all movements that use large and numerous muscle groups. Working these larger muscle groups stimulate the whole body to produce more generalized growth hormone. This will encourage muscle growth throughout the body. So, don't skip out on the leg workout. Isolating smaller muscles is also fine to do. Just try to arrange those sets in your workout so as not to pre-fatigue small muscles that may you need to help perform more compound moments later.

What to Do *between* Sets to Gain Muscle

What you do between sets should not be an afterthought, but instead a planned part of your workout.

How long should I rest? Take shorter rest periods of thirty to ninety seconds between sets. The general rule of thumb is about a minute. Sets may be performed before full recovery has taken place, as long as the repetitions don't drop below the targeted 8 to 15 range. The shorter rest periods and moderate intensity during sets have been shown to result in greater growth hormone responses than heavier loads with longer rest periods.[2] This is good if packing on muscle is your goal.

What should I do during rest time? Performing light aerobic activity and/or some dynamic and active stretches during the rest period has also been shown to be beneficial, and results in mechanical, neural, and metabolic changes that may benefit your training goals.[1] Your rest time between sets should be viewed as active recovery time, not passive rest time spent sitting or texting on your phone.

The low-intensity activity will help with circulation, oxygen delivery, and will help clear the lactic acid from your muscles. Lengthening the muscles through passive stretching has also been shown to promote protein synthesis and muscle growth. Since there are more moderate loads during sets, static stretching would be an appropriate action between these sets, in comparison to a strength or power program where you would want to save them for the end of the workout.

Below is an example of a muscle-building set:

Suspended low or inverted row 5-set pyramid

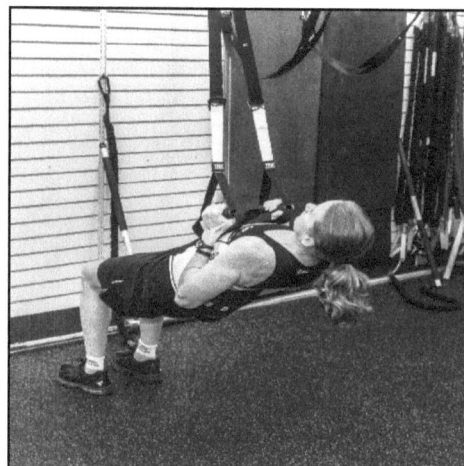

1 x 15 repetitions followed by one minute of dynamic stretching or light cardio.

1 x 12 repetitions followed by one minute of dynamic stretching or light cardio.

1 x 8 repetitions followed by one minute of dynamic stretching or light cardio.

1 x 12 repetitions followed by one minute of dynamic stretching or light cardio.

1 x 8 repetitions immediately followed by 1 x 8 repetitions of a high row (elbows up).

This is just one example. The most important thing is to get the volume at the appropriate load to fatigue you within the target repetition ranges.

Adjust the load to match the target repetition range. You should be increasing the load on the lower repetition ranges and decreasing it on the higher repetition ranges.

Some other approaches to muscle building include:

- Performing multiple sets with the same load and repetition ranges.

- Varying the repetition ranges and loads in ways like the pyramid set above.

- Multiple sets of movement variations focused on the same muscle groups.

- Performing compound sets of different movements targeting the same muscle groups (e.g., a pull-up immediately followed by a row).

- Alternate movements such as a chest movement and a leg movement or a bicep curl and triceps extension.

No matter what approach you come up with, keep the repetition ranges between 8 and 15, and make sure to take your recovery time between sets. Light activity to keep you moving between sets can include light cardio, dynamic stretching, corrective exercises, and static stretching.

Training to Gain Strength

Sets to develop strength are about high load, full recovery, and optimal quality of the movement. The temptation may be to reduce the recovery between these heavy strength sets because you feel ready or want to get more work done. Avoid doing this if strength is indeed your priority. Even if you have caught your breath and feel good, your muscles still need the time to replenish what was used in the previous set - give them what they need to repeat the movement at maximal effort. You can use the time between sets to perform light cardio, corrective exercises, or dynamic stretches. Save the static stretches for after the workout if you're working with heavy-resistance levels (refer to the stretching chapter for more information on why). You may also alternate with moderate-resistance level sets of smaller muscle groups or isolation exercises. If you choose to do this, do not work the same muscles that you're using in the heavy sets. Choose opposing muscles. For example, if you are performing max-effort single-leg squats, performing some moderate triceps extensions or reverse flys between sets is fine. Just remember to focus on which movement is your priority.

What to Do *during* Sets to Gain Strength

Use lower repetitions, ranging from 3 to 8, and higher loads to target maximal strength during your sets. Your goal is to be able to activate as many of your strongest muscle fibers, as quickly as possible, to produce as much force as possible. There is also a neuromuscular component of being able to produce maximum amounts of strength. Since you are trying to perform each repetition at a high intensity, go into each repetition focusing on trying to turn on as many fibers as possible.

> **How to Build Muscle Strength:**
>
> - **Fewer exercises.**
>
> - **Fewer repetitions.**
>
> - **Higher loads.**
>
> - **More rest time between sets.**

Think about accelerating out of each rep to maximize the power you need to create momentum. In other words, be aggressive with your movements, but also maintain total control of your form. Training to increase strength abilities requires high-intensity efforts and optimal quality of movement. With the higher load, form is crucial. You are not doing yourself any favors by squeezing out one or two more repetitions with less-than-optimal form. Focus on fewer movements, and make every set count. The intensity of the sets is taxing on your neuromuscular system as well as the tissues themselves. Focus on the compound movements that target large muscle groups, such as squats (single leg or double), pull-ups, rows, and/or presses.

What to Do *between* Sets to Gain Strength

First off, make sure you are warmed up. I don't just mean ten minutes on the stair climber. That's fine to start with, but then include some low-to-moderate-intensity preparatory movements that will help prime the muscle. This will increase the oxygen level in the muscles, improving the quality of the work to come. Examples of this would be some lower-to-moderate-intensity movements that are similar in focus to the demands of the high-intensity work to follow. I like to use dynamic stretching, bands, or the TRX Rip Trainer® cord system for warm-up circuits before strength sets.

Start each set rested to allow your body to get the most out of it. Take longer rest periods of two to four minutes for sets. Rest between sets is needed to re-establish blood flow, get oxygen to the muscles, replenish energy stores, and remove metabolic end-products that the bout of intensity has created. When training for strength, a longer rest interval results in more reestablishment of your phosphocreatine levels within the muscle, which may result in a higher force production during the next set. Light cardio and dynamic stretches will keep the body moving, keep the circulation of blood and oxygen going to the muscles, and help clear lactate.

So instead of sitting on the bench texting between sets, keep moving by doing some brisk walking, easy cycling, or dynamic stretches such as knee hugs and ankle grabs. You will be adding more efficiency to your workout time as well by doing low-intensity cardio, as it will improve the quality of your intense work and is beneficial for your cardiovascular system. Just be sure to keep the intensity low if this is part of a strength workout.

Pull-Ups

I wanted to give a special shout-out to this movement, as I feel it's one of the best movements to build upper body and core strength. It's also great for improving hand and forearm strength. Most people don't attempt pull-ups often or at all, because they can be difficult to accomplish while maintaining proper form. You are much more likely to see even the hardcore workout buff at the gym at the lat pull-down machine than doing pull-ups. If that's you, consider this a challenge for your next workout.

If your abilities are not quite ready to pull all your body weight up, here is an approach that I use with both clients and myself to help increase strength and ability for this movement. You may use a pull-up bar or a suspended strap anchored high or "super-shortened" to give you sufficient space underneath. You may also use a wide overhand grip (pull-up) or narrow underhand grip (chin-up).

Work the End Ranges

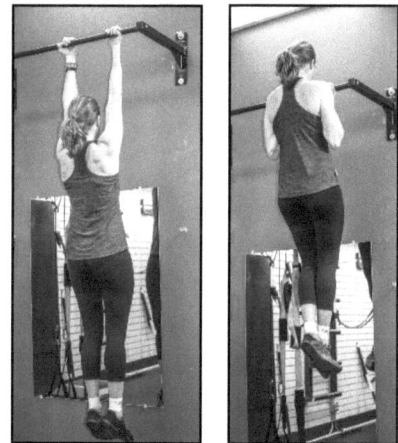

1. Grab the bar or straps and position yourself over the top, holding all your body weight. Focus on tightening your core, remember to breathe, and hold yourself up as long as possible.

2. When you can no longer hold that position, slowly lower yourself down to the bottom, allowing your arms to straighten.

3. Hold that down position for as long as you can maintain with a tight core, shoulders connected, and shoulder blades retracted (no loose shoulders).

Focus on just holding the two end positions of the range of motion of the pull-up. Try to improve the time you can hold yourself. Even if you can only do a few seconds, start there and try to build the duration. Soon you will be surprised by how much easier it is to pull yourself up over the bar. When you can do a few body-weight pull-ups, you may still want to end the set with a "hold" in each end-range position to further develop strength.

Below is an example of a strength-building set:

Push-Ups

Choose the variation that is appropriate for your level and the strength workout objective. This may include hands suspended, feet suspended, traditional, weighted, or spider push-ups.

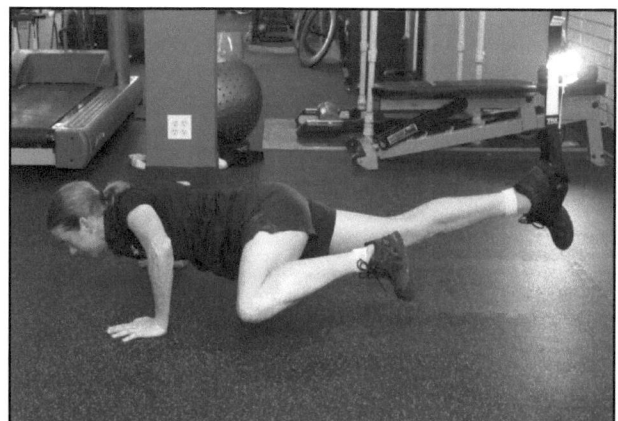

Complete three sets of 5 to 8 hard repetitions through the full range of motion. Keep your plank posture, and focus on going all the way down and driving the movement back up through a tight core.

Take three minutes of rest between sets consisting of light activity, or a dynamic stretch set in between. Strong individuals may need to add weight through

This is an image of the Suspended Spider Push-up. This is just one example. Choose the push-up variation and level of resistance that is appropriate for you.

the use of a weight vest to sufficiently fatigue them at the low-repetition range. When doing the suspended push-up movement with hands suspended, you may also add difficulty by turning to face inward, performing the push-up facing the other way, and positioning your head and shoulders directly under the anchor. Just be sure to obtain an angle that is challenging enough to fatigue you within the 5-to-8-repetition range. Focus on control over the movement throughout each repetition.

Conclusion

Like with any fitness objective, periodize or plan your program into phases during the year. This will help keep your workouts fresh, will contribute to maintaining motivation levels, and keep your body adapting. If you do the same program all year round, you will most likely plateau, and your workouts will stagnate. So even if your primary objective is one thing, changing it up and throwing something new at your body for a few weeks will result in coming back to your original focus stronger, fresher, or in a better place mentally. If an overall elevated level of fitness and great physique is your goal, continue changing things up to force your body to keep adapting.

Chapter 8

Improving Bone Density

You've probably heard of osteoporosis and are aware that bone density is something you should be concerned about, especially as you age. Losing bone density results in an increased risk of fractures, especially at the hip, spine, and wrist areas. It's a progressive condition and often doesn't come with any symptoms until you've broken a bone. Peak bone mass is reached around age thirty, and after that the reabsorption begins to exceed bone formation, resulting in less density and mass in your bones. In the United States, more than fifty-three million people either already have osteoporosis or are at considerable risk due to low bone mass.[1]

Who Is Most at Risk?

Both men and women can suffer bone loss and develop osteoporosis. However, smaller and thinner women are more at risk because they have less bone mass in general. Some additional risk factors that you can't do much about include age, family history, bone structure, and ethnicity. Research has shown that Caucasian and Asian women are more likely to develop osteoporosis. Additionally, hip fractures are twice as likely to occur in Caucasian women than in African American women.[2] Some of the risk factors that you can do something about include: avoiding smoking, limiting alcohol use, improving calcium and vitamin D levels, and increasing activity levels and exercise.

In addition, endurance athletes that participate in low- or no-impact activities (such as cycling) for extended periods of time may also be at risk. Some reasons for this include the long durations spent participating in activities with high energy demands and low forces on the bone, in combination with recovery time of even lower bone forces, and sometimes restricted diets to maintain desired weight levels. Refer to the *bone-health considerations for cyclists* section found later in this chapter for more information on this topic.

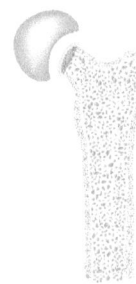

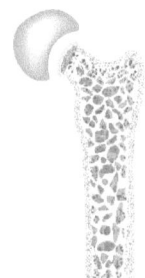

Normal Bone   Bone with Osteoporosis

According to the National Osteoporosis Foundation, "A woman's risk of breaking a hip due to osteoporosis is equal to her risk of breast, ovarian, and uterine cancer combined." Men aged fifty or older are said to be more likely to break a bone due to osteoporosis, than they are to get prostate cancer. That's pretty concerning. However, it's not all bleak and grim when it comes to your bone health as you age. The good news is that osteoporosis and low bone density are both preventable and treatable. Strength training and exercise play a BIG role.

During your peak bone-building years, you can maximize your bone growth by participating in activities that put forces on the bones to stimulate growth. Even if you got a late start participating in activities that develop bone strength, you can still make positive changes. You can strengthen bones and minimize losses through exercise and strength training at any age.

In this chapter, I will show you how to approach strength training and exercise if you're concerned about bone health. Although any form of exercise is good, not all exercise is good for your bones. Cycling is one example of this. Those whose dominant form of cardiovascular exercise is cycling may actually be at greater risk for low bone density despite all of the other benefits that are gained by cycling. Refer to the "Considerations for Cyclists" section at the end of this chapter for more information.

I will discuss ways you can design your workout program (whether you are a cyclist or not) to counteract bone loss. There are also some sample workout circuits at the end of this chapter to give you an idea how to incorporate bone-building exercises into your program.

Put Forces on Your Bones to Make Them Stronger

The aspects that account for bone strength include bone mineral density, content, bone size, and thickness. When muscles contract, they pull on the bones to which they are connected. These forces provide the stimulus for bones to grow both thicker and denser. Maximal strength training and impact forces are the best way to provide this stimulus to your bones. A bone needs to experience a tenth of the amount of force required to break it, in order to be adequately stimulated so it can create increased bone density.[3] Remember this key factor in your strength work.

Don't be afraid to lift relatively heavy weights and add some plyometrics and impact to your program. Jumping rope, box jumps, or even punching a bag for fun provide some impact for your upper body. Adding these elements to your program after developing a foundation will ensure that you are ready for the higher forces these often place on the body (refer to chapter 5).

Strength training results in your body's ability to actually increase the amount of muscle fibers being fired when asked to, as well as how fast they are able to fire. Both of these processes result in the muscles being capable of producing more force, which in turn means more forces exerted on the bones to which they are attached.

In addition to providing greater forces to stimulate bone growth, strength training also reduces risk factors that result in broken bones, by increasing muscle mass and improving balance. This is especially important in older populations of any activity level. If you have better balance, more strength and muscle, and stronger bones, they work synergistically to make you more physically resilient and stable.

You will be better prepared to handle unexpected events, like when your excited puppy darts between your legs, or an unseen slick patch of ground. Your increased athleticism will reduce the chance of falling in scenarios such as these and more. If it happens that you do take a fall, your bones are less likely to fracture from the impact. That's two ways of staying off the injury list.

How to Strength Train for Strong Bones

Put random forces on your bones to stimulate growth. Some research has shown that the best results in the short term come out of subjecting bones to high forces in a more random fashion.[4] Shorter-term training programs of more random high-intensity forces on your muscles and bones have actually been shown to be more effective than programs that progress over time. Now, this is contradictory to a program you might put together for performance gain, but it's still something that should be considered if you're concerned about improving bone strength.

Also, these suggestions are based on short-term results. It doesn't mean you shouldn't periodize your program, it's just that in that case, longer periods may be needed to produce the benefits to bone density. If you are following a periodized program and want to make sure it addresses your bone health, my suggestion is to continue along with what you've begun. However, make sure to include one or two exercises that target bone health regardless of what the overall program goals are. The purpose of these movements is to provide the forces on your bones to stimulate adaptation.

Select exercises that involve large muscle groups. The movements involving the larger muscles or multiple muscle groups are all good choices, assuming an adequate amount of resistance is used. This is because the larger muscles can produce more force than the smaller ones. Multiple muscles working together will also be able to generate more total forces on the bones, as well as provide forces in multiple planes of motion.

Allow for longer rest periods between sets to allow for greater force production. Circuit training is a type of training program where individuals perform movements, one right after the other, with little rest, and then repeat the circuit multiple times. It has not been found to be as effective for bone and muscle growth as a program with longer rest periods and higher resistances. Because the short or absent rest periods in a circuit program don't allow for recovery, the forces you can push are lower. Circuit training may still help with bone health in the long term and is still great exercise. However, if stronger bones are your goal, design a program that involves more strength, higher forces, and longer rest intervals. This will allow for more maximal forces to be produced during the sets.

If you are someone who likes to attend group circuit classes or who is not as comfortable lifting heavy weights or pushing with high force, you should be aware that you are at greater risk for osteoporosis. In addition, if you are a cyclist or long-distance runner who doesn't utilize strength training or doesn't lift heavy weights for whatever reason, you are also at risk. This is particularly the case for lighter and leaner individuals.

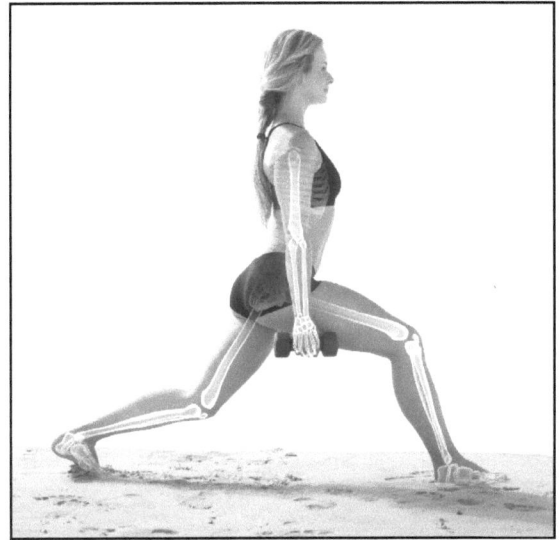

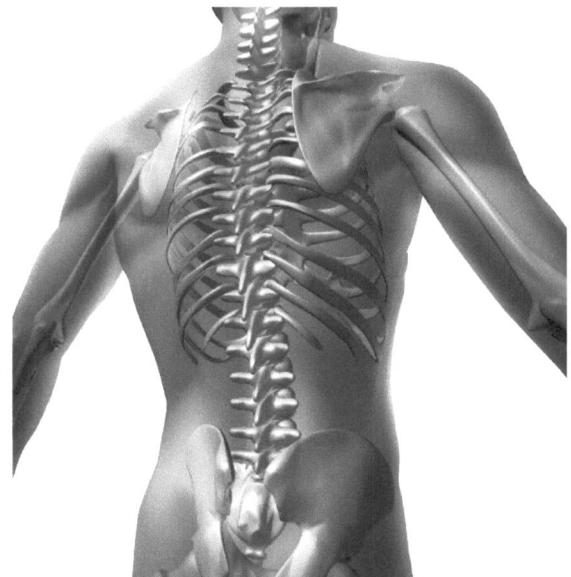

Choose movements to load key areas of the body. The results of multiple studies reveal that bone density is site specific. This means that all of the bicep curls and chest presses in the world will not help you increase bone density in your hips and pelvis, as much as doing lower-body movements that put stress on the hips and pelvis. Lumbar spine stress is achieved by loading weight on the back and spine, such as doing deadlifts or squats with weight (done with proper form) and by performing sit-up-type movements and back extensions. Stress on the femur occurs when legs are put under heavy load or impact forces. Thus, if you want strong bones in your hips, legs, and spine, make sure you include resistance movements that target those areas. Conversely, if you have a particular region of the body you are concerned about, be sure to give that area some more love with additional site-specific exercises.

Include jumping, sprinting, and plyometrics in your program.
Impact movments and movements in which loading is applied at a high rate also provide more stimulus for bone growth. This includes jumping, sprinting and plyometic activities. [5] in addition, if you participate in sports such as tennis, basketball, or other activities that involve jumping, accelerating, or quick changes of direction, you have a definite advantage when it comes to maintaining strong bones. Saying this, devleoping a foundation of strength(chapter 5) in these movements before progressing to more intense jumping and sprinting activities is crucial to ensure your muscles and tendons can handle these high and changing directional forces.

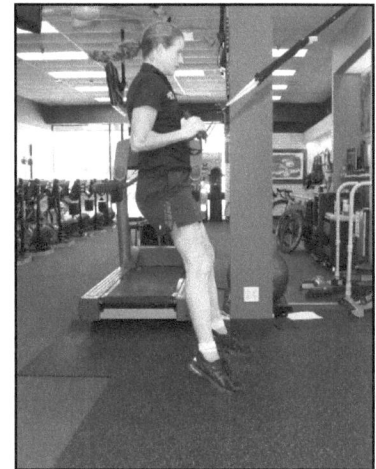

Jump squat using a suspended trainer.

Beyond suspended training. In addition to suspended-training movements, consider adding movements where the spine is placed under load, such as squats with a bag, bar, or a standing machine. Loading up a leg press might be beneficial for the hips, but it will not put the necessary compression forces on the spine needed to stimulate bone growth. The "farmer's walk" (an exercise where you are simply carrying heavy weights); pressing; pulling or lifting heavy kettlebells or dumbbells; barbell work; kicking, punching, or flipping heavy bags; jump roping; pull-ups; high-intensity running, shuffling, or cutting; and jumping are all good additions that will stimulate bone growth. These can supplement your suspended-training program if you have access to additional equipment. An example of this would be performing a suspended squat jump followed by a suspended push-up with high resistance, and a sprint to the end of the block. These would be three extremely beneficial exercises to stimulate bone growth.

Conclusion

If you are concerned about your bone health, it doesn't mean you need to turn your program upside down. Simply include one or two random exercises that stress your legs, hips, and lumbar spine with some impact and force. If you are just starting to strength train or know that you already have low bone density or osteoporosis, the more explosive exercises should be phased in gradually as you improve your strength and fitness level. Always develop the foundation before adding higher intensity or more specific work to your program. Just keep in mind that being consistent and including bone-building activity in your program during the long term, will produce benefits.

Bone Health Considerations for Cyclists

Cycling has a variety of health benefits and is definitely a good activity for your body. However, the research has shown that it does not help create strong bones. In fact, it may even decrease your bone density, depending on the amount of cycling training you do. So, if your sole form of exercise is cycling, you may end up with weaker bones than someone who is not even active! The good news is that you can counteract this with some cross training and strength training.

I also feel that it's important to mention that information in this section is focused on those who participate in outdoor cycling for fitness and competition. Those whose primary form of cardio exercise is "spin" type classes, will still get some good insight from this chapter,

> Adult road cyclists who train regularly have significantly lower bone mineral density in key regions.

but they are less likely to spend extended amounts of time on the bike, and may be at less risk than a cyclist training ten to twenty hours a week. Having said that, bone health is important for everyone, and it's still a good idea to consider it in your fitness program.

Why isn't cycling good for my bones?

There is a lot of research available on bone health and some specific investigations on cycling and bone health. Studies have consistently found several reasons why cyclists have lower-than-normal bone densities...

Cycling is a non-weight-bearing activity. The primary reason for cyclists having low bone density is that it's not a weight-bearing activity. High-level cycling in particular has been shown to have negative effects on bone strength because of the amount of time cyclists spend training and riding. Cyclists spend lot of time seated with no compression forces on the spine and pelvis. Even though it may feel like you are pedaling hard at times, the forces you are putting into the pedals are also not distributed in a way that puts significant strain on your bones, which is needed for bone growth.

Recovery time also non–weight bearing. The necessary recovery time from hard cycling usually involves additional non-weight-bearing activity of sitting or lying down. Most cyclists reported avoiding weight-bearing activities during recovery periods as a way to help enhance recovery from training.

Cyclists generally have lower body mass. Cyclists generally are lighter, and low body mass is another risk factor for osteoporosis and osteopenia. This especially applies to women, who in general have lower body mass, as well as to performance cyclists, who are consistently striving to obtain a low body weight in order to improve performance.

Cyclists have an increased risk of fracture due to crashes or falls. Whether you compete or just ride for fitness and fun, chances are at some point you will take a fall or be involved in a crash. This applies to any level cyclist, whether you ride solo, with friends, in groups, or compete in rallies and races.

Level of Cycling Experience and Bone-Density Risks

If you are a road cyclist, especially if you train hard or have been training for multiple years, you are more likely to develop osteopenia or osteoporosis than the average person. This puts you at a higher risk for fractures, a risk that continues to go up with age and training. In one study, more Masters-Age cyclists were classified as osteoporotic when compared to age-matched non-athletes, and the percentage of those with osteoporosis or osteopenia, increased significantly after a seven-year period.[10] So for those of you in this category (which may be the majority of people reading this), you are not only more likely to be at risk, but the risk factor also gets higher as you get older, and complete more years of cycling training.

In 2012, there was an extensive review of thirty-one studies on the subject of cycling and bone health.[11] The findings showed that adult road cyclists who train regularly have significantly lower bone mineral density in key regions. This was found to be true when comparing cyclists to control populations of both athletes in other sports, as well as non-athletes. Areas of the lumbar spine, pelvic and hip regions and femoral neck were all key areas found to have lower values in road cyclists than in the control groups with which they were compared.

Included in this review were only a few studies involving amateur cyclists or low-level cyclists (versus more experienced and elite cyclists). Differences in bone mass were not found between the cyclists and controls when compared with low-level cyclists. However, studies that examined elite cyclists, or those training at high levels for numerous years, consistently found low bone mineral density. This further supports the idea that the level of training and length of training are strong factors in cyclists being at risk for low bone density.

Junior Cyclists

Most of the research on differences in bone health considered those older than seventeen years of age. It's worth saying that it's believed that cycling in the early years of life does not negatively affect the bones. However, it doesn't positively affect the bones either. Participation in other sports has been shown to positively affect bone growth more than cycling. Translation: allow juniors to train hard and train often, but make sure they are getting some cross training as well to create maximum bone growth.

Differences Found with Different Cycling Disciplines

Road cycling at a competitive level might be more detrimental for bone health than mountain biking and recreational forms of cycling. This is due to all the reasons stated previously: long hours on the bike, non-weight-bearing activity, no impact forces, low forces in general while pedaling, and lots of time off your feet trying to recover from training.

Mountain bikers were found to have higher bone mineral density than road cyclists. One reason given for this was the vibrations endured during off-road riding. Depending on the level of mountain biking, the increased short durations of high force to get over obstacles may also help.

Sprint-trained cyclists have stronger bones than distance-trained cyclists. This makes sense because of the large forces they generate for short periods of time. The leg muscles are creating high forces, which in turn puts high forces on the bones to which they are connected. The high forces for short durations are similar to the demands of weightlifting. However, keep in mind that this is still a non-weight-bearing activity, so as hard as you might go as a sprinter, compression forces on the spine are still not present.

Triathletes and Duathletes do not appear to experience the same negative effects as those who do only cycling training. The combination of cycling and running appears to counteract the negative effects on bone mass that may result from cycling alone.

Cycling and Bone Health Conclusion

Research repeatedly recommends that cycling as a form of exercise should be complemented with cross training and strength training activities to stimulate bone growth. It was also found that cyclists who started weight training and/or plyometric exercises during the long-term studies lost significantly less bone mass. Running has been shown to be beneficial as well due to the impact forces involved. However, both short and long-distance runners will still benefit from including strength work to support overall bone health in their training programs. This is especially true if you have low body weight and run long distances in your training, which requires more nutritional resources. Both long-distance runners and cyclists should take heed and be sure to include strength and cross-training activities that put higher forces on the muscles and bones to keep them strong.

We all want strong bones that are resistant to breaking, especially as we age. This is even more important for a cyclist. Let's face it, a crash or fall at some point in your cycling life is likely to happen. Stacking the odds in your favor by including activities to maintain and stimulate bone strength is your best line of defense against a fracture just in case you do happen to hit the ground at a greater impact than you would like.

Chapter 9

Stretching for Better Movement

Mobility is important. Moving well is important. It's important to feel good. It's also an important aspect of our quality of life as we age. Most of us spend too much of our day sitting down. If you spend a significant amount of time at a desk or in a vehicle, it's especially important to incorporate stretching into your routine. Poor mobility can cause your muscles to feel tight and your posture to suffer. It can also cause imbalances that result in compensations that harm your movement patterns.

Poor mobility and muscle imbalance may lead to aches and pains as well as injuries. This can lead to a downward spiral of inactivity that sometimes goes along with age. When your mobility is poor, it doesn't feel good to move. When it doesn't feel good to move, you move less. When you move less, you lose more of your movement abilities...and so on.

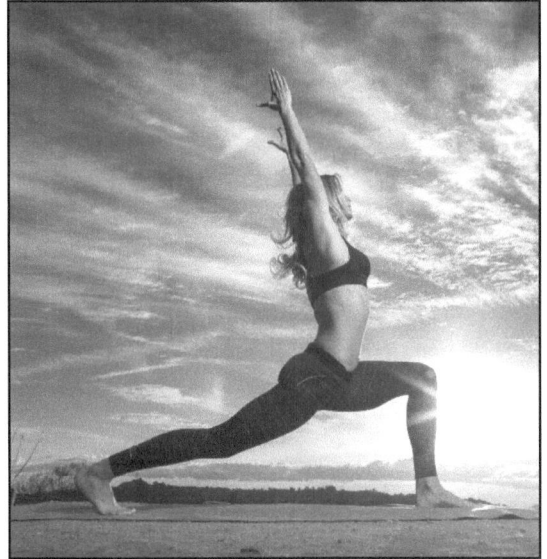

This chapter touches on types of stretching, why stretching is important, and how and when to implement it in your training plan. It also includes a library of stretches, information on having a balanced stretch routine, and key areas of possible tightness to watch out for, depending on your lifestyle. The stretching recommended in this book assumes you are a healthy individual with some tightness or mobility limitations. Those rehabbing from injuries, trauma, or conditions such as osteoarthritis or neuromuscular diseases should refer to their primary care physicians before starting an exercise program.

"Stretching isn't about today's workout, it's about preventing an injury six months down the road."
— Mike Boyle, author of Functional Training for Sports and founder of Mike Boyle Strength and Conditioning

Many of the long-term benefits of stretching are different from the short-term effects. Stretching consistently over several weeks can create an increase in flexibility and lower the tension from the muscle on the joints to which they are connected.[1] Although each individual is different, I've had clients experience reductions in back and neck pain both during daily living and sporting activities, after incorporating stretching into their routines.

Stretching is defined as:

"The application of force to musculotendinous structures, in order to achieve a change in their length, usually for the purposes of improving joint range of motion (ROM), or reducing stiffness or soreness, or preparing for physical activity."[3]

My own personal experience is similar. As a competitive cyclist and personal trainer, I was fortunate enough not to have to spend a lot of time seated and was usually able to stay active during the day. For a long time, I assumed my movement was sufficient just from my daily active lifestyle. I wasn't making stretching a priority. However, I was experiencing aches that would turn into stabbing pains in my lower neck and upper shoulders during long bike rides. After completing the course for my functional movement certification, I realized that my upper spine and torso mobility was not all what I had assumed it was. I added some rotation stretches for that area into and between workouts, and within a few weeks the pain I experienced in my upper shoulders while cycling was greatly reduced. The best part is that although it took some consistent stretching and mobility initially, I can now maintain it and keep the problem at bay with much less effort.

Consistently stretching over days and weeks is much more effective than trying to catch up by doing a long session of a whole bunch of stretch work.

This is good news because it means you don't need to add yet another session requirement to your program. You can work it in between strength movements in your current routine, which can result in tremendous benefits for individuals with mobility limitations or poor flexibility. You can also add stretches as part of a warm-up and/or cooldown. Some of you may need more than others, and some of you may not have to work on this at all. Those that fall into the latter category may be better off focusing on other weak links. But if you feel that doing the stretches in both the dynamic and static stretch library are challenging or results in significant improvement in the targeted areas, it's a good idea to include time for stretching in your program in some way.

Why Stretch?

The primary goal of stretching is to increase and maintain range of motion.

For the purpose of this chapter, there are three primary reasons for stretching, each one having its own objective and place in your workout program.

1. Increasing flexibility and mobility (static stretching) to increase muscle and joint range of motion and bring back and maintain mobility.

2. Preparing for an upcoming training session (dynamic stretching) as part of an active warm-up routine to prepare for the upcoming workout session.

3. Recovering from a previous workout (dynamic stretching). Gentle dynamic stretching can serve as a form of recovery by increasing blood flow and circulation. If you are sore from a previous workout, don't push the stretches. Just move through the range of motion enough to let muscles recover and heal.

Having even one tight area of your body can affect your whole movement chain. An example given in the book "*Stretching for Functional Flexibility*" (Arminger, Martin, 2010) describes a scenario such as this. Someone with shortened calves may have a less-than-optimal ability to bend the ankle, by lifting his or her foot up enough for his or her toes to clear the ground, while walking and running. Because of this, the person needs to compensate by increasing hip flexion to lift the knee higher with every step.

A side effect of this chronic and excessive hip flexion may show us as hip pain.[3] The human muscle and movement chain is complicated. A lack of stretch or mobility in one area affects many others and can result in pain and possible injury anywhere in the chain. Maintaining a program targeting balanced movement can go a long way in preventing aches, pains, and expensive doctors' visits.

There are particularly vulnerable populations who may suffer a lack of mobility due to their daily living activities.

- Do you spend a lot of time seated for your job?

- Do you often wear high heels?

- Do you spend a lot of time in front of a computer?

The most common areas of tightness and poor mobility that I find, are in those who have sedentary jobs, and their pain is in the upper back and hip flexors. If you sit for extended periods of time, both your hip flexors and hamstrings are in a shortened state. Hip extension is important for running and walking. If someone has tightness in their hip flexors, the muscles will at some point in the stride start to resist the extension.

This results in a less-than-optimal stride length or range, as the leg cannot reach the full range of motion to extend behind the body and push off. In addition, other parts of your mechanics may be affected as well (such as appropriate forward lean). Spending a lot of time in high heels means your calves are shortening for long periods of time; they are more likely to get tight and lose mobility. Sitting hunched over a computer is a double whammy. You've probably seen people with rounded shoulders and backs. Chances are, someone who looks like this also lacks mobility in his or her upper spine and is tight in his or her chest and shoulders. The poor posture that results in this can lead to a multitude of other issues. Some of these include less-than-optimal breathing abilities due to less space for the diaphragm to extend, neck and back pain, and muscles being asked to perform tasks they were not designed to do.

Refer to the stretch libraries found in this book for specific stretches you can do if you have a sedentary job.

What Types of Stretches Are There?

We are going to focus on two types of stretching: Static and Dynamic.

Static stretching. When people think about the concept of stretching, it's often static stretching that comes to mind. Static stretching can be defined as passively stretching a muscle to the point of tension or mild discomfort. It's stretching the muscle to its farthest point away from where it attaches for an extended period of time.

Performing static stretching consistently over time will improve your range of motion and mobility. To achieve initial gains, it's recommended you initially commit to performing your stretch routine several times a week. After you have achieved some improvement, you may reduce the sessions or the durations to maintain your improvements. However, don't end up reducing them so much that they fall out of your program altogether. Make sure you make stretching a part of your lifestyle so as to not revert and lose the gains you've made.

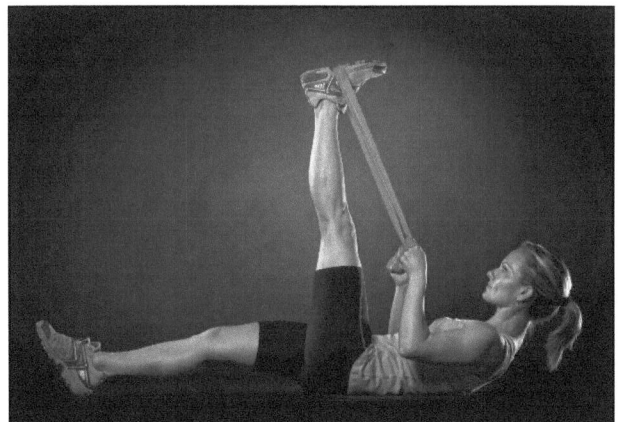

How long should I hold static stretches? The literature supports holding static stretches for twenty to thirty seconds maximum. The reason for this is because most of the stress relaxation occurs in the first fifteen to twenty seconds of the stretch.[1] This means that after fifteen to twenty seconds, your muscle starts to relax, and you can provide less force to hold the stretch in the same position.

How hard should I push static stretches? Perform these static stretches slowly, and don't go so far into them that it hurts. Start with a light stretch, and increase as you feel comfortable doing so. If the speed or the force of the stretch is too high, sensors in the muscles may respond by tightening up as a protective mechanism. Ease into the stretch until you feel some tension. If you feel any discomfort or pain, reset and start again. You may find that during the second or third repeat, you'll be able to go farther into the stretch as your muscles loosen up.

When should I do static stretches? Static stretching is great for improving flexibility and maintaining good movement abilities. However, you may have heard the advice not to stretch before hard workout sessions. The reason for this is that stretching for twenty to thirty seconds or longer causes a temporary reduction in strength and power generation in some of the fibers. Your muscle fibers have elastic properties to them. When they are stretched, and the stretch is held, this causes the muscle to temporarily lose some of its tension, much like if you would stretch and hold a rubber band. This is temporary and is not at all harmful. The elasticity comes back, and your muscles are on their way to have an increased ROM and more flexibility.

However, this means that doing static stretches before intense workouts involving maximal strength efforts, jumping, or sprinting, may affect what you can do during those activities. If you're more of a novice when it comes to fitness, or flexibility is one of your priorities, don't worry about this when performing static stretching. Just stretch, and do it consistently. Your workouts are not designed for power development, but for better movement and fitness abilities. The health benefits you will get from stretching far outweigh any temporary decrease of force capabilities.

If you are doing more advanced or intense workouts, though, this temporary decrease in elastic tension and force capabilities is something you might want to consider. Keep static stretches as part of your cooldown if you're planning on doing a workout geared toward strength or power development, or plyometric and jump movements.

Dynamic stretching. These are moving stretches that often mimic the motion that will eventually be performed afterward during the workout session. This type of stretching is good for both cooldown and warm-up sessions. Using dynamic stretching as part of the warm-up will help prepare and loosen muscles for the demand that will be placed on them.

They will lower resistance in the muscles you are about to work out, improve oxygen delivery, increase metabolic reactivity, and may result in you having a more effective workout. A workout may even consist of a series of dynamic stretches and nothing more! Dynamic stretches as a cooldown will circulate blood, help clear waste products from the muscles, and allow for better circulation as your heart rate comes down, all which prevent pooling of blood from happening.

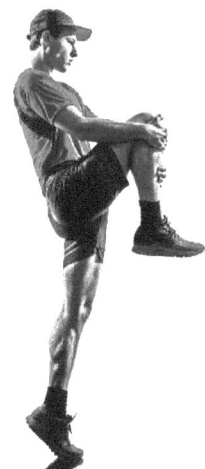

How long should I do dynamic stretches? Hold the end-point of each position for just one or two seconds. Keep moving through the set. Most of the dynamic stretches will either have you moving your extremities through a range of motion, one side at a time, or alternating sides. A ballpark number of repetitions is in the range of 8 to 12 on each side, or 10 repetitions total if the stretch is targeting both sides of the body. The number of repetitions of course depends on the movements being performed. Rest as needed between sets—you may be surprised how much work these movements can feel like if you're working through tight muscles.

How hard should I push static stretches? Perform these static stretches slowly, and don't go so far into them that it hurts. Go into the range of motion until you feel a light stretch, and push it from there as you feel comfortable. Never bounce or push so hard that it's painful.

Research currently recommends an active warm-up routine that mimics the upcoming workout. Dynamic stretching fits right into that. The dynamic stretch movements not only work your muscle and joints through your full range of motion, they will also increase circulation and heart rate and get you mentally and physically ready for the upcoming workout.

When to Stretch

Dynamic stretching can be done any time you can fit it into your schedule. It can serve as a warm-up before a workout or a cooldown after. It can also be performed as an active recovery workout, light workout, or recovery day. Performing some of the dynamic stretches after a long day of travel or a long workday will help to balance your muscles out and will probably help you feel a lot better. Beginning the day with some dynamic stretches will help you start off on the right foot and get you moving. They don't have to be intense. They don't have to even take more than a few minutes. But they will set the tone for your day and help keep your body and muscles feeling good.

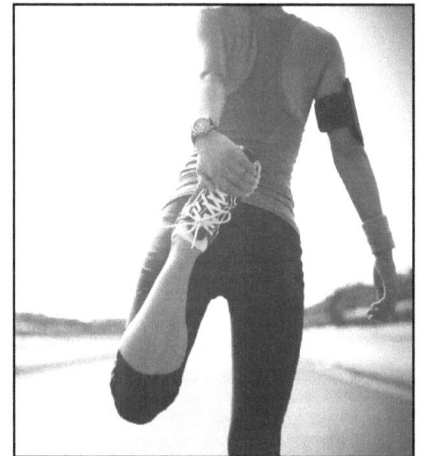

Static stretching can also be done at any available time. However, if you are training at high intensities or attempting to increase power and maximal strength abilities, refer to the "Static Stretching" section. Static stretching and intense stretching of prime movers should not be done prior to events that require a max strength output or power production. If this applies to your program, you would be better off doing dynamic stretches before and during your workout, and saving the static stretch for afterward and recovery days.

For most readers, if you were to add some static stretching before and/or during your workout, that would be perfectly OK. When it comes to general fitness and health, the benefits most people get from stretching outweigh any lag time that might result in a slight difference in power production.

Conclusion

In summary, understanding why stretching is beneficial, determining how to incorporate it into your program, and learning the stretches for each muscle group, are important aspects of a complete training program. You can be the strongest and fittest person in almost every way, but your weakest link may be hurting the quality of your movement. This applies to both daily living activities and recreational or competitive endeavors. Making sure your freedom of movement is allowing for optimal efficiency, ensures that you're getting the most from your workout and recovery sessions.

A note to those who are hypermobile: If you are someone who is naturally flexible or even excessively flexible, stretching doesn't really need to be a priority for you. It may feel good, and doing it for recovery or after long periods of inactivity is still a good thing. Studies have found that higher rates of injury can occur in those not flexible enough, as well as in those who are too flexible. In addition, joint stability and mobility are inversely related. If you or someone you are working with falls into this hypermobile category, my suggestion is to focus on developing stability and strength over flexibility. Choose movements from the "Exercises Library" detailed later on in this book, and spend your workout time with that in mind.

Stretching Considerations for Cyclists and Triathletes

Cyclists often suffer from some of the same tight areas as someone with a sedentary desk job. Cyclists who also have a desk job during the day and who train hard in the evenings and on weekends are even more at risk for developing imbalances. The reason for this is that cyclists are spending long periods of time seated on a bike and over the handlebars. This results in the hip flexors and front of the body developing tightness. Triathletes who train in the aero position are at risk as well. Triathletes have the unique demand of needing optimal mobility coming off a hard (and sometimes long) bike ride to be able to perform well in the run. Tight hip flexors and a tight front of the body can restrict breathing, zap your performance, and counteract hours of hard training. The good news is that this issue is generally an easy fix. It just takes adding some stretches to your cooldown or warm-up to balance out the time you spend on the bike. If you spend a lot of time riding, make sure to focus on stretches that lengthen the hip flexors, open up the chest and shoulders, and target the upper and lower torso to achieve this balance.

Chapter 10

Library of Stretches

Static Stretches

Hip-Hinge Stretch, Wide Stance Static

Targeted Area: Back of the legs and calves as well as the inner thigh, due to the wide stance.

Setup: Straps fully extended

A great stretch, especially if you spend a lot of time seated during the day.

1. Start facing inward with a wide foot stance. Hold the handles and straighten your arms out in front of you.

2. Bend over by hinging at the hips and reaching with the arms in front of you while keeping your back in a flat position.

3. Hold for roughly thirty seconds and return to starting position.

Note: Remember to breathe! Take continuous deep breaths during the stretch.

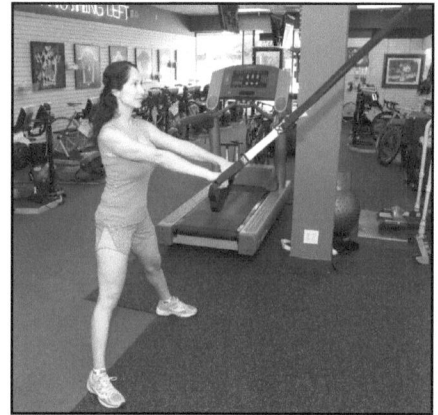

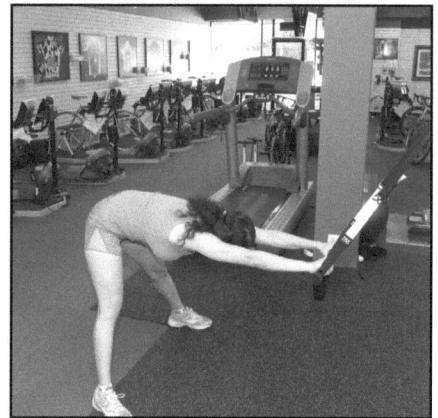

Behind-the-Back Shoulder Stretch Static

Targeted Area: Chest and shoulders

Setup: Straps fully extended to shortened

This stretch opens up the front of the body and improves posture. If you spend a lot of time seated or in a vehicle during the day, this is especially important.

1. Start facing outward with the suspended training strap hanging directly behind you.

2. Reach back and grab the strap with one arm behind your head and the other behind your lower back.

3. Inch your hands closer together along the strap until you feel the stretch in your shoulders. Hold for twenty to thirty seconds.

Note: Maintain a good, tall posture, and try to keep the back of your head, upper spine, and sacrum all in contact with the strap during the stretch. Focus on keeping the top elbow back to give you a better stretch.

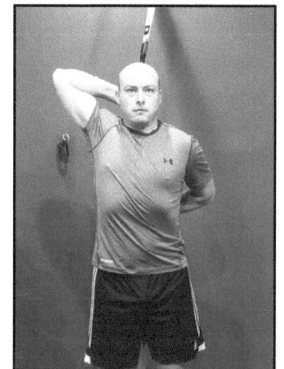

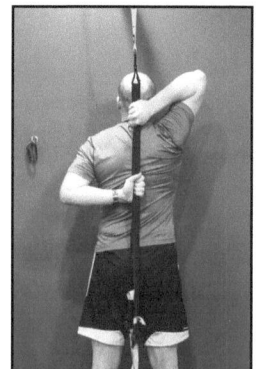

Calf Stretch Static

Targeted Area: Calves

Setup: Straps fully extended

This stretch is good for your walk and run gait because it develops adequate ankle mobility.

1. Start facing outward with the straps under your armpits and arms close to your side, bent at the elbows. Lean forward into the straps.

2. Push your heels into the floor until you feel a stretch in your calves. Step back farther and lean more into the straps to increase the amount of stretch.

3. Hold for roughly thirty seconds.

Note: You may also stretch one leg at a time in the same manner. Just keep the other foot forward.

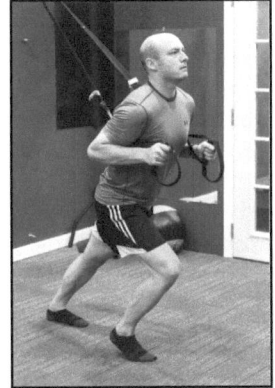

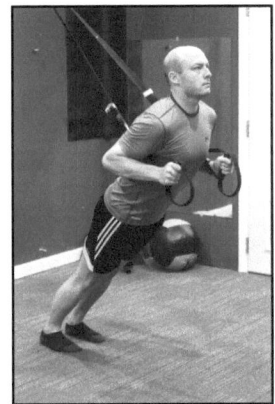

Back and Hamstring Stretch Static

Targeted Area: Hamstrings and back

Setup: Straps fully extended

This stretch targets the entire chain of muscles on the back side of the body.

1. Face toward the straps, holding the handles.

2. Lean back by pushing your hips behind you and extending your arms. Keep a slight bend in the knees.

3. Hold for roughly thirty seconds.

Note: Fully extend your arms and squeeze your ears to obtain a good stretch of the large back muscles.

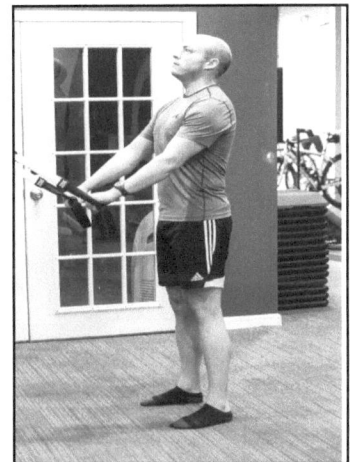

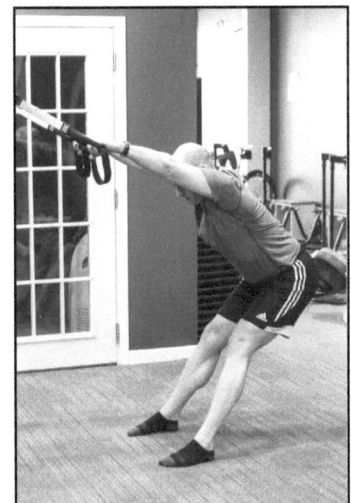

Hip Flexor Stretch (Half Kneeling) Static

Targeted Area: Hip flexors and the front of the thighs.

Setup: Straps fully extended

These are two variations of a great stretch for both the quads and hip flexors. It's good for those who spend a lot of time seated at a desk or behind a wheel, or cyclists who spend a lot of time on the bike. Use a pad or towel under the downed knee for comfort. You will be stretching the front of the leg of the downed knee.

1. Focus on good posture and making yourself tall. Reach upward toward the ceiling with the same hand as the knee you are kneeling on to increase the stretch. You should feel a stretch in the upper part of the front of that thigh.

2. Add the arm extension to increase the stretch and lengthen out the upper torso.

3. Hold for thirty seconds on one side, and then switch sides.

Note: If you don't feel the stretch, you may elevate your back foot more, which will increase the stretch. You may also reach back if you are flexible enough and grab the back foot with your opposite hand.

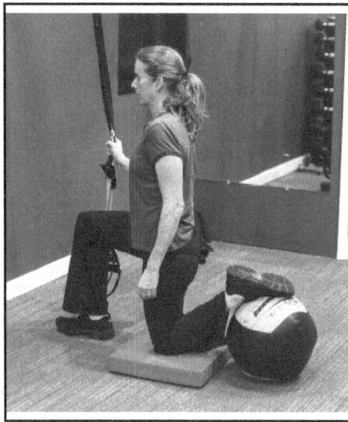

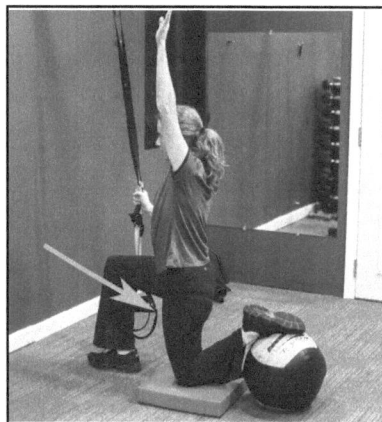

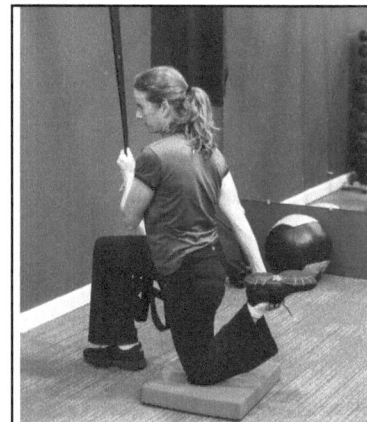

*You don't need a suspended trainer for this version, but you may use one for balance.

To the right is a version of the same hip flexor stretch with the back foot suspended. Increase the height of the suspended trainer by shortening the straps. This will increase the height of the back foot and the amount of stretch.

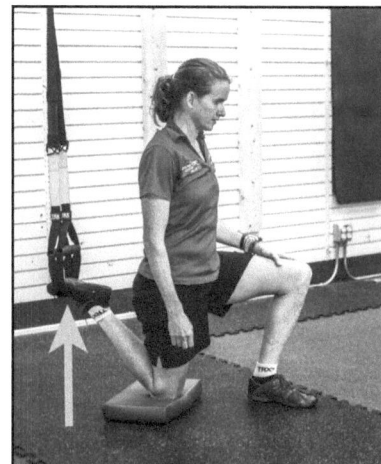

Arm Bar Stretch Static

Targeted Area: Shoulders

Setup: Straps fully extended

1. Stand facing outward, holding one of the straps in each hand, and extend your arms straight out to the side from your shoulders. There should be tension on the straps.

2. Bring one arm across the front of your body while keeping it extended.

3. Adjust your position forward until you feel a gentle stretch in the shoulder of the arm that is crossed in front of you. Hold for thirty seconds on one side, and then switch sides.

Note: Stay tall and keep good posture during this stretch.

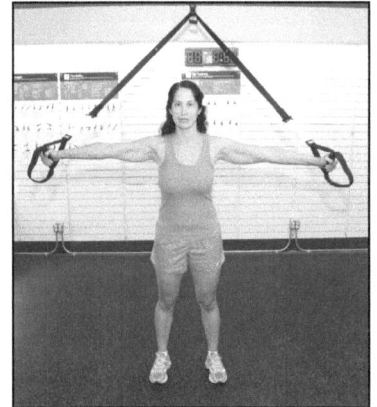

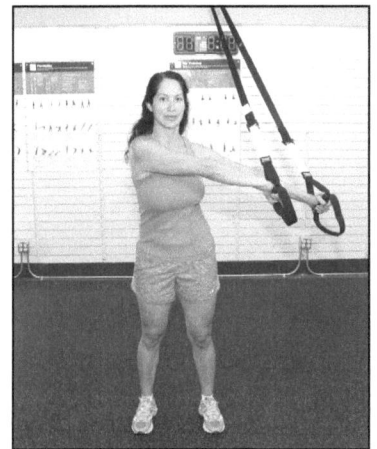

Hip Flexor and Chest Stretch Static

Targeted Area: Hip flexors and chest

Setup: Straps fully extended

This stretch will open up your chest and lengthen your hip flexors at the same time—great for those who spend a lot of time behind a desk. It's also a good stretch for cyclists because your position on the bike results in the hip flexors and front of the upper torso being in a shortened position for much of the time.

1. Stand facing outward, holding one of the straps in each hand.

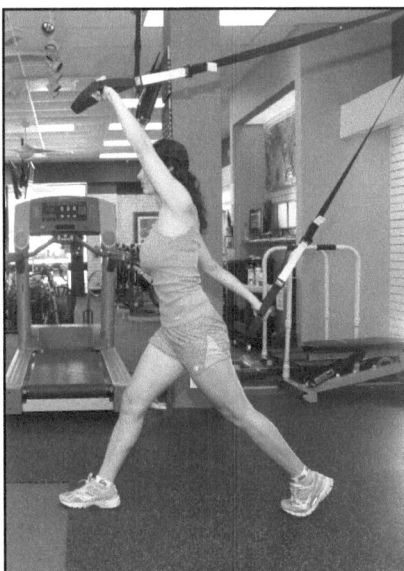

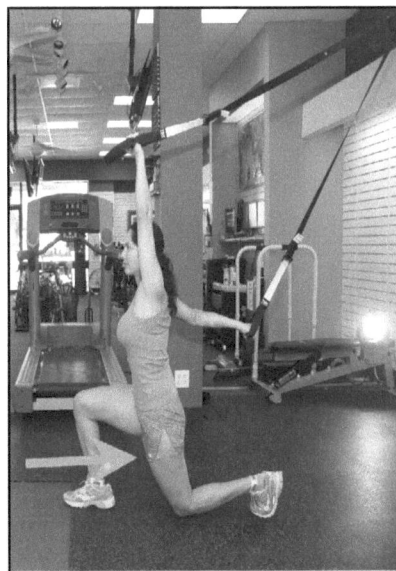

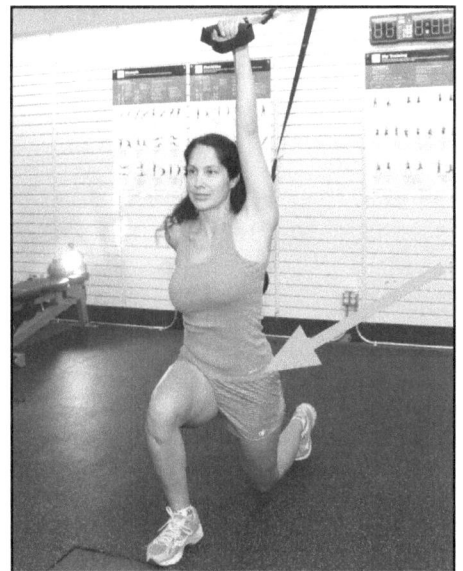

Continued on next page....

2. Move forward until you have tension on the straps. Reach up and extend one arm toward the ceiling and the other down toward the floor. Kneel down on the knee that is on the same side as the raised arm.

3. Adjust your position forward or backward until you feel a gentle stretch in the front of your upper thigh and in your chest area. Hold for thirty seconds on one side, and then switch sides.

Note: Contract your abdominals prior to and during the stretch to set your pelvis in the correct position and prevent your back from arching.

Hip and Inner Thigh Stretch Static

Targeted Area: Hips and inner thighs

Setup: Straps fully extended

1. Stand facing inward while holding onto the handles. Make sure to take a wide stance with your feet far apart from each other.

2. Sway to one side, allow that knee to bend, and lower yourself down while keeping the other leg extended.

3. Allow yourself to sink down into the bent leg. Go only as low as you are comfortable with, and then switch sides.

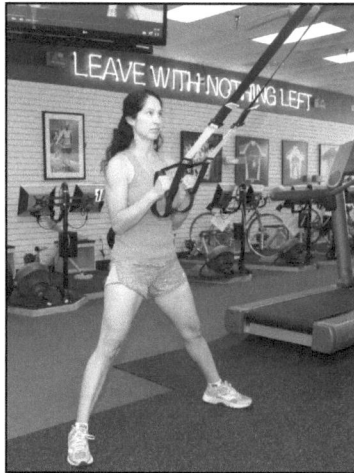

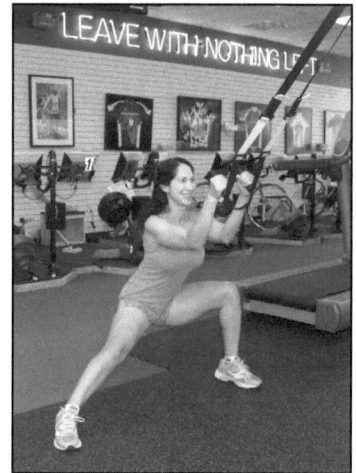

Note: You may feel this in your hips on the side you're leaning toward, or in your inner thigh on the extended leg, depending on your individual flexibility.

Upper-Torso Stretch Static

Targeted Area: Upper body and torso

Setup: Straps fully extended

The elongation of the body through the torso will help improve posture and breathing for those tight in the upper torso.

1. Stand facing inward while holding onto the handles.

2. Turn toward one side while extending your arms up and over that shoulder. Your head may turn in the direction you are reaching.

3. Keep your arms extended by reaching toward the ceiling and allowing the rotation to come from your torso. Hold for thirty seconds on one side, and then switch sides.

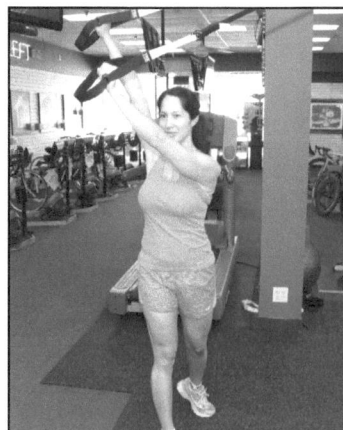

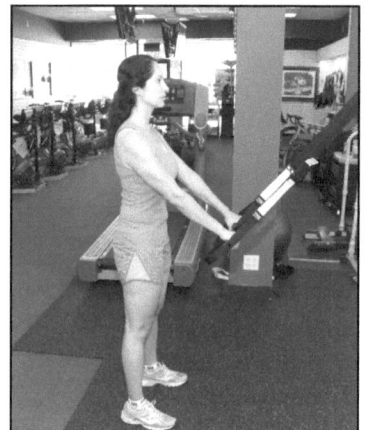

Note: Stay tall, turn yourself into the rotation, and lean into the straps until you feel the stretch.

Lower-Torso Stretch Static

Targeted Area: Torso and hips

Setup: Straps fully extended

You will be pleasantly surprised at how good this stretch feels both during and after, if done correctly. Elongation of the body through the torso during this effort will help maintain mobility in the shoulder and torso. It will also stretch the hamstring of the straightened leg. Try to stay relaxed and loose and allow your body to accept the stretch.

1. Stand facing inward while holding onto the handles.

2. Allow yourself to bend at the waist, pushing your hips back behind you. You will be somewhat hanging on the straps.

3. Turn to one side while keeping that leg straight and allowing the other to bend. Rotate to that side until you feel an adequate stretch. Hold for thirty seconds on one side, and then switch sides.

Note: You may turn your head and look in the direction toward which you are stretching.

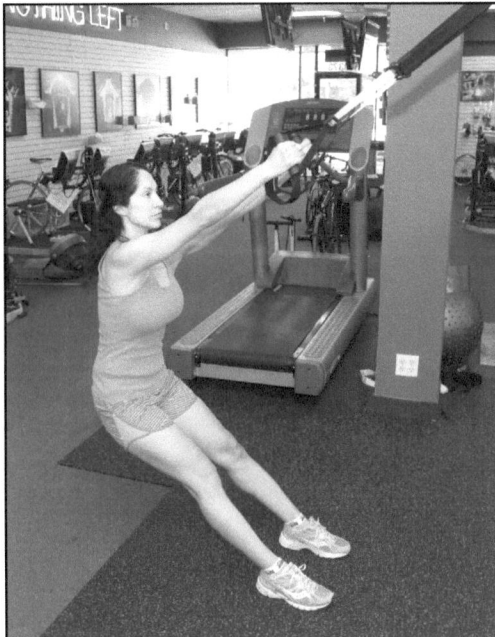

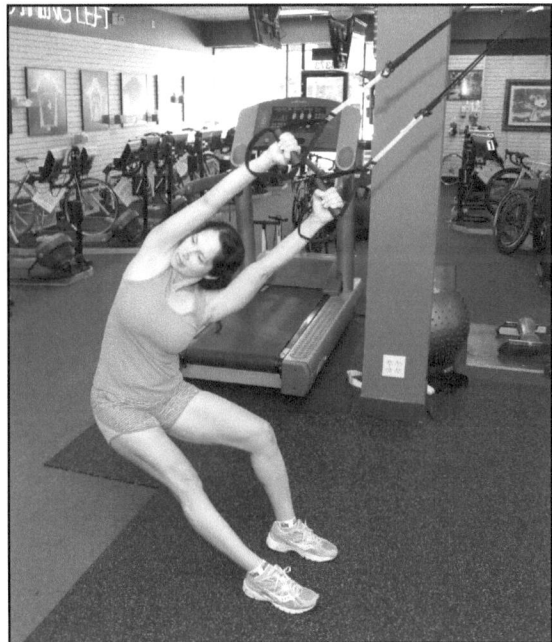

Hip-Drop Stretch Static

Targeted Area: Hips and inner thighs

Setup: Straps fully extended or shortened to mid-length.

1. Stand facing inward while holding onto the handles with your feet shoulder-width apart.

2. Drop your hips down to the floor as you lift one foot and place it on the opposite knee.

3. Allow yourself to go down until you feel a stretch in the hip of the leg that is elevated. Go only as low as you are comfortable with, and then switch sides.

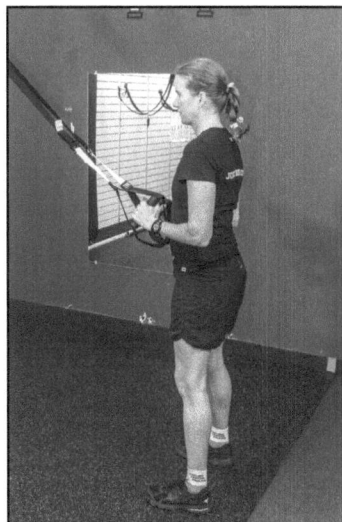

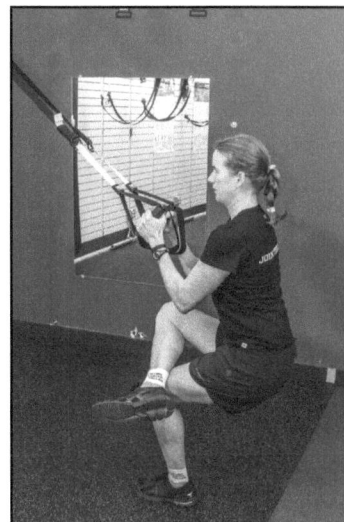

Note: Those with adequate hip mobility will be able to descend a lot lower than those without such mobility.

Chest Stretch Static

Targeted Area: Front of chest and shoulders.

Setup: Straps fully extended or shortened to mid-length.

A good exercise for those who have jobs requiring a lot of time bent over a desk or computer, which is a position that tends to close off the front of the body. Keeping the mobility in the shoulders and chest may also improve posture and breathing abilities.

1. Start facing outward, and put your forearms through the foot cradles.

2. Raise your arms so that your upper arm is parallel with the floor and your elbow is bent to ninety degrees.

3. Move forward until you feel a gentle stretch in your chest and shoulders.

Note: A slight forward lean to increase the stretch is OK.

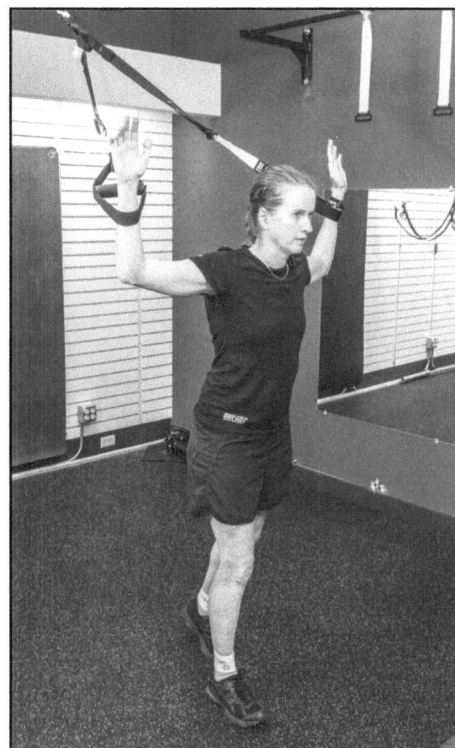

Golf Stretch Static

Targeted Area: Upper torso

Setup: Straps fully extended.

Keeping the mobility in the upper torso and spine will help improve posture and breathing abilities.

1. Start facing forward, holding the handles and standing with a slight bend of your knees.

2. Keep one arm in place, and reach up and slightly behind you with the other arm, rotating your torso and looking in the same direction.

3. Extend into the rotation until you feel the stretch and you feel like you're working the upper torso to hold the position. Hold for thirty seconds and switch sides.

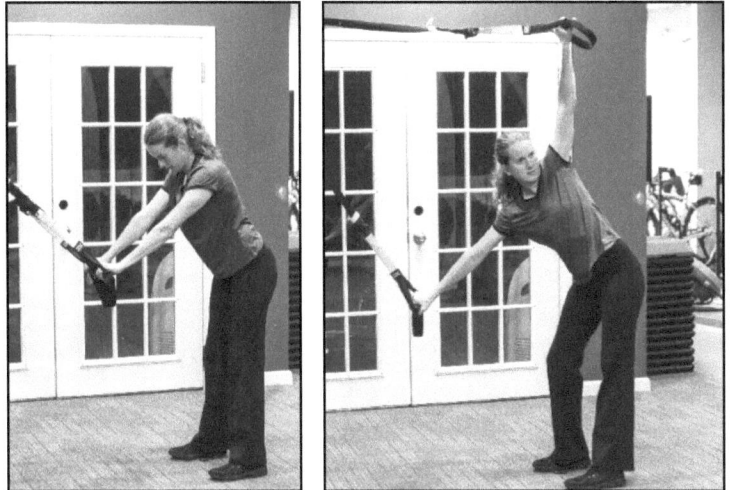

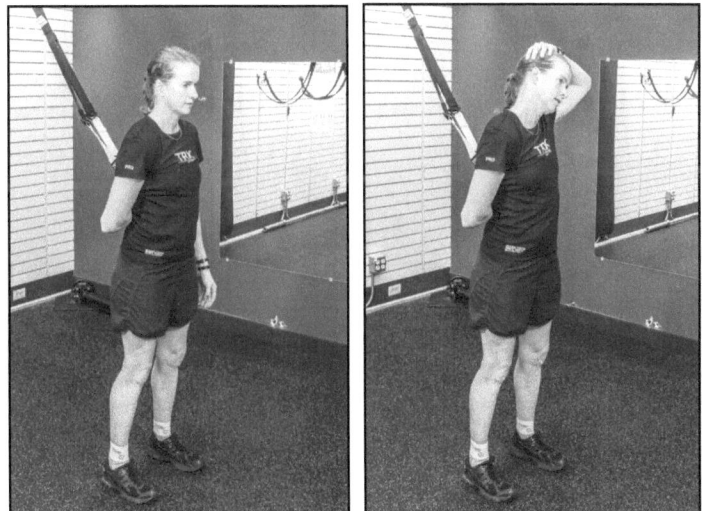

Note: You may allow the leg to straighten on the side toward which you're rotating, but try to keep the knees pointed forward.

Neck Stretch Static

Targeted Area: Neck and shoulders

Setup: Straps shortened to mid-length or fully shortened.

This stretch will keep things loose in the neck and upper torso, especially if you feel like your upper back and neck tend to get tight.

1. Start facing away. Reach behind your back with one arm, and hold either the handles or the straps themselves. Position yourself so your hand is at the midline of your back and also as high up as you are able to reach.

2. Keep that arm in place, and with your other hand, gently pull your head to the side until you feel a stretch in the neck and upper shoulder muscles.

3. Hold for thirty seconds and switch sides.

Note: Stay tall and maintain good posture.

Thoracic-Spine Stretch (Suspended) Static

Targeted Area: Upper torso

Setup: Straps fully extended or shortened to mid-length.

This is a good one for those who have jobs requiring a lot of time bent over a desk or computer, which tends to create a hunched-over position of the body. It will improve posture and breathing abilities.

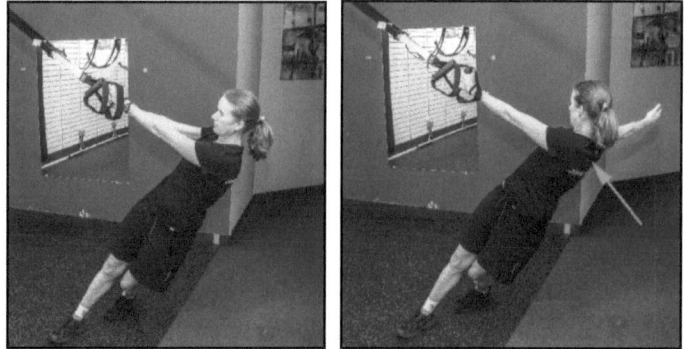

1. Start facing sideways, holding onto one handle. You may use single-handle mode, or simply hold one handle and let the other hang loose.

2. Allow your body to lean away from the straps while keeping it straight like a board. Your feet should continue to face sideways.

3. Rotate through the torso until your shoulders are now facing forward.

4. Continue to rotate, release your outside arm, and reach away from you in the direction of your rotation. Hold for twenty to thirty seconds on each side.

Note: You may turn your head and look toward the direction in which you're rotating and reaching toward.

Hamstring Stretch Static

Targeted Area: Neck and shoulders

Setup: Straps fully lengthened

A good stretch for people who feel they're tight in the back of the legs and hips.

1. Start facing toward the straps with a shoulder-width stance, holding one strap in each hand.

2. Keeping only a slight bend in your knees, hinge at the hip, bend forward, and push the straps out in front of you. Go down deep enough so you feel a gentle stretch in the back of your legs.

3. Hold for thirty seconds.

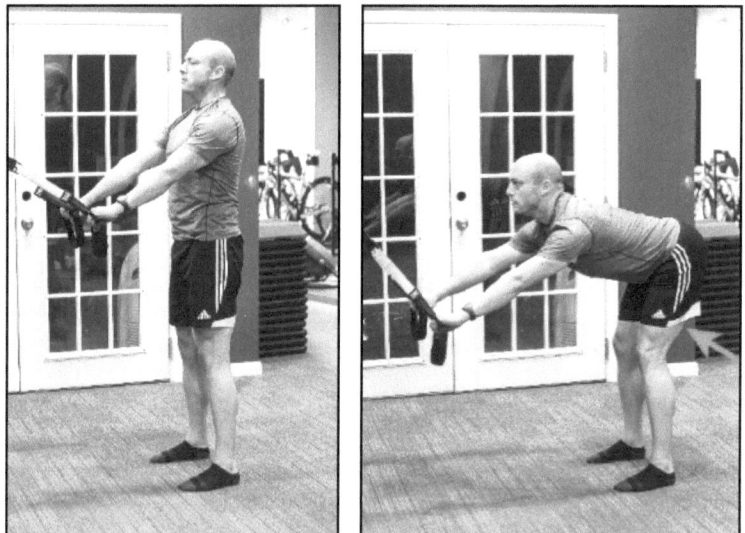

Note: Maintain a slight bend in your knees, just enough so they're not locked. Don't allow them to bend more during the stretch.

Squat Stretch Static

Targeted Area: Hips, calves, and inner thighs

Setup: Straps fully lengthened

A good all-purpose stretch that develops mobility in multiple areas of the hips and legs.

1. Start facing either toward the straps or on the side of the straps facing sideways.

2. Squat down toward the floor while holding onto the straps to allow you to maintain your balance, an upright torso, and good posture.

3. Hold for thirty seconds.

Note: Push your hips and heels down toward the floor to facilitate the calf stretch. Push your knees outward with your elbows to facilitate the inner thigh stretch.

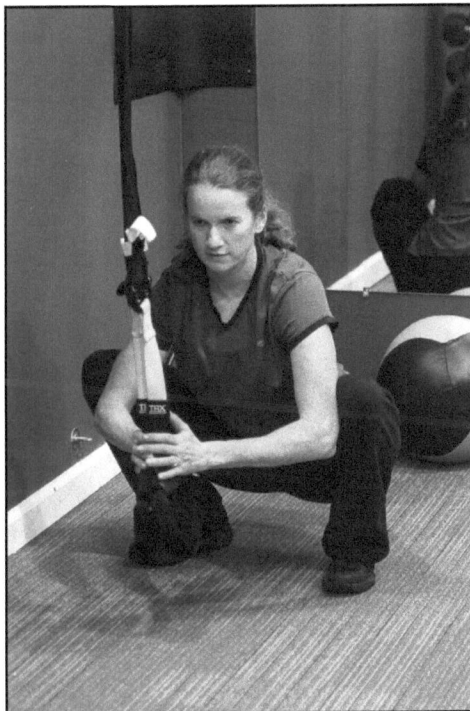

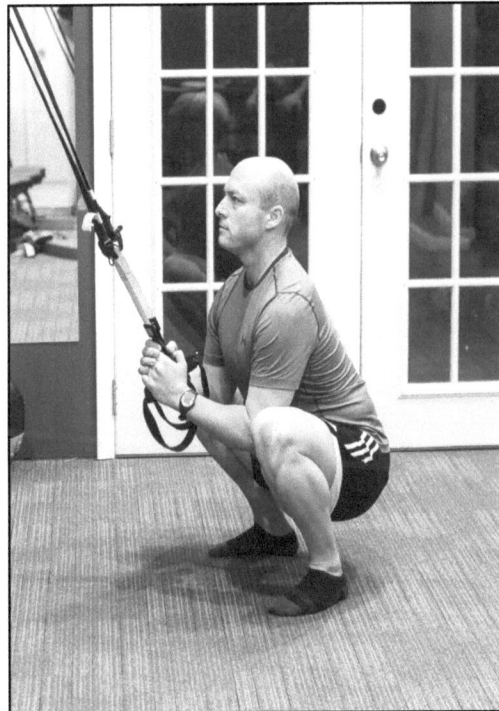

Thoracic-Spine Stretch (Lying Down) Static

Targeted Area: Upper torso and thoracic spine

One of my all-time favorites: This stretch is especially relevant to those who spend a lot of time sitting at a desk or computer, behind the wheel, or on a bicycle.

1. Lie down on your side with one arm under your head and the other at your side.

2. Grab your ribs with your top hand and roll backward. Envision trying to place your top shoulder blade on the floor behind you.

3. Once you have rolled back as far as you're able to go, extend your top arm out toward the wall and your bottom arm toward the ceiling.

4. Take several deep breaths, and relax as much as you can in this position. Hold for twenty to thirty seconds.

Note: A foam roller is used in the picture, but it's not needed to do this stretch. You may use a rolled-up towel or any type of small block or firm pillow.

The reason for using something here is to anchor the knee down. This prevents the hip from opening up during the rotation and makes sure the mobility to achieve the movement is coming from the upper torso area.

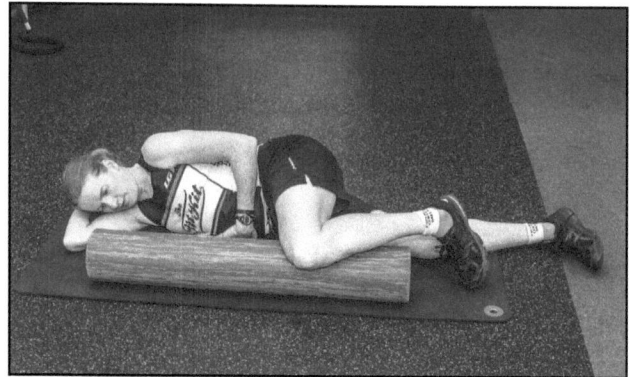

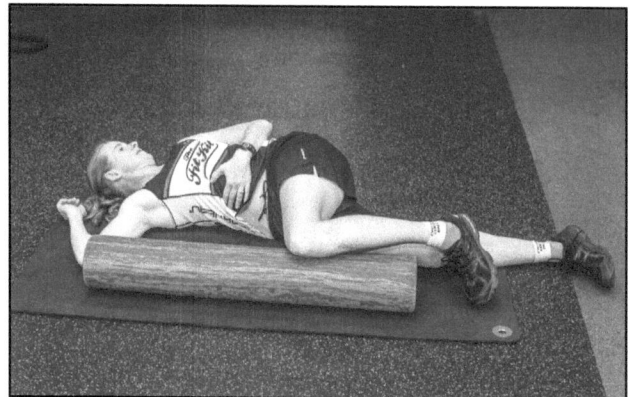

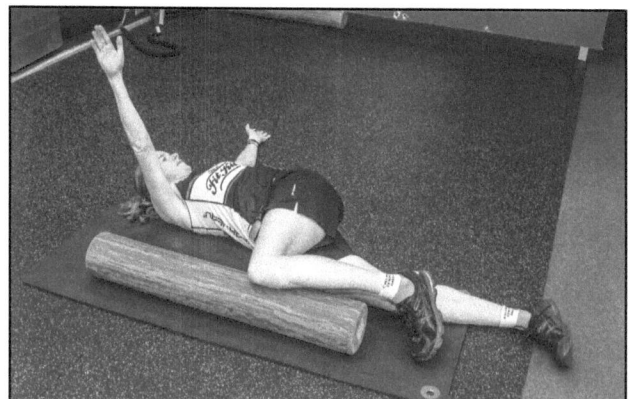

Suspended Spider Stretch

Targeted Area: Hips

Setup: Straps fully lengthened.

You should feel this one in your hips and inner thigh. You will also get a little core work during this stretch, from supporting your body weight with your arms and torso. Remember to hold your plank!

1. Start on your hands and knees, facing out, and place one foot in both cradles.

2. Extend the suspended leg, and bring the free leg forward toward same side hand. That foot should be next to and just outside the hand on the same side.

3. Take several deep breaths, and relax as much as you can in this position. Hold for twenty to thirty seconds. Switch sides and repeat.

Note: Actively extend the suspended leg back behind you by squeezing your glutes and hamstrings, and see if you can feel how the stretch changes in the hip area after you activate the muscles in that leg!

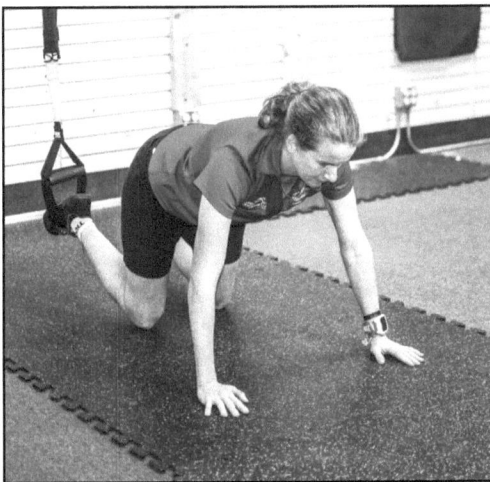

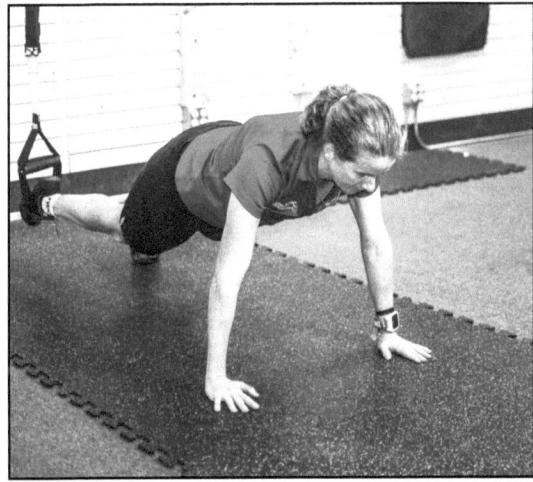

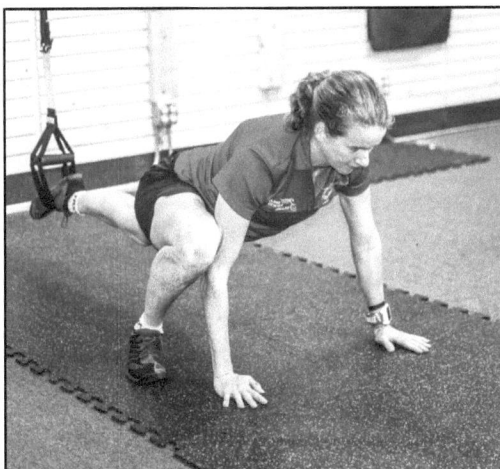

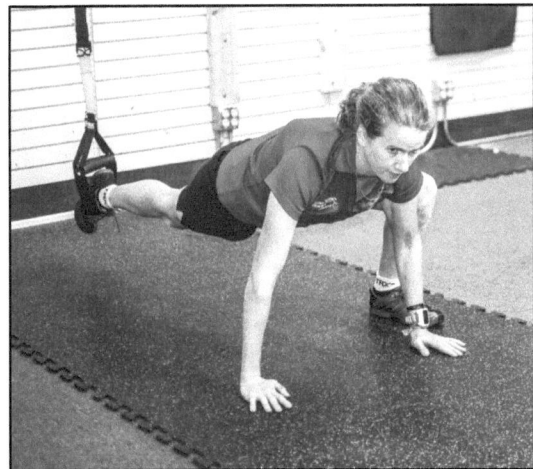

Dynamic Stretches

Walking Quad Stretch (Ankle Grabs) Dynamic

Targeted Area: Quadriceps (front of thigh) and hip flexors

No equipment needed

This movement develops both balance and stability on the supporting leg and mobility on the side being stretched. This is because you have to balance in the single-leg stance for a moment during each step while stretching the opposite leg.

1. This is a walking dynamic stretch. With each step, kick your heel toward your butt and grab your ankle with the opposite hand.

2. Hold onto that ankle, but don't pull with your hand. Instead, squeeze your glutes and hamstrings to actively bring the knee back until you feel a stretch in the front of the thigh and front of the hips.

3. Hold the stretch for just one or two seconds, and then switch legs.

Note: Using your opposite hand will prevent pulling the knee outward and instead direct the angle of the stretch behind you.

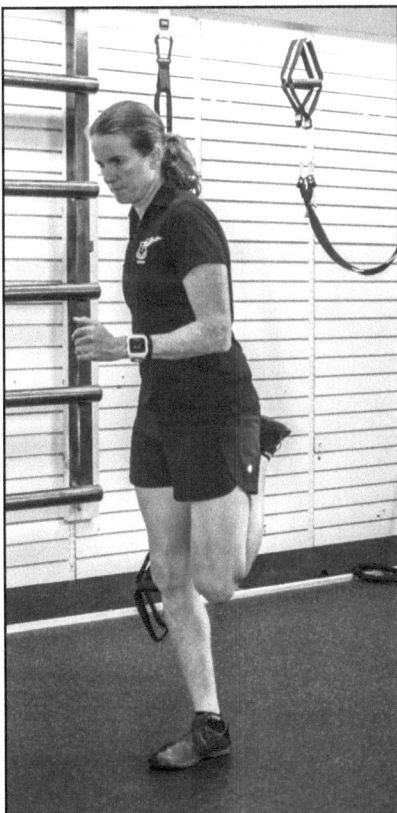

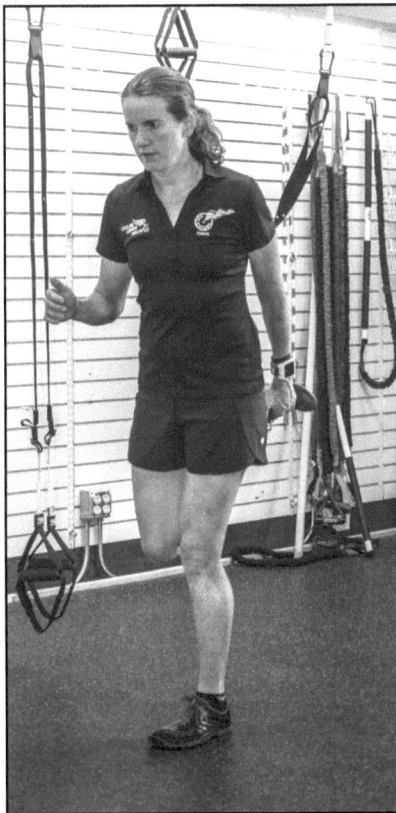

Modification: You may hold onto the suspended straps if you find it hard to keep your balance. Still, hold the stretch for just a second, turning as needed to allow the free hand to grab on to the strap. As you gain stability and flexibility by doing this, you can then graduate to the walking stretch.

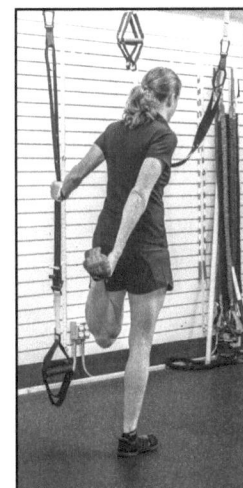

Squat-and-Rotate Stretch Dynamic

Targeted Area: Upper torso, arms

Setup: Straps fully lengthened.

Warms up the legs while loosening up the upper torso area.

1. Start facing toward the straps and begin to squat.

2. As you come back up, rotate and reach behind you and up toward the sky as far as possible.

3. Hold for one or two seconds, return to the start position, and repeat on the opposite side.

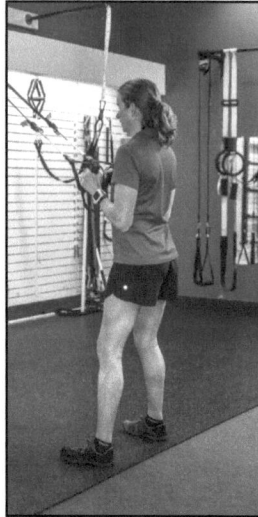

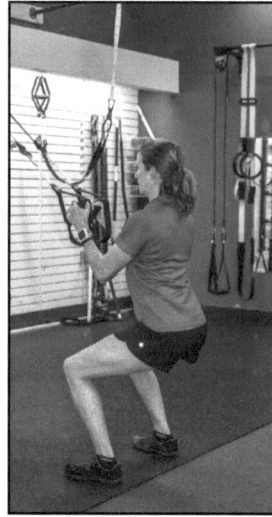

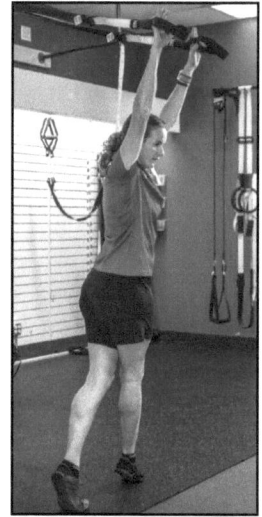

Note: Squeeze your ears with your arms and fully extend them during your reach.

Knee-to-Chest Walk Dynamic

Targeted Area: Hips

No equipment needed

This stretch develops mobility in the hips and improves balance and stability in the supporting-stance leg.

1. With good posture and keeping a slight bend in the supporting leg, lift the knee as high as possible and gently hug it to your chest.

2. Hold for one to two seconds, step forward, and repeat with the opposite leg.

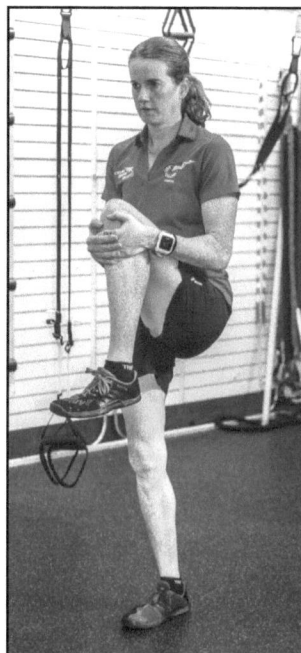

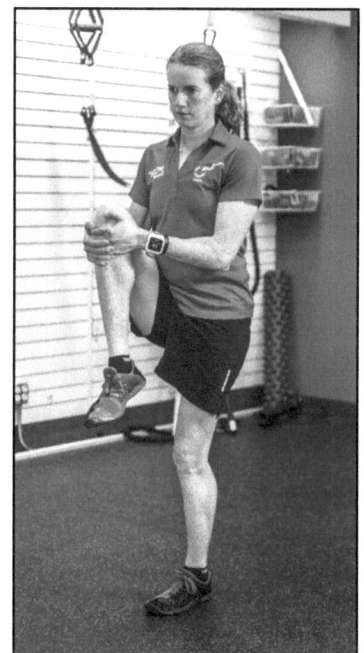

Note: Always keep just a slight bend in the supporting leg. Don't lock it out.

Ankle-to-Chest Walk Dynamic

Targeted Area: Hips

No equipment needed

This one develops mobility in the hips and improves balance and stability in the supporting-stance leg.

1. With good posture and keeping a slight bend in the supporting leg, lift the knee as high as possible, allowing it to rotate outward as you grab the knee and ankle.

2. Gently hug your leg to your chest, pulling upward just above the ankle to bring it closer to your chest.

3. Hold for one to two seconds, step forward, and repeat with the opposite leg.

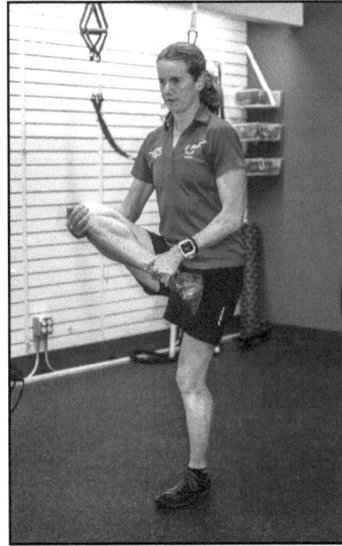

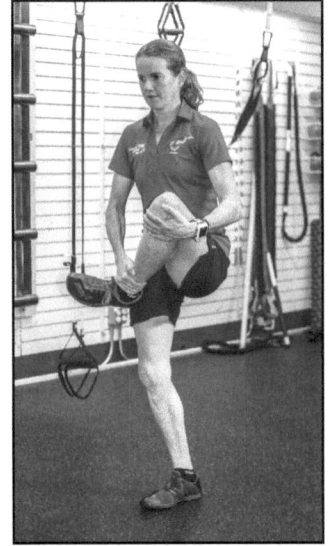

Note: Always keep just a slight bend in the supporting leg. Don't lock it out.

Scarecrow Stretch Dynamic

Targeted Area: Upper torso, chest

No equipment needed

This is a good all-purpose stretch that develops mobility in the thoracic spine area and also opens up the front of the body with a gentle chest stretch.

1. Stand tall with your elbows bent to ninety degrees, raised, and in line with your shoulders (scarecrow position).

2. Maintain this position and rotate as far as you are able toward one side.

3. Hold for one to two seconds, and switch sides.

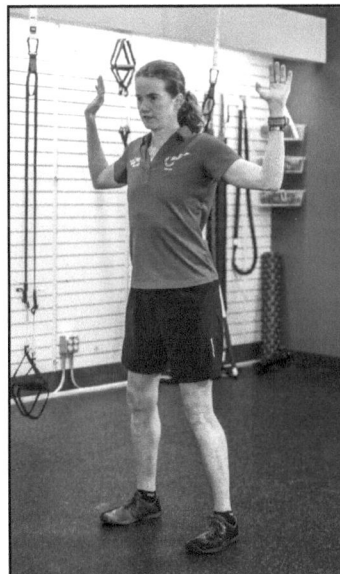

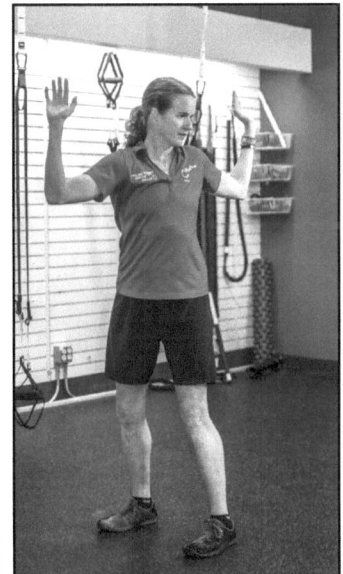

Note: Make yourself tall, and think about leading the rotation with the shoulder blade of the shoulder you are rotating toward. Keep your elbows back.

Monster Walk Dynamic

Targeted Area: Hips and hamstrings

No equipment needed

Develops mobility in the hip and hamstrings and improves balance and stability in the supporting-stance leg.

1. Keeping a slight bend in the supporting leg, kick the opposite leg upward while keeping it straight. Swing the opposite arm around to meet the foot of the leg in front of you.

2. Switch sides, and continue to alternate.

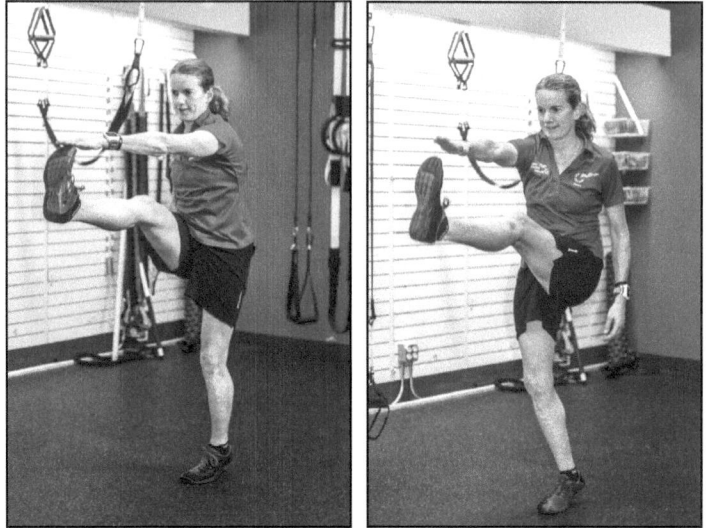

Note: You may not be able to touch your toe to your fingers in front of you, and that's OK. Work on increasing the height you can kick the leg up to while keeping it straight.

Hip-Drop Stretch Dynamic

Targeted Area: Hips and glutes

Setup: Straps fully lengthened.

This stretch loosens up the hip on one side while building stability in and warming up the supporting leg.

1. Start facing toward the straps.

2. Cross one foot over the opposite knee, and drop your hips down toward the floor.

3. Hold for one to two seconds, and switch sides.

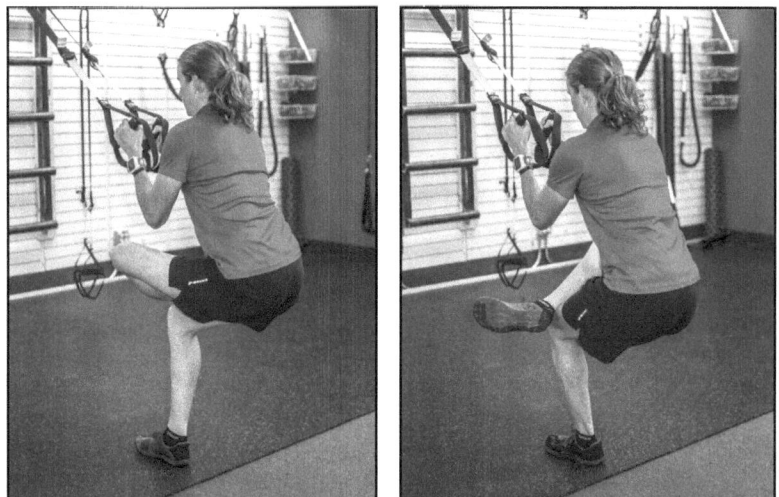

Note: Keep good posture in your torso and upper body.

Lunge-and-Rotate Stretch (Suspended) Dynamic

Targeted Area: Torso and arms

Setup: Straps fully lengthened.

The lunge pattern will build strength and stability as well as warm up the legs for upcoming work. The rotation increases the mobility of the torso while teaching the hips to stabilize during the upper-body movement. This is a more advanced movement. Master the split squat movement(p. 168) or the lunge movement(p.169) before adding the lunge and rotate dynamic stretch to your program.

1. Start facing outward, holding the handles with your arms straight out in front of you.

2. Take a step forward, and drop the back knee down toward the floor.

3. Rotate your arms and torso toward the leg in front. Hold for one to two seconds.

4. Push back up, switch sides, and repeat.

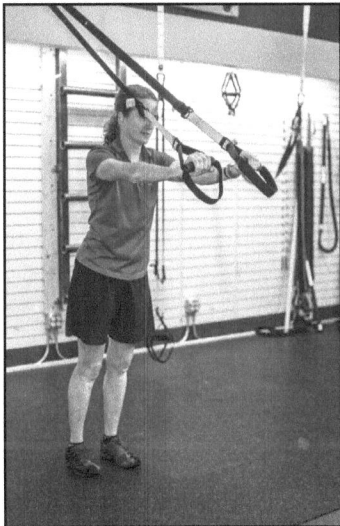

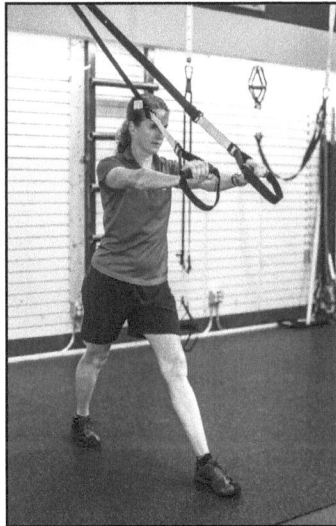

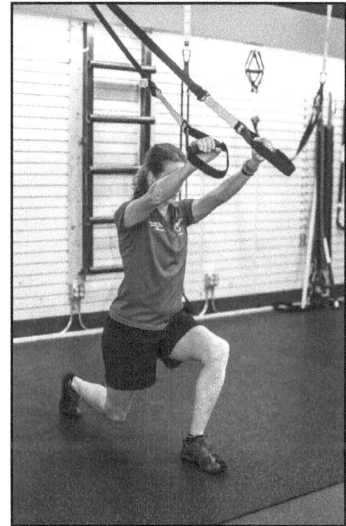

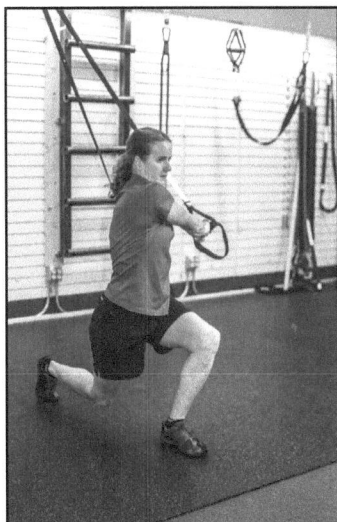

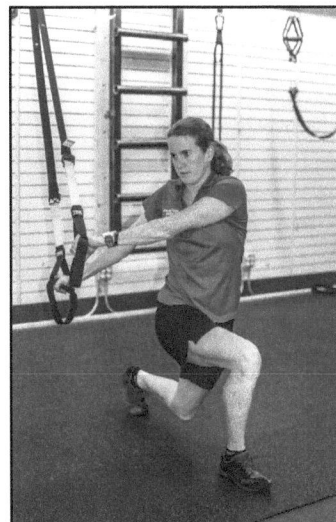

Note: *Keep your torso vertical and front knee over the front foot when dropping down into the lunge position. Relax your shoulders and envision pulling your shoulder blades down to your pockets during the rotation.*

Spider Walk Dynamic

Targeted Area: Hips, inner thighs

No equipment needed

A more advanced movement. This will work the core, and you'll really feel it in the inner-thigh area.

1. Start in the straight-arm plank position.

2. Keep your body straight like a board. Bring your right foot up to the outside of your right hand.

3. Bring your left foot up to the outside of your left hand.

4. Hold for one to two seconds, and then walk your hands out until you are back in the straight-arm plank position.

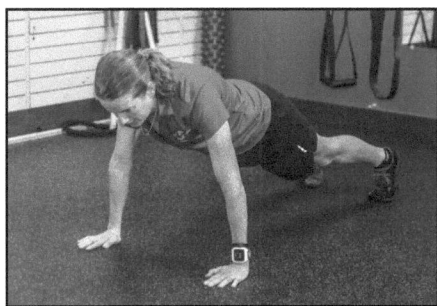
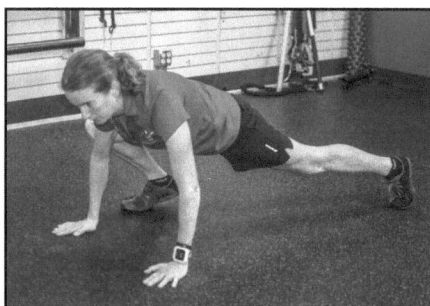
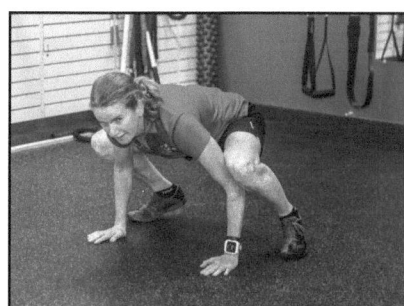

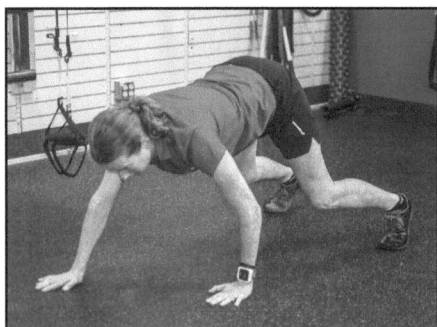
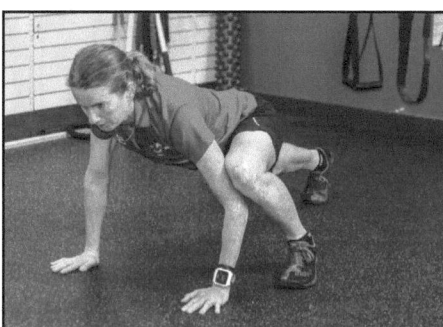

Note: *Gently push the elbow into the inside knee of the forward leg to increase the inner thigh stretch.*

Lunge-and-Rotate Walk Dynamic

Targeted Area: Upper torso, chest, and hips

No equipment needed

A good all-purpose stretch that develops mobility in the upper torso area. It will also open up the front of the body with a nice chest stretch while requiring you to maintain stability in your hips during the walking lunge. This is a more advanced movement. Master the split squat movement(p. 168) or the lunge movement(p.169) before adding the lunge and rotate to your program.

1. Stand tall with your elbows bent to ninety degrees, raised, and in line with your shoulders (scarecrow position).

2. Take a large step forward, and drop the back knee down toward the floor.

3. When you reach the bottom of the lunge, maintain the scarecrow position and rotate as far as you are able toward the front leg. Hold the rotation for one to two seconds, and then return to the front-facing scarecrow position.

4. Push through the back leg to come back to the starting position. Switch sides and repeat.

Note: As you become more proficient with the movement, you may progress by stepping through the starting position, immediately going into the next lunge step.

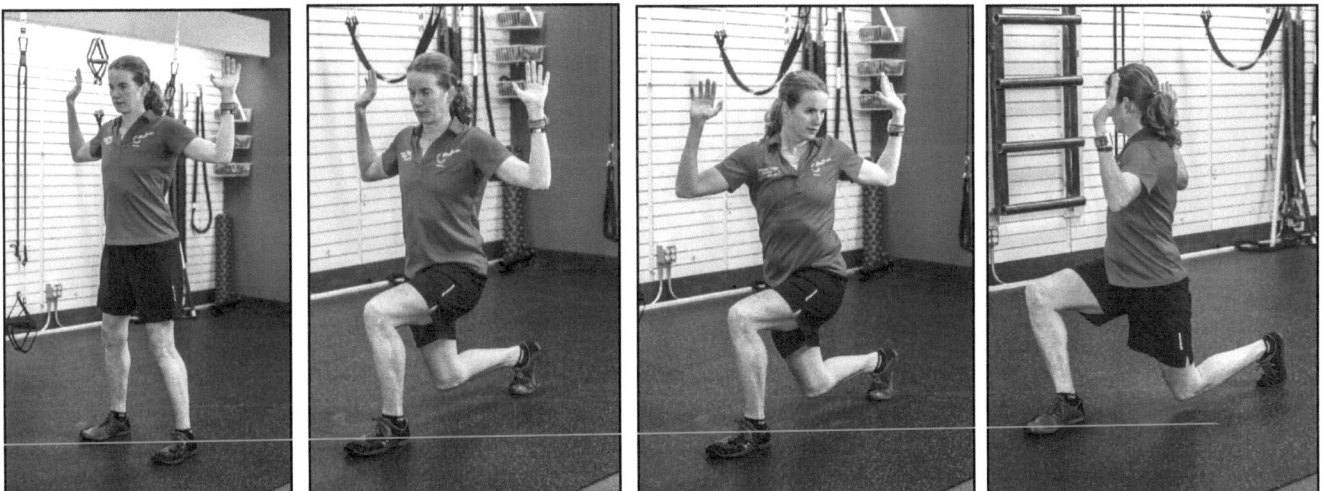

Inchworm Walk Dynamic

Targeted Area: Hamstrings, calves, and core

No equipment needed

A catchall movement that builds core and arm strength, as well as flexibility of the lower back, hamstrings, and calves.

1. Stand straight with a slight bend in your knees. Bend at the waist by hinging at the hip, keeping your back flat.

2. When you have reached the end of your hip hinge, only then allow your knees to bend so you can place your hands on the floor.

3. Walk your hands forward until you are in a straight-arm plank position.

4. Walk your feet as close to your hands as you can, keeping your legs straightened. When you can't get your feet any closer, walk forward once again with your hands.

Note: Press your heels down toward the floor to facilitate the calf stretch.

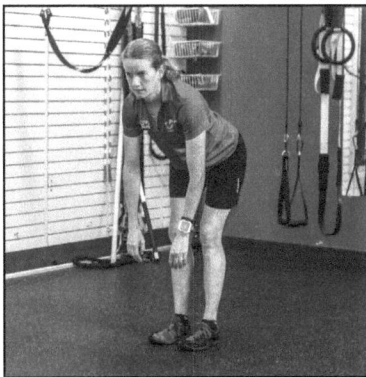

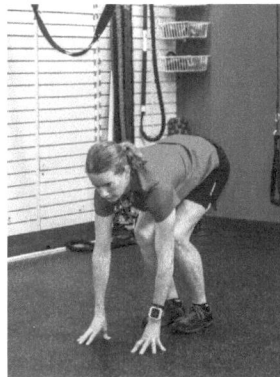

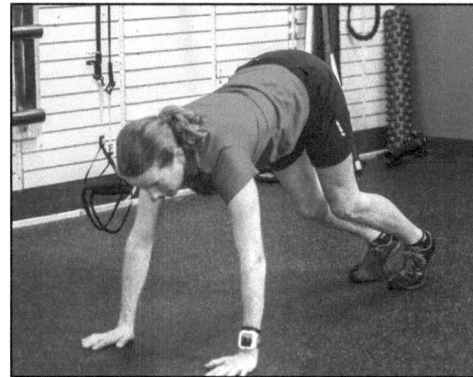

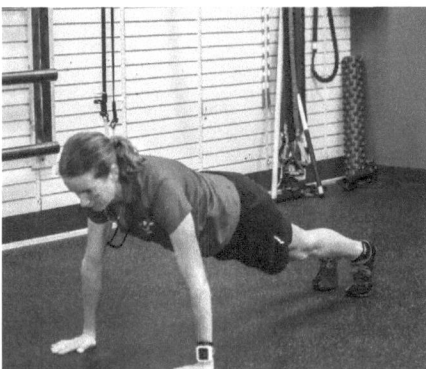

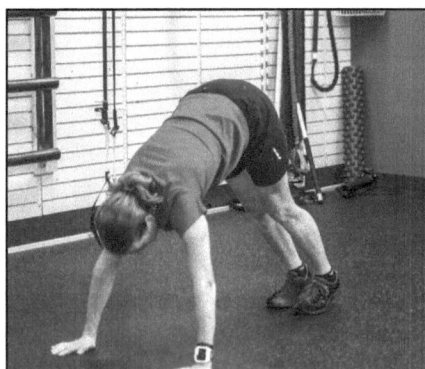

Scorpion Stretch

Targeted Area: Hips and torso

No equipment needed

Loosens up the hamstring in the back of the leg through the leg raise, and the it loosens the hip and glute when you bring the leg across your body.

1. Lie down flat on your back with your legs straight, and pull your toes toward you.

2. Keep one leg straight and down on the floor. Keep the other leg straight and raise it straight up as high as you can.

3. When it's as high as you can get it, bring it across your body and toward the floor on the opposite side as far as you can comfortably go.

4. Come right back up, repeat all repetitions on one side, and then switch sides.

Note: Your arms may be at your side or extended out away from you on the floor. Keep both shoulders and shoulder blades on the floor as you bring the leg across.

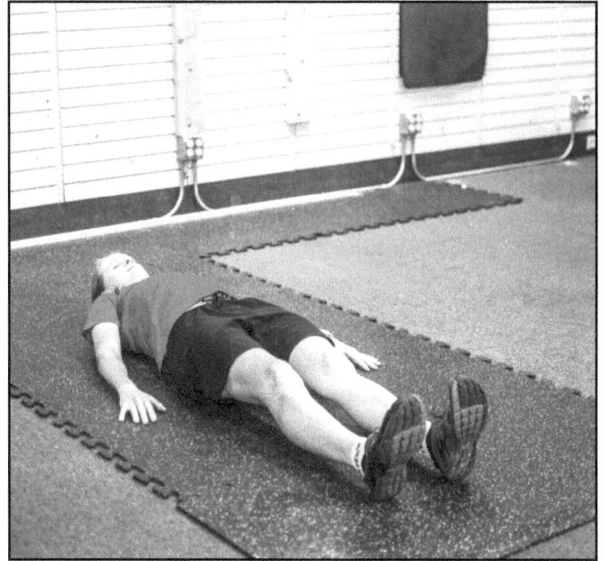

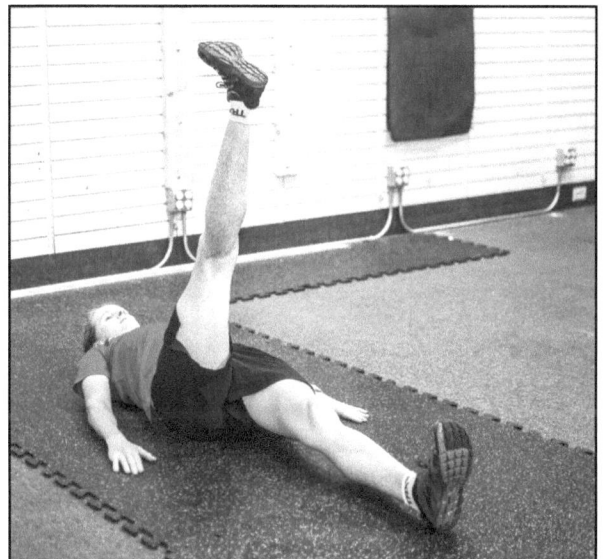

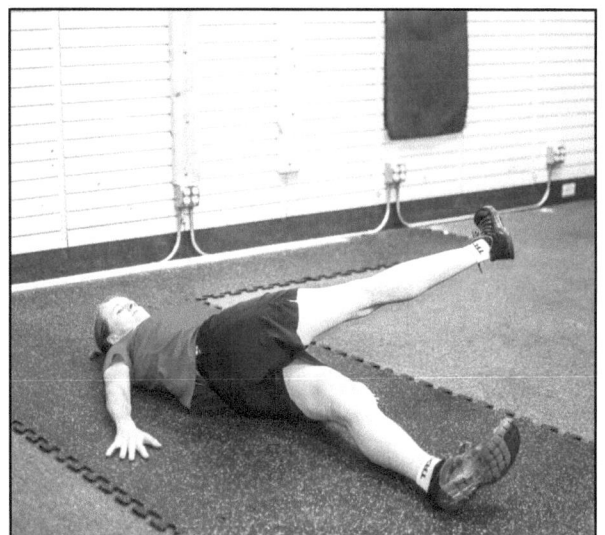

Chapter 11

Strength Training for Cycling

Can Strength Training Really Help Me Be a Better Cyclist?

For some, cycling is a passion and part of who they are. For others, it's just an occasional endeavor for fun, exercise, or to see the world from a different perspective. Whether you enjoy casual rides or hardcore competition, having more strength and stability will result in a more enjoyable ride.

This chapter will tell you why this is true and how to achieve it through the right approach. I examine details and findings from studies about which aspects of cycling can benefit from performing strength training. For those interested in increasing their cycling abilities through better strength and stability, I also discuss making strength training more specific to the demands of cycling, and more importantly, to the specific type of cycling you do.

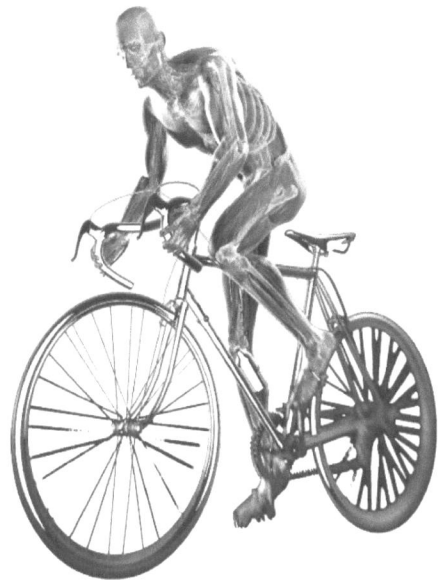

The studies discussed in the following section all focus on outdoor cyclists. The experience levels of cyclists as well as the different types of cycling should be considered when performing strength training with the goal of improving your cycling performance. An index of cycling-specific movements that can be performed on a suspended trainer is included in this section for reference. Depending on your level of cycling experience and the type of cycling you're most interested in focusing on, this chapter will help you identify your needs and effectively add strength work to your program.

As noted in the bone density and cycling section (chapter 8), it's important to mention that information in this chapter is focused on those who participate in outdoor cycling for recreation, health, fun, and competition. Those whose primary form of cardio exercise is spin classes will still get some good insight from this chapter, however, and it would be most appropriate to place themselves in the category of recreational cyclist.

What the Studies Say about Strength Training for Cycling

I'll start by reviewing literature on strength training for cycling performance. This section is certainly not required reading, but for some of you, a greater insight will lead to increased yield from workout sessions.

While literature on strength training in cycling is abundant, studies on suspension training and cycling are scarce, as are independent studies of suspension training itself. Most published studies in my review used traditional methods, such as back squats and leg presses, for their strength training programs. I have also attempted to identify studies that use body-weight exercises, or exercises similar to some of the suspension training exercises. Many of the studies compare a control group utilizing a cycling-only training program to an experimental group using the same cycling program in conjunction with a resistance-training program.

Coming from a weight-training background, I was not surprised to see that a majority of the studies support resistance training as a supplement to cycling performance. Yet it was exciting to note just how many different positive performance adaptations come from resistance training.

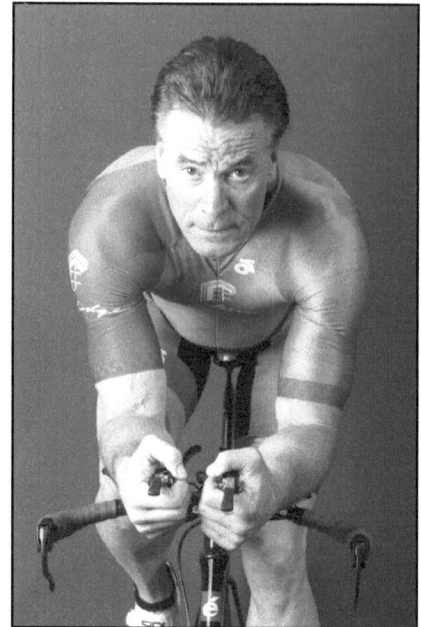

Resistance Training and Road-Cycling Performance Studies

Let's start with a review of five independent studies that added a strength training program to cycling training. This was published in the *Journal of Strength and Conditioning Research* in 2010.[1] The studies in this review consisted of different strength exercises, populations, and cycling-training programs but tied things together with a common goal of looking at effects on cycling performance with the addition of a strength training program.

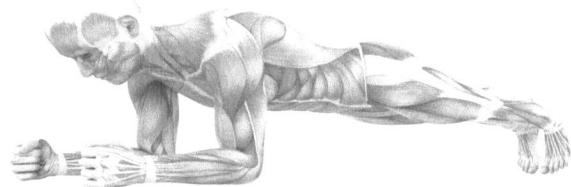

In this review, three of the five studies observed significant performance benefits. These three replaced a portion of the athletes' cycling training with resistance training in the control group[2,4,6] versus piling resistance on top of the existing cycling program. Additionally, two of the three employed high-intensity, explosive-type resistance exercises versus traditional sets of moderately paced repetitions.

The remaining two studies did not show significant performance benefits. Both used traditional, non-cycling-specific strength exercises, such as back squats, leg presses, and machine hamstring curls. Both programs also added resistance-training work on top of existing cycling regimens.[3,5] The study in this review, which I found to be most relevant to the competitive cyclist, combined both explosive training and high-resistance interval training to the programs of already trained competitive cyclists.[2]

Previous studies have shown explosive resistance training provides performance benefits, but most of these studies were done during non-competitive season phases. Just one was performed during the competitive season. It combined explosive step-ups with on-bike interval sets of thirty seconds on and thirty seconds off, and it showed impressive results. Performance gains were demonstrated in peak power, which is the highest amount of power they could produce, as well as the average power during both a one-kilometer and four-kilometer maximal effort test. There were also decreases in how much oxygen was needed at a given workload.

> "It is likely that replacing a cyclist's endurance training with resistance training will result in improved time trial performance and maximal power."

Based on this review, you could conclude the following:

1. **Replacing a portion of cycling training with resistance training while keeping overall training volume static, may be more beneficial than merely adding resistance training to an existing program.** This is great news for time-pressed amateur cyclists. Adding quality strength training is shown to be beneficial for cycling performance, and extending training time to include it is unnecessary. More is not always better (the type A's out there should pay attention). Increasing both volume and intensity of workouts by adding strength work to already challenging cycling regimens, creates a higher risk of fatigue or overtraining, which may cancel any gains. So, cyclists may find reducing their cycling time to add a little strength work is worth the trade-off in performance benefits.

2. **Explosive movements replicating cycling action are more likely to produce on-bike gains than non-specific exercises such as back squats or leg presses.** Weight training is typically symmetrical, whereas cycling is not. In cycling, the rider pushes down with one leg while pulling up, or at least unweighting, with the other. And it's the same for the arms. Add in the associated work of muscles in and around the pelvis, spine, and shoulders, and symmetrical weight training begins to have less relevance to cycling's overall body movement patterns. The study that combined strength training with a cycling regimen in the form of explosive single-leg step-ups (similar to sprinter starts), recorded significant gains, whereas the two studies that assigned movements of primary symmetrical, non-body-weight movements did not show significant results.

Results from More Studies on the Effects of Strength Training on Cycling Performance

Pedal Efficiency Increases. This study on cycling, strength training, and pedaling efficiency compared two groups of cyclists over twenty-five weeks.[7] One group performed heavy strength training; the other did not. The strength training program used included a squat movement plus two single-leg and hip movements. The group that strength-trained showed more improvement at the end of the twenty-five weeks than the group that did not. The total training time between the two groups was kept equal during the program. The greater improvements in a forty-kilometer individual time trial (ITT) performance in the strength training group were attributed to peak force occurring earlier in the pedal stroke.

Strength Can Be Maintained with Fewer Sessions. The same pedaling efficiency study also supported this idea. The initial ten weeks required twice-weekly sessions with heavy resistance and multiple sets of several lifting exercises. Afterward, sessions were reduced to once every seven to ten days with slightly reduced resistance. Not only did the strength training group experience greater strength gains and performance improvements in peak power, but their mean power during a forty-kilometer ITT was also greater than the control group's after fifteen more weeks of the less-frequent and less-intense program (twenty-five weeks total). This supports the approach that once additional strength is gained, it can be maintained with fewer, less-intense sessions, allowing focus to turn to other training aspects.

Upper Body Strength Matters. Another study looked at results in cycling performance after adding upper body strength work.[8] Force applied to handlebars during starting, climbing, and sprinting, as well as force transfer through the trunk to the pedals, was enhanced by an increase in upper body and core strength. Greater rigidity in the core also translates into more efficient transfer of arm and shoulder forces to the legs during pedaling action. Hill climbs and other strenuous exertions, such as attempting to stay with the peloton or opening a gap on other cyclists, highlight the improvement. Often the moments that matter the most, occur when trying to stay or open a gap with other riders. The extra power you can generate through the core and upper body might just make or break your desired outcome.

Additional Considerations

Without continuing to go into detail on the results of every study out there (which would make this a very long book), I want to highlight some general trends in the literature. These are adaptations that you might experience with the addition of some strength work.

Greater oxygen economy was often observed in a steady-state cycling effort after adding strength training. Applied to you, this would mean your body would need less oxygen at a given workload. This would make you more efficient at producing the same amount of work, which allows you to save energy for later in the race, or perhaps for the running portion of a triathlon. It may also give you the ability to push harder and go faster in any particular effort than you could before, because now you have that extra reserve.

A greater maximum strength of your muscles results in a smaller percent of the muscle's max strength having to be used with each pedal stroke to obtain the same force. This again allows for less demand on your body during the same workload.

Positive adaptations in neuromuscular activation and rate of force development. Strength training is a high-intensity activity that requires your neuromuscular system to learn to use its strongest muscle fibers, and more of them. Your muscles learning how to fire more fibers, and at a faster rate, can result in more power when sprinting, climbing, accelerating out of corners, or catching or leaving behind a competitor.

Conclusion of Research Section

I hope you now understand why strength training should be included in your program. I also hope you now have more incentive to do it. We learned that you don't need to add extra time or a multitude of exercises to your training program. You do, however, need to put a little thought into your program design if you want to achieve cycling-specific benefits from strength training. Although studies on suspension training and cycling were basically nonexistent at the time of writing this book, there were enough body-weight movements included in cycling-specific studies to support the benefits of including this type of strength training in your program. Since suspension training is body-weight training, I think it's fair to assume, for the purpose of designing a strength training program to improve cycling abilities, that suspension training is an acceptable (if not ideal) mode of strength training.

So how do you add strength training to your cycling program in the way that is most effective for you? Your level of cycling, cycling goals, and cycling discipline are all things to consider. The next section will get into more detail on how to select cycling-specific movements and will lay out the best program for you as an individual.

Designing a Suspended-Training Strength Program for Cyclists

Making Strength Training Cycling Specific

The SAID principle is a widely known and accepted principle in athletics. SAID stands for "Specific Adaptations to Imposed Demands," and it basically means that your body will adapt to the demands placed on it in the same way that those demands are placed on it. It's pretty simple. If you train with a lot of fast and short intervals, you will develop speed. If you ride for long durations at a slower pace, that is the focus upon which you will be adept. The same thing applies to strength training.

Knowing this, select movements can be included that are relevant to cycling.

Basic cycling demands include:

- Generating power through the legs and hips
- Legs working in sync but independently
- Balance
- Adequate mobility of the hips and torso
- Power transfer from the upper body to the lower body through the core
- Control of both internal and external factors through the core

There are additional, more specific demands if you're focusing on a specific cycling discipline, and I will cover those shortly.

The following is a list of suspension training movements that are specifically beneficial to cycling. This list is designed to give you some choices when putting together your own program. Level 1 movements are more basic and offer a good place to start for beginners. These can be progressed as you get stronger and your abilities develop.

Level 2 movements are more advanced and/or complex movements. These are merely suggestions on good movements that are relevant to the demands of cycling, so don't feel like you need to limit yourself to only these, or even to only suspension training. Give some thought to what movements in general are most relevant to cycling, or to the type of cyclist you are. Focus on your specific goals, and apply them to all methods of resistance training you choose to use. The next sections talk more about things to consider based on both your ability level, and the type of cycling discipline in which you participate.

Level 1 Movements

- Bicycle Kicks
- Plank
- Split Squat
- Reverse Lunge
- Hip Hinge
- Push-Up (Hands Suspended)
- Row
- Half-Kneeling Roll-out
- Half Get-Up
- Suspended Get-Up
- Sprinter Starts
- Hip Raises
- Triceps Extensions

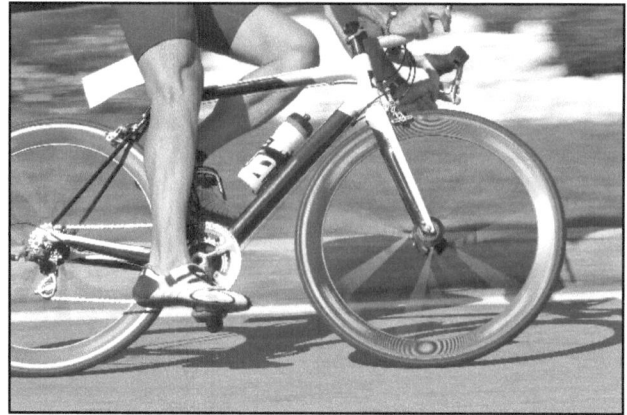

Level 2 Movements

- Single-Leg Squat
- Suspended Reverse Lunge
- Suspended Power Lunge
- Push-Up (Feet Suspended)
- Atomic Crunches
- Mountain Climbers
- Suspended Side Plank
- Tall Kneeling Roll-out
- Inverted Row
- Pull-Ups or Assisted Suspended Pull-Ups
- Overhead Squat

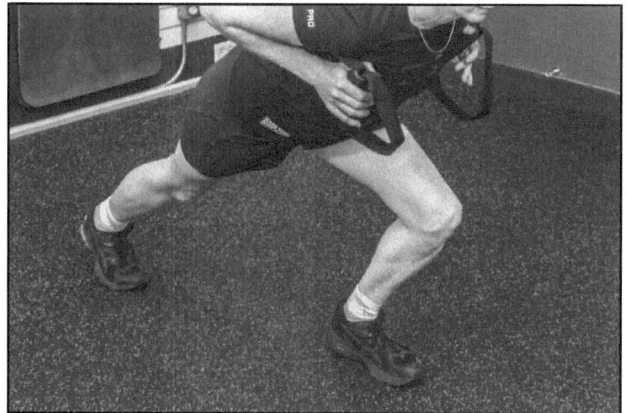

Although all the suspension training movements listed in this section are cycling specific, not every exercise will yield maximum benefit to every cyclist. This is because different types of cyclists have different sets of demands on their bodies. They are also coming from different levels of fitness and ability. A recreational cyclist may need to increase overall strength and stability to allow for more comfortable and enjoyable rides, while a track cyclist may need a program for increased power development. The first thing to consider is…what type of cyclist are you?

Three broad types of cyclists are covered in this book: recreational, fitness, and competitive. Each of these requires its own level of fitness and has demands specific to that discipline. Each may also attract individuals with much different levels of ability and exercise experience. Suspension training can play a part in helping all three of these types of cyclists achieve their goals.

No matter what category a cyclist falls into, he or she will benefit from a solid general foundation of strength and stability. Building that foundation during the first block of a strength training program is crucial, and this is true for all categories of cyclists, from beginner to elite. The level 1 or 2 foundation workouts located on pages 212 and 215 are a good place to start for anyone who is beginning a strength program for the first time or someone coming back to strength training after a break.

Recreational and Fitness Cyclists

Cycling experience and objectives:	Areas to work on:
• Beginner-level cyclists • Cycling for enjoyment • Cycling for exercise • Improving cyclist	• Stability in gusting crosswinds • Handling unexpected obstacles • Maintenance of correct posture • Increasing comfort on the bike • Reducing fatigue to enjoy the ride longer

You want to have fun on your bike, feel healthy and strong, and enjoy being out in the open air. Maybe you're getting into cycling for the first time, or maybe you have been riding for years. Most cyclists in this group have no desire to keep pace with anyone other than for good company. It's sufficient to feel strong on your bike and complete a ride without becoming unduly fatigued. This category may include beginner or intermediate-level cyclists and exercisers.

Developing a strong torso and core will delay the onset of fatigue and provide assistance if fatigue does set in. This requirement applies very much to cycling, where controlled pelvic movement is at the center of the activity. Fatigue and loss of posture may cause discomfort along the spine in the lower back due to lack of conditioning in the muscles supporting the stomach, spine, and pelvis—in other words, lack of core strength. Additionally, working on correct movement patterns will help maintain good mechanics during pedal stroke, and increase endurance levels when the rider is confronted with a steep hill…or when turning a corner and realizing the tailwind that was such a friend on the first part of the ride is suddenly an adversary.

Comfort is crucial. If you are not comfortable on your bike, it's not going to be enjoyable. A proper bike fit is important for this aspect. Adequate mobility in your own body is equally important. It supports greater comfort during rides and can prevent excessive physical strain due to riding position.

Fitness and Fast Recreational Cyclists

Cycling experience and objectives:	Areas to work on:
• Intermediate-level cyclist • Experienced cyclist • Cyclists who ride with a group and in rallies • Former racing cyclist who rides strong but no longer has specific competition demands	• Stability in gusting crosswinds • Handling unexpected obstacles • Maintenance of correct posture • Maintenance of efficient pedal stroke • Increasing power and speed • Lowering overall fatigue

You ride hard and like to push yourself. It's important to you to keep up with your riding buddies and groups, and to survive tough hills, surges, periods of high pace, and long rides or rallies. You want the same increased strength and stability as a recreational rider, but you may already have a higher level of fitness thanks to your more intensive training. This category may also include seasoned cyclists who are not training at competition level in terms of structure, volume, or intensity.

You don't have to worry as much about specific demands and periods of competition as a competitive cyclist does, but you would still benefit from building up your abilities on a suspended trainer to the more advanced progressions and movements.

Designing a Program for Recreational and Fitness Cyclists

Recreational and fitness cyclists generally benefit most by selecting exercises that emphasize building a foundation appropriate to their ability levels. Make it a priority to focus on form and proper progression of the difficulty level because:

1. Recreational cyclists may be coming from a beginner's fitness and ability level, and would benefit most from developing functional strength and balance to support their cycling.

2. Fitness cyclists may have a strong level of fitness, but lack a history of strength training.

3. The fitness cyclist who has a high level of both cycling fitness and strength training may progress quickly to the more advanced movements, but will always benefit from the basics.

Competitive Cyclists

Cycling experience and objectives:	Areas to work on:
• High level of cycling fitness • Currently in competition or training to compete • Focused on a specific cycling discipline • Riding with fast groups and pacelines (road or track) • Training solo with specific goals • Usually follows a structured regular training plan	• Rapid accelerations and force generation • Stability in gusting crosswinds • Handling unexpected obstacles • Targeting specific demands of the discipline • Maintenance of efficient pedal stroke • Fatigue resistance under high intensities • Obtaining high power numbers specific to the discipline

Competitive cyclists train hard to be able to perform at their best for specific types of events. They need to consider the demands of their events as well as have an overall plan that will have them riding strongest when it matters most.

Subcategories of competitive cyclists include off-road, triathlon, mountain, track, and cyclo-cross. Each of these disciplines requires a solid foundation of strength and stability, and has a specific set of demands.

Any suspension exercise under the recreational and fitness categories will also benefit competitive cyclists in any sub-discipline. I highly recommend beginning a strength training program by following the recommendations found in chapter 5 or by selecting from the exercises detailed later in this book and mastering, at minimum, a three to four week program. During this initial block, focus on mastering the technique and progressing the difficultly level of each exercise. Stick with the same movements, but vary the difficulty level as you get stronger. This will also allow adaptation to training demands on a neuromuscular level as well as develop the strength and structure in your muscle tissues necessary to handle the demands of more advanced movements that will come later.

Competitive cyclists with a strong fitness background will be more likely to progress to more advanced exercises and progressions. Many are more complex and require more stability and strength, while some are plyometric in nature. Following are a few things to consider for each discipline when selecting exercises to augment an already established program.

Triathletes. Top priorities are mobility and fatigue resistance. Triathletes need a strong, stable, and fatigue-resistant pedal stroke. They also have to maintain an aerodynamic position on the bike for extended periods of time. Transitioning from the bike to running with efficient mechanics, requires optimal mobility from muscles that may have been in a shortened position during the bike leg.

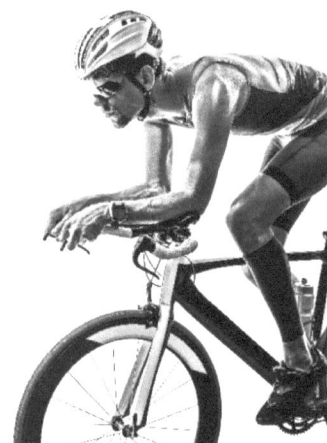

The need for short bursts of acceleration for a few seconds at a time is also beneficial for gaining momentum out of corners and passing competitors within the time allowance. Think about choosing movements that develop the core and upper body to hold the aero position, as well as to train the hip, knee, and ankle to remain in alignment during both the pedal stroke and single-leg run stance.

Include some stretches to ensure adequate mobility in all areas.

Road. Top priorities here are fatigue resistance and overall strength and stability. Racers need to maintain a solid, efficient pedal stroke through repeated anaerobic efforts and adverse conditions.

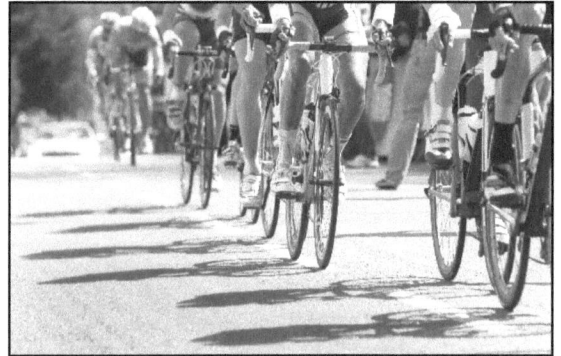

A strong torso is crucial for providing a solid center to transfer force to the pedals during accelerations, climbing, and sprinting. Upper body strength is part of this strong center and can help with the push-pull dynamics that generate transfer force to the pedals in climbing and sprinting. Think about choosing movements that develop stability of the hips, knees, and ankles, as well as movements that require full-body strength where the core stabilizes through the center.

Track. Top priorities are power and repeatability of short, hard efforts at high speeds. The demands of track racing include activating as many muscle fibers as possible, as fast as possible to create maximum acceleration as soon as possible. Track cyclists need to be able to repeat multiple short, hard sprints with periods of high-threshold intensity in-between. They also need a very high leg speed to achieve high cadences while producing large amounts of force.

Choose exercises that emphasize power development and have an explosive or plyometric component to them. These exercises will develop the neuromuscular systems as well as the large-muscle fibers that are responsible for quickly generating high amounts of force.

Mountain. Top priorities are stability and repeatability of short, hard efforts. Mountain bikers need full-body strength and stability to control the bike on rough terrain. They also need strength and proper alignment in their pedal stroke across a wide range of RPMs.

The hand position during mountain biking is pronated, which is different from the other disciplines, and is something to think about mimicking when selecting exercises to develop strength through the wrist and arms.

Mountain bikers often need to be able to lift up the front of the bike while stabilizing the back of the bike. This requirement of having strength on top of the unstable platform of the bike on rough terrain makes suspension training ideal for developing strength. The platform of many movements on a suspended trainer is a very similar type of instability. Upper body, core, and full-body strength can be developed to also handle extreme instability during the strength movement. Choose full-body movements that involve the core stabilizing through the center. Progress to single-leg movements that require force generation and stability during hip and knee extension and flexion. Some work on unstable surfaces may also benefit this discipline.

Cyclo-cross. Top priorities are overall stability, mobility, and repeatability of hard efforts. This discipline requires a variety of demands. CX riders need strength in their pedal stroke, as well as strong torsos to transfer force and control the bike on adverse terrain.

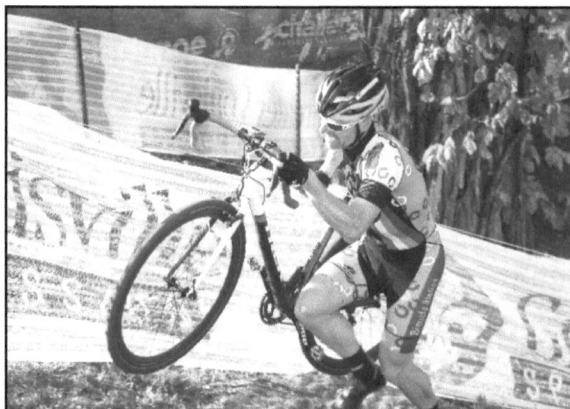

Cyclo-cross often requires lifting up the front of the bike over obstacles or dismounting and carrying the entire bike while running (often over soft and unstable ground), climbing, or hurdling barriers. A strong core that can handle asymmetrical loads is crucial. Running up steep inclines, over barriers, or through sand pits requires hip and knee stability and fatigue resistance. In addition, adequate hip mobility is needed for hurdling barriers and remounting the bike.

Choose full-body movements that involve core stabilization and transfer of power through the center of mass, and single-leg movements that require explosive extension and hip stabilization. Also include some upper body and core exercises that require the body to move or stabilize with one side only.

Ultradistance. This may include ultradistance racing or long-distance touring. Fatigue resistance and comfort on the bike over extreme durations of time, are your top priorities. Proper pedaling biomechanics and core stamina are also extremely important and must be maintained for long durations of time.

Choose both dynamic and static stretches to make sure you have adequate mobility of the ankles, hips, torso, and upper body. Choose core as well as full-body movements that require stabilization and power transfer through the core.

Sidebar: A Cautionary Note for Competitive Cyclists

This chapter assumes you are at a high level of fitness and ability. Thus, some advanced suspension exercises are included, and these require high levels of body awareness, strength, and stability. If you are a racing cyclist but not yet skilled in suspension training, ease your way in. One of the biggest mistakes I see is people who immediately jump into the most advanced exercises when starting a suspension-training program. Some of these individuals can just about manage the movements but usually have incorrect form and are unable to execute the full range of the movement.

It's a bit like doing anaerobic intervals on the bike before you've established your endurance base. Not only will you not achieve your potential, but compensations occurring to complete the movement can likely result in negative forces on the body.

No matter what your cycling level is, I strongly recommend you start with the intermediate movements and progress to the advanced movements when your skill level allows for it.

When to Strength Train for Cycling

If you are a competitive cyclist, you probably have a training plan that focuses on a racing season. Even if you don't race, there are still times of year that are better for cycling no matter where you live. You may want to be at your best fitness for a cycling trip or particular rally.

The *Hotter'N Hell Hundred* is the largest sanctioned century bicycle ride in the country and takes place in Wichita Falls, Texas, in August. Too many times I've had clients who want to start training for this or other similar events but start too late in the game, and end up paying the price on event day (and sometimes for weeks after).

There isn't really a time not to resistance train. However, if you have a structured plan, there may be an optimal way to select what exercises to do, and incorporate them into your training schedule.

Off-season or preseason is the time when most cyclists start thinking about strength work. One of my goals in writing this book is to help more people actually perform strength work to supplement their cycling, as well as to make it easier to include in their training plans. For those who are not really sure what to do in terms of strength training, I have given a little direction below to refer to when planning your workout. If you're following a plan targeting one or a series of competition events, the basic rule is as follows:

General/Specific Maintenance

Start with a general program to give you a chance to build a foundation and master the movements. After that, get more specific with the movements you're selecting and executing, and consider the demands required by your type of cycling. As you approach your event or the peak of your competition season, transition into a maintenance program you can use on a more infrequent basis. This allows for the majority of focus to be on competition events, or on-bike training sessions, while maintaining the strength and stability obtained.

Preseason Program

This is a more generalized program that will give you a foundation of strength and stability, as well as more comfort with using the suspension trainer. The strength and control you will develop with this program will create an important foundation necessary to support the next phase. This consists of a balanced program of upper body, lower body, and core movements. Refer to the level 1 and level 2 foundation workouts on pages 212 and 215 for an example of this program. Because the focus is general strength and stability, the workouts are appropriate for a wide range of people who may have different goals and abilities they will be considering after obtaining a strong foundation.

Do this program twice a week for four to six weeks. You may progress during this time by adding resistance, or moving to the next progression for any given movement. However, continue to build on the similar movement patterns. This allows for strength to be built upon the gains made in previous workouts. You may also add a third strength or cross-training workout of your choice, depending on how well you feel you're recovering from the workouts, and what you're doing in addition to your strength program.

Early Season Program

Progress to more difficult exercises, complex movements, or higher intensity and explosive movements.

Consider the individual demands of your chosen cycling discipline. Is it your priority to develop short-term power, increased stability, or fatigue resistance? Think hard about the things your chosen cycling discipline requires from you when selecting movements, as well as when executing them in your workout. Refer to the previous sections for each discipline to spur some ideas for exercise selection.

Competition Season Maintenance Program

Back off the intensity and focus on stability and maintenance of the strength you developed in the previous program(s). According to the study referenced earlier in this chapter, strength gains can be maintained with a frequency of as little as one session every ten days. In addition, this session need not be of maximum intensity. This will allow you to go into your race-specific intervals, or races themselves, with more freshness, but still with the strength and stability you obtained in the previous training blocks. In this phase, I suggest putting on-bike work first in your program, and focusing on race-specific fitness. Remember, the goal is simply to maintain the strength and stability gains you have made due to the hard work you have done over the last several months.

During a taper or the week preceding a key competition event, I suggest leaving strength training out of your program altogether. This will ensure optimal freshness during that event. If you are undergoing a multi-week taper for an endurance event such as an Ironman or ultradistance event, you may want to keep it in until the final week of the taper, but be sure to reduce the intensity and focus on the stability component. Strength training during this time should not leave you too sore, as you should not be increasing the intensity during this time or shifting the types of movements you are doing. Stick with movements you have been doing in the weeks preceding, and remember that the goal of a taper or the week preceding competition is to allow your body to recover and rebuild from previous training.

Conclusion

Use the information in this chapter to help you decide what type of strength training would be most beneficial to you, and how to incorporate it into your individual program. If you're working with a coach, you may want to discuss how to best incorporate it into the training plan you're establishing.

The index of exercises can be used as a reference when selecting movements. However, available exercises are not limited to that index, and don't be afraid to expand from it. Also, although suspension training is ideal for developing cycling-specific strength, that doesn't mean you need to limit yourself to suspension training either. There are a variety of methods to develop strength and stability to enhance your cycling. No matter what method or tools you're using, remember to consider what you're trying to do in relation to your cycling experience level, the demands of your cycling discipline, and where you are in your competitive season. This will give you the direction to get the most out of adding strength work to your program.

Chapter 12

Strength Training for Running

Can Strength Training Really Help Me Be a Better Runner?

This chapter is for runners as well as anyone who participates in any activity that involves running. If you are a runner, you will gain much from the information in this chapter. If you don't consider yourself a runner but play soccer, basketball, tennis, or engage in any type of activity that includes running, this chapter is for you as well.

There is a ton of research out there to support the idea that strength training is beneficial to run performance. But again, the research on suspension training and run performance is scarce, and badly needed. However, I did find some studies that used body-weight and explosive-type exercises that I felt were very similar to some of the exercises using a suspended trainer that can be found in the exercise library. I also listed these movements in the running-specific workouts that can be found at the end of this chapter.

Often, runners and endurance athletes refrain from resistance training to avoid gaining muscle mass that might translate to extra weight to carry during runs. However, studies have shown that muscle strength can be improved without increases in weight.

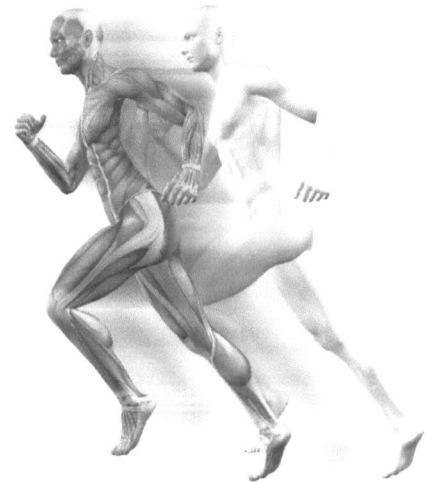

What Makes a Strong Runner?

Imagine a runner who lacks solid stance or good posture. When he or she is running, you may see the person sink a little with each step. You may notice his or her hips drop on one side each time he or she lands on the other leg. The person's core may be soft, like a bowl of jelly, and provide no stability for the lower extremities to push off. The core may also poorly transfer force from the upper body and provide little support from good posture. You have probably seen this person running. You might be this person.

Now imagine the person with strength and stability in his or her hips and legs. There is no sinking or softness when the person's foot makes contact with the ground. The ankle, leg, and hip stay perfectly aligned and absorb that energy to release to aid in the push-off. The person's core is like a rock-solid piece of concrete that transfers the drive from the arms and gives a solid platform for the lower extremities from which to push. His or her posture allows for maximum room for the diaphragm to expand during breathing. This person looks better, feels better, and runs faster and more efficiently.

What Studies Say about Strength Training for Running

1. **Strength training improves running economy.** The term running economy basically refers to the amount of oxygen you need at a given submaximal pace. For example, say you run an eight-minute mile on a flat grade for a certain duration. If you improve your running economy, you will be able to run the same eight-minute mile but need less oxygen to do so. By improving your running economy, you become a more efficient runner because you lower your energy cost at a given speed.

   Running economy measurements and tests are done with the runner performing at a submaximal level. Most of the studies I researched looked at the effect strength training has on running economy in experienced runners. [1,2,6,8,9] The pace used was based on each runner's individual pace for a predetermined distance that depended on the experience level of the group being tested. The same run at the same pace for each runner was performed before and after a six-to-eight-week training block. Runners who performed strength training during this time were compared to those who didn't. Oxygen use was measured during this run. The consistent results in the literature show that the strength training group needed less oxygen to perform that exact same effort after adding strength training to their running program compared to the groups who only performed run training. The amount of improvement was in the range of 5 percent.

2. **Strength training improves time to exhaustion.** The tests measuring time to exhaustion were generally a graded treadmill test where the speed was increased every three minutes until the runner was too tired to continue. A time-to-exhaustion test was also performed and measured before and after the training block in the studies previously mentioned (as well as many others). The group that performed strength training showed greater improvements in this test as well. They could continue further into the test, and achieve higher peak speeds before reaching exhaustion.

3. **VO_2 max values did not improve, but performance did.** VO_2 max is the maximum amount of oxygen that can be used and is usually measured with harder efforts of increasing intensity. It's interesting that VO_2 max values did not change after strength training was added and the runners were retested. This means that the strength training did not raise the ceiling of the amount of oxygen that could be used, yet the runners still became more efficient and were able to perform more work. One possible reason for this is the increased efficiency, including the ability to store and release elastic energy during the run stride, which I talk about in the following section.

Why Does Strength Training Improve Running?

The reasons why adaptations from strength training resulted in better running were consistent throughout the literature. They included the following:

1. **Improved motor requirement patterns and neural adaptations.** The neural muscular system may become more efficient in terms of which muscles to turn on, and exactly when to turn them on. When landing on one leg during the stance phase, the strongest, largest muscles need to be ready to both control and stabilize (prime movers), and then accelerate body weight. What is equally important is that before the prime movers can do their job, the smaller muscles that are needed to stabilize the joint (stabilizers), need to contract in a way that gives the prime movers the optimal platform from which to create force. Strength training may benefit running by improving the timing and coordination within these muscles. In addition, being able to more effectively turn

off muscles not needed at any given time is a plus.

2. **Strength training results in improved relative intensities.** With each step during your run, you're using a given amount of the maximum strength you can produce. After performing a block of strength training, this maximum amount of strength is now a higher number. With this increase, a lower percentage of the maximum strength available is needed during each stride to obtain that same workload. This may lower the actual number of motor neurons recruited and result in less overall demand. The same changes occur in cycling when considering the forces produced during the pedal stroke.

3. **Strength training increases muscle stiffness and the ability to absorb and release energy.** There is an elastic component in muscle that is very important in running. When contact is made with the ground, some of the energy from the impact can be stored like a spring, and released during push-off. Imagine stretching a rubber band. As you stretch it, it becomes tight and full of stored energy. When you let go, that energy releases and causes the band to snap back. The elastic component of your muscle fibers stores energy in a similar way. When the foot makes contact with the ground, the muscle fibers initially lengthen as they contract to control and decelerate your momentum. When you transition, some of the energy that was stored (like the rubber band) is given back. This gives a slight aid in the movement forward. During running, it's not a huge amount, but over the course of thousands of steps, it adds up. This results in less energy you need to generate to run at the same pace.

4. **Strength training may shorten time to peak force.** This suggestion was given in a study on maximal strength and running economy in distance runners.[2] I thought it was extremely insightful and wanted to make sure to mention it in this chapter. It was stated that if the peak force of the muscle contraction occurs earlier, the relaxation after the contraction time in each stride will be increased. The blood flow to exercising muscles occurs almost exclusively between muscle contractions. [2]As a result of this, better circulatory flow through the working muscles during the relaxation time should allow more oxygen and needed substrates to reach the muscle fibers. This increased recovery between contractions could lead to a longer time to exhaustion.

Some Additional Benefits of Strength Training

Improved core strength equals faster running. A study on recreational and competitive runners added a core-training program, resulting in significantly faster five-thousand-meter run times over six weeks versus the control group that did not do extra core training.[3] Some of the runners were more conscious of using their core to stabilize their run form, and had a better understanding of body position and posture while running.

Both strength and performance benefits can be obtained and maintained with one to two sessions per week. The sessions also don't have to be long. But they do have to be done at the intensity needed to result in the adaptations, and the selected exercises must target relevant muscle groups.

Strength training reduces age-related performance declines. A study from 2013 examined running economy and strength training in Masters runners.[2] In addition to the running performance benefits, the study found that adding strength training to the Masters runners program may help reduce age-related declines in performance. Therefore, if you are in that demographic and want to hold onto your run times as you get older, consider adding some strength training to your program.

Strength training reduces loss of stride length. As you get tired, your stride shortens, and this results in you going slower. Strength training has been shown to prevent or delay this shortening of stride that comes with fatigue. A study from 2008[4] compared three groups of middle-distance trained runners.

Stride length loss at race speed was measured in all groups by having all the runners do a series of repetitions at race pace and measuring the difference of stride length in the third repetition compared to the last repetition.

Figure 12.1. To the right is a comparison of the mean percentage of stride length (cm)/speed (SLS) loss between the three study groups. Periodized = periodized strength training group; nonperiodized = nonperiodized strength training group; control = no strength training group. The Journal of Strength and Conditioning Research Vol. 22 (July 2008):1176–1183.[4]

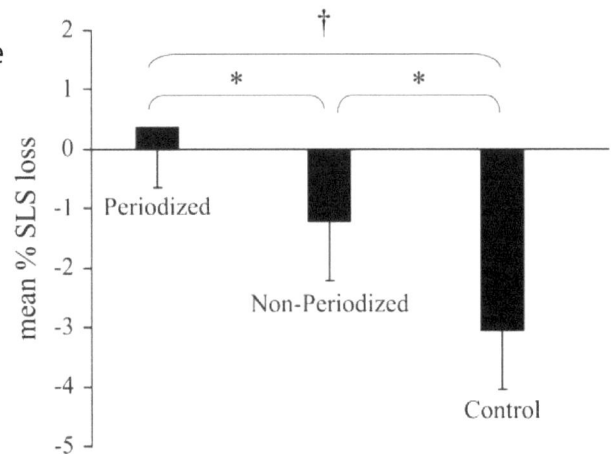

One group performed an eight-week periodized strength training program starting with circuit training and light loads and transitioning to explosive movements, including plyometrics and higher-intensity, run-specific movements. The non-periodized group performed the same type of exercise, but with no progression or week-to-week variation. The third group did not strength train. All three groups performed the same run program during this time. When the same intervals were performed after the strength training periods, the group who had performed the periodized strength program was able to maintain their stride length during the intervals as they fatigued. The non-periodized program group experienced some stride-length loss with fatigue, but not nearly as much as the group who did not incorporate any strength training.

This is great information to keep in mind, especially for those who compete in running or run-related sports. One of my personal mentors in triathlon coaching likes to say that *"The race is won by the person who slows down the least,"* and that truly applies to the results of this study.

How You Strength Train Matters

What you do in your program in terms of the type of strength training, exercise selection, and intensity of the movements, can affect the performance gains transported to run activities. Several studies not only looked at the effects of strength training on running, but also compared the type of strength training performed to see if one way of doing it produced better performance gains than another. In most of the research, strength training fell into one of three categories listed in the following pages.

The type or category of strength training performed in the studies did appear to have different levels of benefit to run performance.

Maximum Strength Training. This involved heavy loads and low repetitions. The resistance was in the range of 80 percent of the maximum amount that could be performed one time (1RM), and the repetitions were in the range of 4 to 8.

Circuit Training or Endurance Strength Training. The program design of these groups was a little more varied, but all consisted of lighter loads and more repetitions or timed sets.

Explosive or Plyometric Training. These types of training consisted of lighter loads but higher peak forces. The objective of this method of strength training is to accelerate the weight (or body) as fast as possible, generating as much force as possible in the shortest amount of time. Now, I need to point out that although explosive and plyometric training methods are similar, and I have put them into the same category for the purpose of this book, they are not exactly the same.

Plyometrics are explosive movements in which the deceleration of your body weight is controlled and transitioned to acceleration as quickly as possible. The muscle is contracting eccentrically on the descent because it is lengthening as it contracts to control the weight. The muscle then contracts concentrically as it shortens and accelerates the weight. The elastic component described earlier comes into play with these types of movements because it allows energy to be stored as the muscles are stretched and released as they contract.

For example, if you did a squat jump starting from the squat position and jumped as high as possible, that would be an explosive movement. However, if you did the same squat jump but started from a standing position, dropped into the squat, and then immediately exploded into the jump, that would also be explosive, but it would be considered a plyometric movement. In the plyometric movement, energy is stored during the deceleration and used during the subsequent jump, which results in a higher jump due to the stored elastic energy. More examples of plyometric movements in the exercise library include skaters, lunge hops, and ski jumps.

More running performance gains were found with maximal strength efforts and explosive movements. The studies mentioned in the above section, that showed the most increase in running economy and time to exhaustion, used maximal strength training. Adding any type of strength training in general has been shown to benefit running, however, the studies comparing maximal efforts and explosive/plyometric movements tended to show stronger improvements in run performance or improvements over a wider range of variables.[4,5,6] These variables included a three-kilometer time trial, peak running performance on a graded treadmill test, before-and-after oxygen use at a given speed, and perceived exertion.

When the plyometric training was compared to explosive training with concentric contractions only, both programs resulted in improvements in running performance.[5] The plyometric training group showed the most gains, with a 7 percent improvement in run economy, and the explosive, concentric group showed a 4 percent improvement. On top of that, these improvements were obtained with just one strength training session per week!

The circuit training groups in the studies still made significant but smaller improvements in the run performance variables measured.

These improvements in strength and running performance came with no increase in body weight. This should come as good news for runners concerned about extra weight that may come with building muscle. The reason given for this is that with the minimal and explosive-type weight training, much of the strength gains come from neuromuscular adaptations, versus an increase in muscle mass. Also, remember that during the training periods studied, the run groups were all still doing their endurance-training program, which may have contributed to maintaining weight as well.

Conclusion of Research Section

As you can see, there is a multitude of reasons to perform strength training if you want to be a better runner. Hopefully, having a better understanding of what exactly these performance benefits are and why they result in better running, will give you more reasons to include strength training in your own program.

The next section will go into even greater detail on how to design a run-specific strength program. This will include what exercises to select and why, things to consider based on what type of running you do, and why stability is just as important as strength when it comes to running. I also touch on why it's important to your run form to have adequate mobility, and how to achieve that as well.

Making Strength Training Running Specific

Specific adaptations to the imposed demands principle (SAID), that I covered in the cycling chapter, apply to running as well. Your body will adapt to the demands placed on it in the same way those demands are placed on it. So when it comes to running, if you train with a lot of fast and short intervals, you will develop speed. If you run for long durations at a slower pace, that's what you will be good at. The same thing applies to strength training.

Knowing this, include movements that are relevant to your running goals.

Basic demands that apply to running include:

- Stability and strength of the ankle, knee, and hip

- Ability to support and control body weight on one leg for many repetitions

- Adequate mobility of the hips, ankles, and torso

- The ability to slow your momentum and then accelerate it again during the push-off

- Upper-body strength and arm drive to add power to the stride

- Good posture and torso mobility to allow for maximal breath capabilities

Below is a list of suspension training movements that are running specific. This list is designed to give you some choices when putting together your own program. Level 1 movements are more basic and good ones with which to start. These can be progressed as you get stronger and your abilities develop. Level 2 movements are more advanced and/or complex movements. Also give some thought to what movements in general are most relevant to running or the type of activity that you participate in that involves running. Although all the suspension training movements listed in this section are running specific, not every exercise will yield maximum benefit to every runner. If you're a recreational jogger, you may have different strength, stability, and flexibility needs than a soccer player or a triathlete.

In addition, keep in mind that these are merely suggestions for good movements that are relevant to the demands of running, so don't feel like you need to limit yourself to only these or even to only suspension training. Give some thought to what movements in general are most relevant to the type of runner you are and to your specific goals, and apply that to all methods of resistance training you choose to use.

Level 1 Movements

- Bicycle Kicks
- Plank
- Split Squat
- Reverse Lunge
- Push-Up (Hands Suspended)
- Row
- Hip Hinge
- Half-Kneeling Rollout
- Half Get-Up
- Suspended Get-Up
- Sprinter Starts
- Ski Jumps

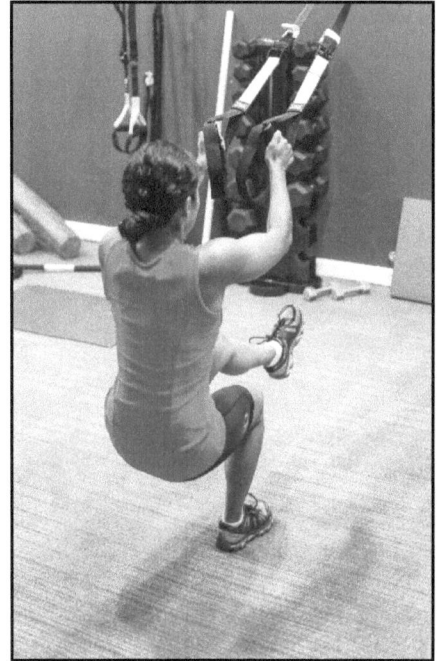

Level 2 Movements

- Single-Leg Squat
- Suspended Reverse Lunge
- Suspended Power Lunge
- Split-Squat Jump
- Push-Up (Feet Suspended)
- Atomic Crunches
- Suspended Side Plank
- Pull-Ups or Assisted Suspended Pull-Ups
- Tall Kneeling Rollout
- Suspended Burpee
- Squat-Press Jumps
- Skaters
- Sprinter Starts with Hop

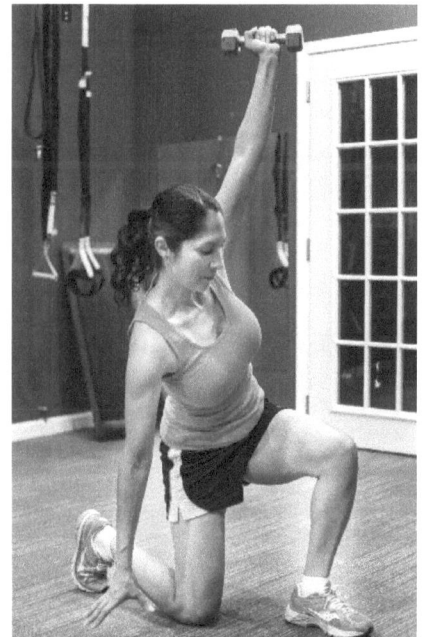

Why you choose to run for exercise is personal to you. You may run for health and fitness, fun, competition, or to support the training demands of another activity. There is a variety of both run disciplines and activities involving running, each having its own specific demands. Even if you don't label yourself a runner, running may still be a big component in other activities in which you participate. Below you will find some examples of activities that would benefit from a run-specific strength program, and some of the specific running demands of each type.

Recreational jogging: Balance, injury prevention, and comfort with the activity.

Short distance: Speed and optimal run mechanics.

Long distance: Fatigue resistance and optimal mechanics over long durations.

Trail and off-road running: Stability to handle uneven surfaces and unexpected obstacles.

Adventure racing and "Tough Mudders": Sustained running, occasional accelerations to the next obstacle, uneven terrain, and total-body fatigue resistance.

Triathlon: Mobility of the hips after being on the bike for long durations. Fatigue resistance, since the running portion is at the end of the race.

Multidirectional running sports: Frequent changes in movement, speed, and direction, and the possibility of impact or collisions that may occur. Soccer, basketball, tennis, softball, floor hockey, and Ultimate Frisbee are all included in this category.

Earlier in this chapter, I talked about basic demands of running on the legs and hips, and what exercises to include to build strength for those demands. I also touched on the variety of activities that involve running, and how the benefits to developing strength for running apply to more than just those who consider themselves runners. Now, I will give you one more reason: strength training as a means of injury prevention. Even if you have zero interest in improving performance, staying injury-free will keep you happier, healthier, and is also much easier on your wallet in the long run.

Injury Prevention

Running performance is about more than just running in one direction. Most of this next section will target the multidirectional sports listed above that require frequent changes in speed and direction and have the possibility of impact. I'm going to talk about a study done on soccer players, but I also believe it applies to similar sports such as basketball, tennis, and Ultimate Frisbee.

This study looked at injury rates among fifty-two elite youth soccer players divided into two groups.[9] One group performed twelve weeks of a periodized, progressive strength training plan that included plyometrics. The other did not strength train. Seventeen injuries were recorded throughout the season. Most of them involved the lower limbs. There were four injuries in the group that strength

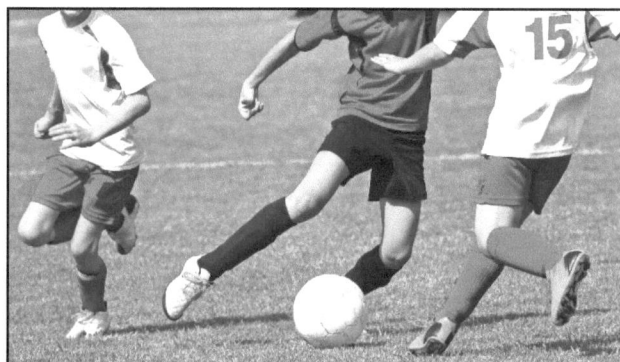

trained, and thirteen injuries in the group that did not. It was said that during the season, 50 percent of the players in the control group sustained an injury during the season, and only 15 percent of the players in the group that performed strength training sustained an injury.

Soccer injuries come in a wide variety, but most affect the lower extremities, including the upper leg, knee, and ankle. This particular study also referenced additional studies that have demonstrated that increasing hamstring strength reduced risk of injuries in a variety of populations of soccer players.

The study showed that stabilization training improves coordination within muscles, and between muscles. Strength training will also strengthen muscles as well as the tendons and ligaments around them. This will increase the forces that the muscles themselves can sustain, increase joint stability, and increase bone density. Now, none of this guarantees your invincibility when your competition slams into the side of your knee while diving for the ball, but it can at least increase your chances of being able to handle the impact or the quick, forceful change of direction you make when you see it coming.

I also wanted to mention that this specific study was done on younger players from thirteen to fourteen years old. The authors suggest that younger players who have the opportunity to strength train early will be more likely to develop the prerequisite abilities to allow them to participate at higher levels. One concern with young athletes is that when they strength train, it can be detrimental to use weights that are too heavy. The reason for this is that their growth plates may not have fully finished developing yet, and subjecting the bones to heavy weight could be damaging to those areas. Body-weight and suspension training is an ideal approach for younger athletes, however, as it will develop both coordination and strength without the risk of injury from training with heavy plates, bars, and dumbbells.

This study, and most other studies that I have read involving strength training, include what was usually referred to as a preparatory or familiarization phase in the experimental group that performed a strength training program. This was generally a phase of three to four weeks where subjects performed more general, lower-intensity movements in order to develop an initial foundation, and both neural and muscular adaptations to the strength movements. The more specific and higher-intensity movements were performed in the training phase that followed. This goes back to developing a foundation, which is discussed in chapter 5. I want to emphasize again the importance of using a similar approach when you start a strength training program yourself.

In addition to the research in the previous section, the following are some things to consider when adding strength training to your program to enhance your running abilities.

Stability Matters in Running

Resistance training specific to running is about more than just being able to push and control weight. It's about developing the motor patterns and neuromuscular control to maintain proper alignment of the ankles, knees, and hips, as well as the upper torso during extended training sessions and competition events. The stability training is something that machines such as the

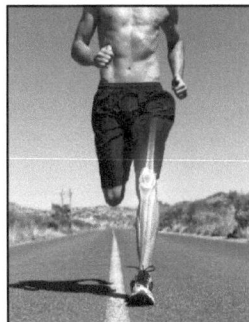

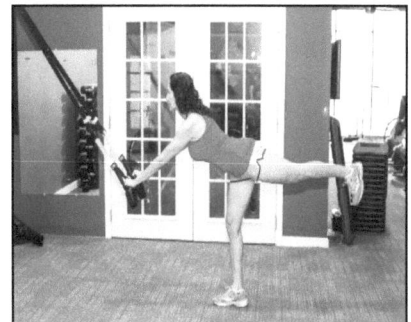

leg press, leg extensions, and other isolation machines don't provide. Strengthening stabilizers with hip abduction exercises or side planks is a good start, but simply strengthening stabilizers will still not teach them when they need to fire. With stabilizers, it's about timing. Muscles responsible for stabilizing need to know exactly when and where to fire to create a stable platform necessary for prime movers to do their job. This is especially true for maintaining strong mechanics with proper alignment of hips, knees, and ankles during the single-leg stance during the run. As soon as you start to lose that stability in your running, the integrity of your mechanics and your efficiency both suffer. You are also putting harmful stress on your muscles, joints, and ligaments that could result in injuries.

Everything Is Connected. When your hip stabilizers fail to do their job, your hips may start to drop with each stride. That may lead to your knees caving inward instead of staying in line with the hip and ankle. When the knees cave inward, it puts increased stress on that joint as well as increased rotational force on the bones that connect to the ankle joint. This is just one example.

With stability in mind, think about the exercises you select in your program and how they are executed. Being a runner, your strength program should incorporate at least one or two single-leg movements. These should be movements that challenge stability and balance as well as strength. The hip hinge and single-leg squat are two examples of good lower-extremity exercises for runners. When you're executing these movements, the goal should be maximum control of the movement. Take a second to pause at each end-of-range motion of that movement, and make sure you have 100 percent control of it. The level should be challenging and slightly out of your comfort zone but doable. If you're struggling to maintain balance through your repetitions, back it off a bit until you find a level that is still challenging, but one you can do successfully.

> *Master Your End Zones*
>
> *When doing your strength training movements, obtain 100 percent control over each end-of-range motion of a movement with a slight pause. This approach is helpful in developing optimal stability and control of the movement.*

Mobility Matters in Running

We want to create strong, resilient muscles, and flexibility in those same muscles. Having the ability to move through all the required ranges of motion is important to run mechanics. If you're tight in one area of the chain, you're fighting against resistance from your own muscles just to move through the range of motion. In addition, one tight muscle may not only limit your movement with that muscle, it may also affect what the muscles around it are supposed to do. The good news is that most mobility issues resulting from tight muscles are fixable with a little work.

Following are three areas in which I commonly see mobility issues affecting run stride, and some stretches to help fix them. Spending time working on flexibility isn't necessarily something everyone needs to do. If you have great mobility, your time is better spent elsewhere. However, I've found that the majority of the people who live in today's world, especially those that sit for long periods in cars and at desks, have developed some limitations and/or imbalances that negatively affect both general posture and run mechanics.

Hips

Our hips must have adequate mobility to be able to reach the range of motion we need to achieve the best and most efficient mechanics. The hip flexors are responsible for swinging the leg back during your run stride. Strong hip flexors are necessary for a strong knee drive. They also need to be mobile enough to allow you to achieve full extension during the push-off of the run phase.

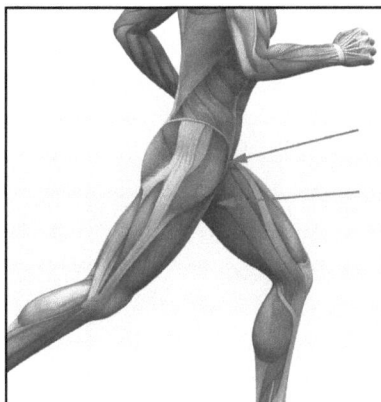

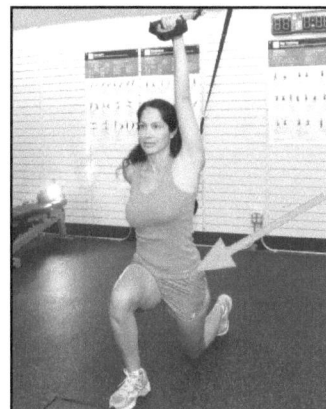

A hip flexor stretch

One of the most common running limiters I encounter in clients is tight hip flexors. This is especially true for working professionals who have careers that require them to spend a lot of time sitting. Long durations spent sitting mean the hip flexors and hamstrings are shortened for extended periods of time. This results in mobility issues that affect your run stride. If you can't get into proper extension, you may be losing out on length in your run stride. You also may be losing out on forward propulsion from the glutes and hip extensors.

Ankles

You need strong calves to absorb impact, as well as to push off and propel you forward. You also need mobility to be able to pull your toe up (dorsiflex) and shorten the lever that you're pulling back to achieve the most efficient swing through. Lack of mobility in the ankle can also limit your extension and push-off, because you will not have the range of motion to allow the ankle to bend sufficiently in order to get the leg behind you to set up the foot for the push-off.

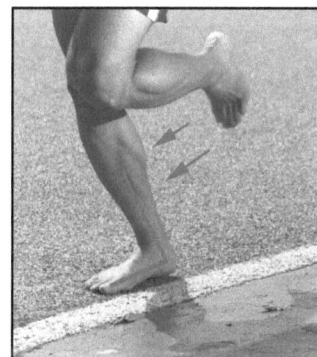

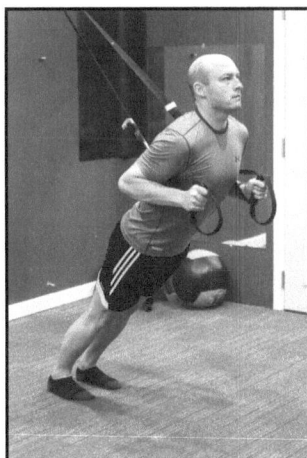

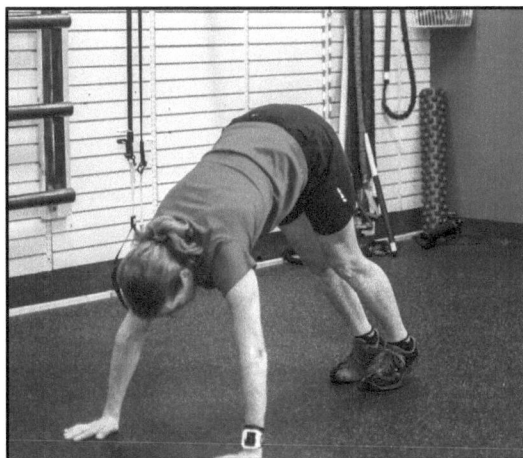

To the left are two examples of stretches for your calves. The first one is a static calf stretch, and the second one is the inchworm dynamic stretch.

Upper Body

We run with our legs, so why would upper body flexibility matter in running? Well, there is actually a huge upper-body component to running. The first and biggest issue is breathing. Again, those who spend a lot of time sitting are especially affected by this. The thoracic (upper) part of your spine is made to be mobile. But spending hours over the course of days, weeks, and even years sitting at a desk, or behind the wheel, can chip away at this mobility.

Some of the effects of that confinement are restrictions in the amount of room your diaphragm has to expand, along with limitations in arm movement and overall posture. Have you ever seen someone run with a stiff torso or hunched-over upper back? If this sounds like you, you are leaving a lot of potential performance gains sitting on the table. The two stretches above are great for developing mobility in the upper spine and opening up the chest and shoulders to allow for improved posture overall, and during running.

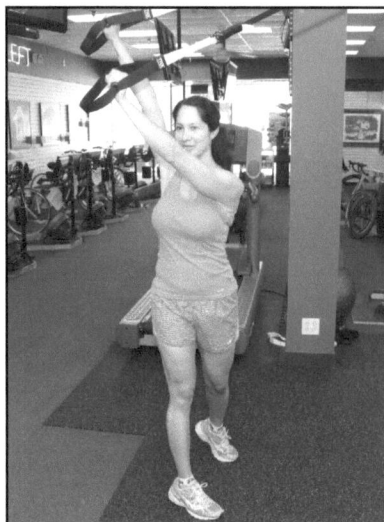

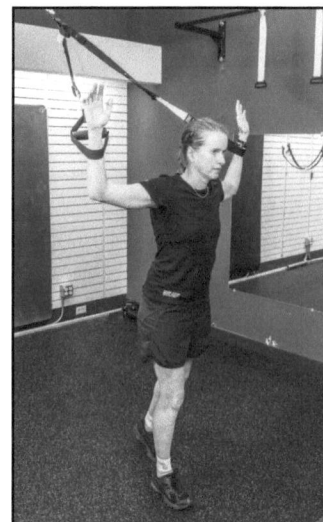

The T-spine stretch (left) targets the upper spine, and the chest stretch (right) targets the chest and front of the shoulders.

Conclusion

Whether you run for competition, fun, health and fitness, or as a part of another sport, adding a run-specific strength program can both improve your running abilities, and help keep you injury-free.

Studies overwhelmingly show that strength training can help you be a stronger, more efficient runner. This includes extending time to exhaustion at a given pace, becoming more efficient through improved run mechanics, and the ability to store and release elastic energy during the run stride. Strength training also helps running by improving the requirement of muscles that are in charge of controlling, stabilizing, and accelerating your body weight on a single leg.

In addition, it will enable you to maintain the strength to perform this movement many times over long durations, while retaining strong form and mechanics. It can help you prevent injuries, hold onto your abilities as you age, and be more aware of your mechanics. You don't need to devote a lot of time to a strength training program, but you do need to design a program that is run-specific if supporting and improving run abilities is your goal. This includes the type of exercises you select, how you progress them, and the intensity at which you program them.

Keeping these things at the forefront in your workout program and staying consistent with it, will help keep you running strong, feeling strong, and participating in the activities you love.

Section 3

Tools
Exercise Libraries
Sample Workouts

Chapter 13

Toolbox

Grab Some Tools and Get Started!

This chapter is designed to be a toolbox of approaches to jump-start your workouts, and keep things interesting. It includes solutions for when you're working out with a partner, when you're on the road without equipment, when you may be short on time, or when you just want to feel better after a long day at work. The workouts are designed to be a random mix of things you can make use of depending on what situation you might be in at any given time. They're also designed to make it easier for you to get started and stay consistent while having more fun!

"I really want this, but I just can't find the time these days."

"I am so tired and just not into it today."

"Ugh, I have to travel for work this week… again."

"I am ready to do it, but I'm having a workout mind block and can't decide what I should do!"

If you have ever thought these things to yourself, this chapter has the solutions for you!

Exercise Pairing

Just like wine and cheese, certain movements pair well together. This is because they target complementary areas of the body. So, while one part of the body works, the other gets a little recovery. An example would be to pair a pushing movement with a pulling movement or an upper-body movement with a lower-body movement. Alternating opposite muscle groups allows you to accomplish more work in less time. It also develops the cardiovascular system as your heart continues to pump and provide the overall oxygen needed, as you shift the workload around to different areas of the body. The following chart gives you some suggestions as to which categories movements fall into based on what part of the body is being targeted, as well as the difficulty level of the movement.

Level 1 movements are the most beginner-friendly, but that doesn't necessarily mean that they're the easiest—most movements can be as hard as you decide to make them based on the resistance you choose. They can, however, be easily adjusted to a resistance level that is appropriate for those at beginner strength through experienced level.

Level 2 movements are more intermediate in ability level, and may require more strength and body coordination.

Level 3 movements are the most advanced, and require optimal levels of strength, core stability, and coordination.

	Pushing	Pulling	Core	Lower Body	Full Body
Level 1	Push-Up (Hands Suspended) Tricep Extension Fly	Row Bicep Curl Reverse Fly	Plank Bicycle Kicks Half Get-Up	Squat Split Squat Hip Raise Hip Hinge	Squat Press Squat Row Run in Place
Level 2	Push-Up (Feet Suspended) Power Push-Ups Plank to Push-Up Position	Assisted Pull-Up Inverted Row Single-Arm Row Back Extensions	Sit-Up/Crunch Suspended Side Plank Tall Kneeling Rollout	Reverse Lunge Hamstring Curl Skaters Sprinter Starts	Suspended Get-Up Squat-Press Jump Bear Crawl Squat to Reverse Fly
Level 3	Spider Push-Up Swim Pull Assisted Dips	Chin-Up Swim Pull Inverted Row with Wide Grip	Pike Atomic Crunch Suspended Saw	Suspended Power Lunge Single-Leg Squat Suspended Lateral Lunge	Suspended Burpee Full Get-Up Overhead Squat

What If...

Here are some quick tips on what you can do if you find yourself in these situations.

You're short on time and only have a few minutes:

- ○ First select one movement from each column of the chart above.
- ○ Increase the intensity of the workout sets to make up for the decrease in time.
- ○ Do thirty seconds of each movement with zero to fifteen seconds of rest between movements.
- ○ How many repetitions can you perform of each movement in thirty seconds?
- ○ How many rounds can you do in five minutes? Ten minutes? Fifteen minutes?

You've been sitting all day:

Maybe you have been stuck at a desk all day for work or just got done with a plane flight or car ride.

Your hamstrings, quads, and the front of your upper torso are probably tight from being in a shortened position. Perform one to two sets of these stretches on the suspended trainer to bring them back to life, and restore balance to your body and muscles.

- o Upper- or lower-torso stretch (pp. 64, 65)

- o Hip flexor and chest stretch (pp. 62, 63)

- o Hamstring and back stretch (p. 61)

You're traveling without any equipment:

There are a variety of body-weight-only movements in the exercise library. In addition, many movements that are shown using a suspension trainer can be adjusted and performed without one. Just pay extra attention to form, and if needed, place a hand on the wall or a stable surface next to you for balance.

The planks, sit-ups, crunches, mountain climbers, squats, hip hinges, split squats, reverse lunges, jump squats, and skaters in the library, are all suspended-trainer movements that can be modified and performed without a suspension trainer if needed.

Below are two examples for a body-weight-only circuit if you are in a crunch, and want to stay consistent or blow off some steam. These can be done anywhere, including a small hotel room, conference room, or outdoor patio.

- o **Body-Weight Circuit Level 1: Three to five sets of thirty seconds each, with thirty seconds of rest**
  Run in place, modified push-ups, split squats, half get-ups, ski jumps, lateral hip raises

- o **Body-Weight Circuit Level 2: Three to five sets of thirty seconds each, with thirty seconds of rest**
  Skaters, push-ups, reverse lunges, full get-ups, burpees, side planks

You're just not motivated:

Follow the ten-minute rule! There are days where it's just harder to get excited about working out. We all have them. You want to do it, you know you should, but the momentum to get going is just not there. Give yourself ten minutes for a good solid warm-up. This should include a couple of dynamic stretches, and a light or full-body movement or two.

If you're still tired or you're not feeling good, and you're just not into it after ten minutes, give yourself permission to postpone the workout for a day, guilt free. The catch is that those ten minutes of exercise are critical. More often than not, you will get warmed up and feel better about continuing. If that's not the case, you may actually need the rest time, and you'll have at least given yourself some light exercise that will serve as active recovery, and leave you better off for the workout the next day.

Working Out with a Partner?

If you like to work out with a friend or significant other, here are some tools you can use to make your workouts more exciting, fun, and challenging! Whether you have just one suspended trainer for more than one person, or each person has his or her own, there are many ways to bring teamwork into your workout. Here are a few things you can do for camaraderie, or to get the competitive juices flowing.

○ **Tag Team.** Choose two movements and a duration or targeted rep range. Partner 1 starts with one movement while partner 2 starts with the other. After the reps or time goal, switch movements. Decide before you start how many rounds you will do. No stopping early and leaving your partner hanging!

○ **Go Down the Ladder.** Pick one movement and a starting number of repetitions. Partner 1 starts the exercises by performing that number of repetitions while partner 2 rests. When partner 1 finishes, partner 2 performs that same number while partner 1 rests. The next set is done with one less repetition, and so on until the last set is only one rep.

○ **Rotating Stations.** Create a circuit that includes one or more body-weight-only movements, and some cardio movements (see index below). Perform timed sets and rotate through the circuit so each person has a chance to do each exercise.

Tag Team

Partner 1	Partner 2
Rows for 30 seconds	Squats for 30 seconds
Rest 15 seconds	Rest 15 seconds
Squats for 30 seconds	Rows for 30 seconds
Rest 15 seconds	Rest 15 seconds

Go Down The Ladder

Partner 1	Partner 2
Set 1: 5 repetitions	Rest
Rest	Set 1: 5 repetitions
Set 2: 4 repetitions	Rest
Rest	Set 2: 4 repetitions
Set 3: 3 repetitions	Rest
Rest	Set 3: 3 repetitions
Set 4: 2 repetitions	Rest
Rest	Set 4: 2 repetitions
Set 5: 1 repetition	Rest
Rest	Set 5: 1 repetition

Rotating Stations Example

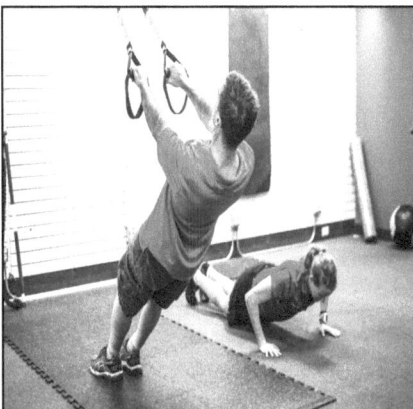

- Station #1: Pick a suspended trainer exercise.

- Station #2: Pick a body-weight movement.

- Station #3: Pick a cardio exercise from the cardio section (run in place, jump rope, jumping jacks, and so on).

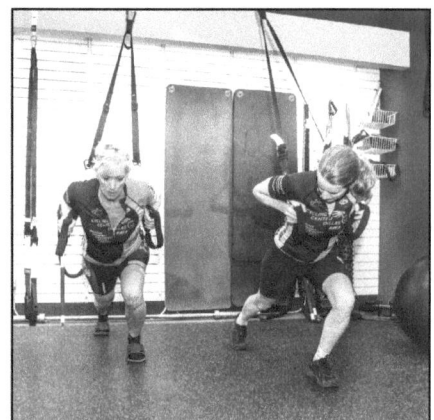

Use anywhere from two to five stations depending on how many people, suspended trainers, and space you have. Write down each station on a piece of paper, Post-it note, or anything you have available! Use either a set time, such as thirty seconds per station, or a repetition number that each person must complete at each station. Rotate through each station two to five times.

Progress Challenges

Want to know for sure that you're improving? Here are a couple of tests you can do. Start a block of training with one of the challenges below, record the results, and repeat in a few weeks to see how you have improved. Seeing results is motivating!

One-Minute Endurance Challenge: Perform as many repetitions of a movement as you can in one minute. You may rest as needed when the sixty seconds are up. Choose a push-up, leg movement, or row, or test all three! Make sure you mark where your feet are if you are doing a suspended version of a movement so you can perform the follow-up test at the same angle.

Push/Pull Strength Challenge: Mark a spot directly under the anchor with a piece of tape, or have a partner stand with his or her feet on that spot.

- Push-ups: Place your toes on the mark.

- Rows: Place your heels on the mark.

Perform as many consecutive reps as possible. Record your repetitions and retest in few weeks.

*As you advance, you may want to do this same test using feet-suspended push-ups and pull-ups.

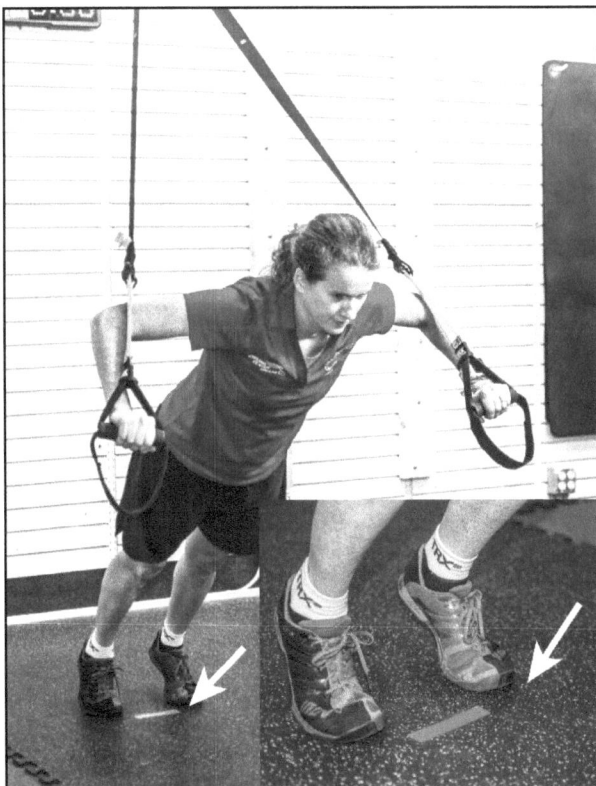

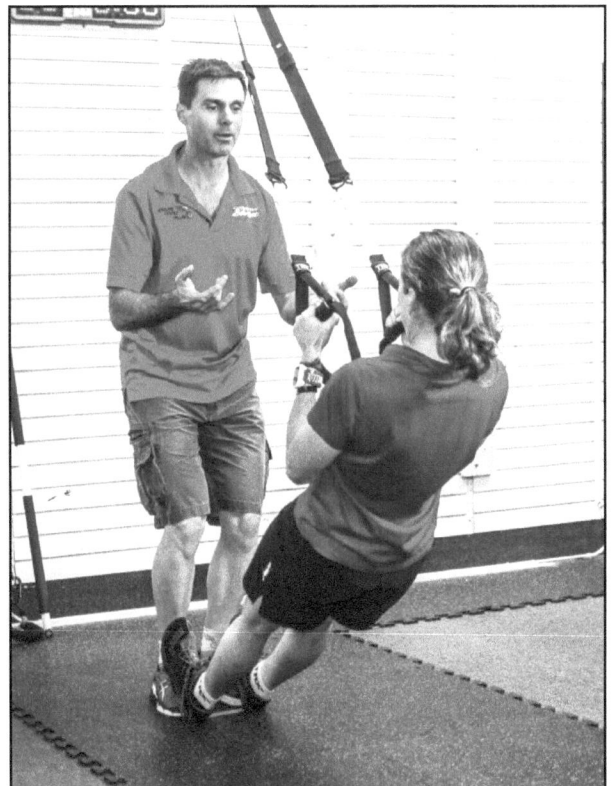

Additional Tools with Which You Can Combine Suspension Training

You may have access to additional equipment at a gym, or have some of your own. Design workouts combining what you have available to add even more variety! Here are some ideas:

- Free weights (barbells or dumbbells)
- Machines
- Battling ropes
- Elastic bands
- Sandbags
- BOSU ball or stability disc
- Medicine balls
- Kettlebells
- Balance boards
- Jump ropes
- Stationary cardio machines (treadmill, rowing machine, elliptical, and stair stepper)
- Strength machines
- Active motion bar

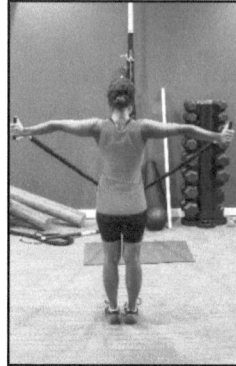
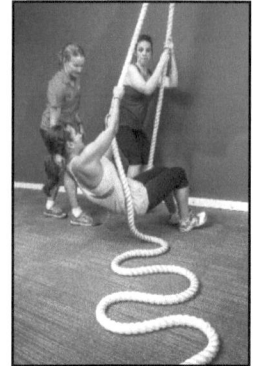
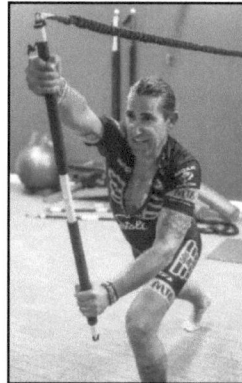
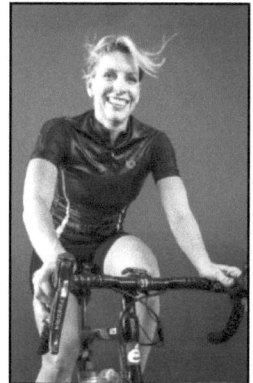

Conclusion

A suspended trainer is an extremely useful, functional, and fun tool that can add so much to your fitness and health program. Combining the use of one, as well as a variety of things you can do with your body weight alone, can give you a complete, dynamic, and effective program for just about any goal, ability, or lifestyle. However, keep in mind that the suspended trainer is just that—a tool to make it easy and more interesting to get in better shape, and be healthier and stronger. Don't feel like you need to limit yourself to only this type of training. It can certainly improve your abilities and transfer over to other methods or tools you may want to include in your workouts as well.

Suspension training is a great place to start for beginners, or those just getting back into things after a break because, of the ease of adjusting the difficulty levels. For those who may have seen these hanging at your gym, or thought about trying out a small group class in your area, I hope this book has given you the confidence to give it a try for the first time, or to try some new movements.

For those already comfortable with training with suspension and other methods, I hope I was able to give you some ideas of both movements and workout designs to add to your programs.

If you prefer to work out at home, you travel frequently, or you are a cyclist, runner, or triathlete who needs a strength program that can easily fit into other workouts, you may want to consider investing in your own equipment. There are many brands at many different price points, and new products are coming out every day. The suspended trainers used in this book are the TRX® brand, and I feel they're among the best-quality suspended trainers available at the time of publication.

They're a staple in most of my workout programs, for both me and my clients. There are also cheaper suspended trainers available, many of which are just fine for personal use. In addition to the TRX® trainers, I use the Primal 7 System® and the CrossCore 180®. Both have some unique features to them, but I find them to be a little more challenging to set up anywhere and adjust. I encourage you to do some research, read reviews, and decide how much you're willing to invest, and where you'll be using the trainers.

Chapter 14

Exercise Libraries

Core Movements

Grounded Plank Positions

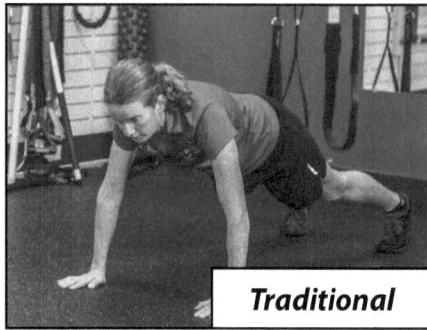
Traditional

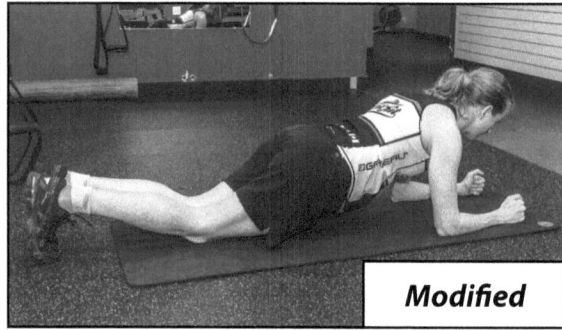
Modified

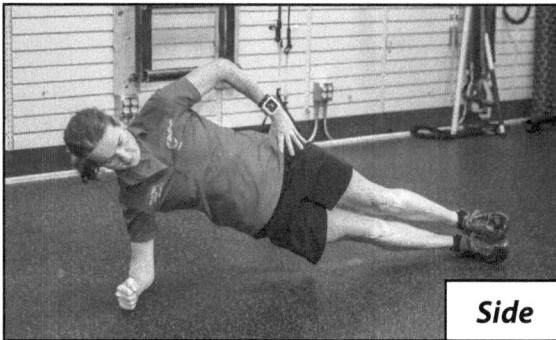
Side

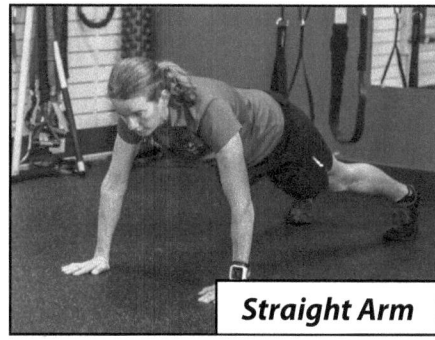
Straight Arm

Cross-Body Crunch

An alternating crunch movement that targets the core, while also working flexibility of the hamstrings through the straight-leg raise.

Primary Focus: Core

Secondary Focus: Hip flexors

1. Lie on your back with your legs straight, one arm extended above you, and the other arm at your side.

2. Simultaneously, raise the extended arm and the opposite leg to meet in the middle above your body. Keep both legs straight during the movement. The down leg should not come up or bend.

Repeat all repetitions on one side, and then switch sides.

Starting Position　　　　　　　　　　　　　　　　　　**Finishing Position**

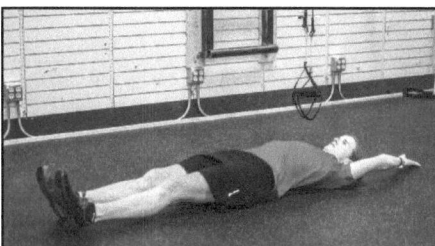
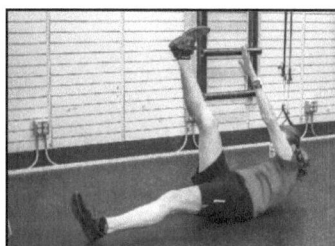
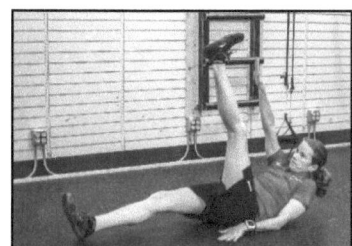

Note: *Lift the shoulder blade of the moving arm off the floor as high as you can when you bring the arm forward to meet the leg. As you gain strength in your core, you will be able to lift that shoulder higher.*

Supine March

A basic but important movement that will strengthen both the back side of the core and the hip flexor that lifts the leg up.

Primary Focus: Glutes, hamstrings

Secondary Focus: Hip flexors

1. Lie on your back with your knees bent and your feet flat on the floor.

2. Push through your feet and squeeze your butt to lift your hips off the floor.

3. Keeping your hips up, lift one leg off the floor and bring your knee to your chest, continuing to press hard into the floor with the opposite leg, to keep your hips elevated.

4. Bring the leg back down and switch sides, keeping the hips up the whole time. Alternate sides and repeat for the targeted number of repetitions.

Starting Position   **Finishing Position**

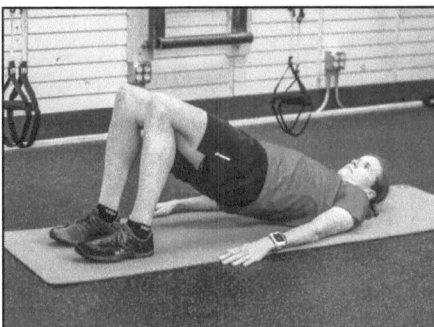

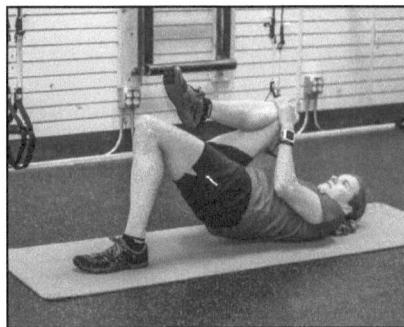

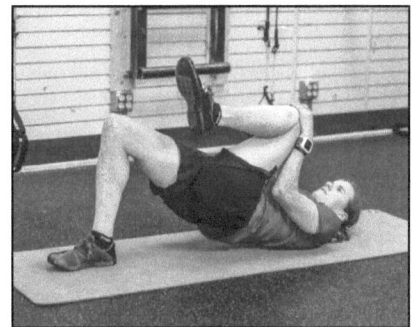

Note: *As you lift one leg, your hips will want to drop down or rotate to the inside. Don't let them! Push hard with the downed leg as you lift the other off the floor.*

Tips and Progressions:

- To make it easier, place your hands on the floor and away from you, and gently push into the floor to give you more stability and assistance with the movement.

- To make it harder, straighten your arms and point your hands to the ceiling right above your chest. Press your hands together, squeezing your chest muscles, and hold this position during the movement.

Mountain Climbers

You are basically adding a leg movement to a straight-arm plank. There are also two more variations using the suspended trainer: one with your hands suspended, and one with your feet suspended.

Primary Focus: Core

Secondary Focus: Hip flexors and arms

1. Get into a straight-arm plank position.

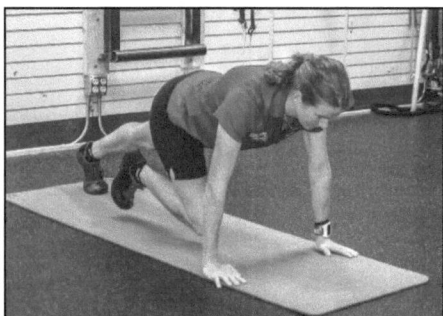

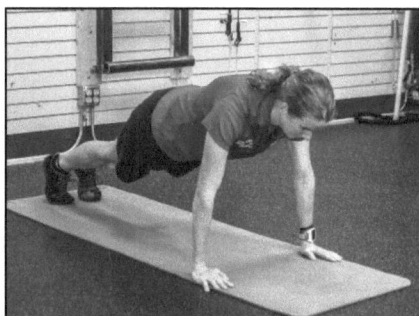

2. Maintain your body position to be straight like a surfboard and alternate pulling your knees toward your chest, one at a time.

3. Repeat for targeted repetitions or time.

Starting Position   **Finishing Position**

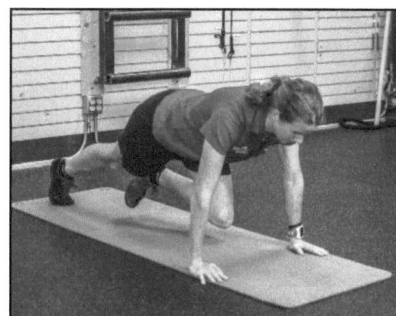

Note: *Keep your butt down and body straight! A common thing I see is that when people get tired they end up lifting their hips higher and higher because it makes it easier. Don't do it.*

Tips and Progressions:

- To make it harder, increase the speed until you are simultaneously bringing one leg forward and the other back. Your feet will touch the ground on both ends of the range of motion on this version.

Lateral Hip Raise

This is an excellent movement to strengthen hip stabilizers, which are important for strong hip and gait mechanics during walking and running.

Primary Focus: Core and obliques (lateral part of the core)

Secondary Focus: Arms, glutes

1. Get on your side, supporting yourself through your forearm by placing the elbow directly below your shoulder. The bottom knee should be bent and inline with your elbow, and the upper leg should be straight.

2. Push your hips off the ground through your downed knee, and simultaneously lift your top leg while keeping it straight.

3. Descend back down and repeat for the targeted amount of repetitions or time.

Starting Position   **Finishing Position**

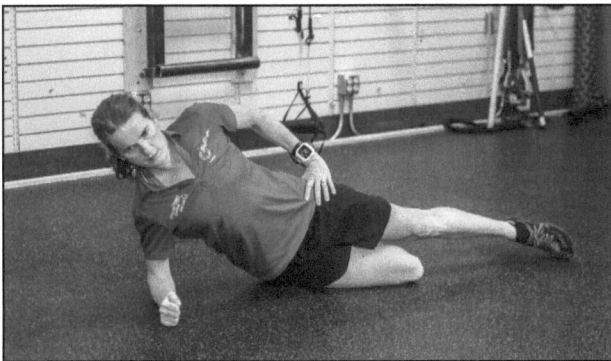

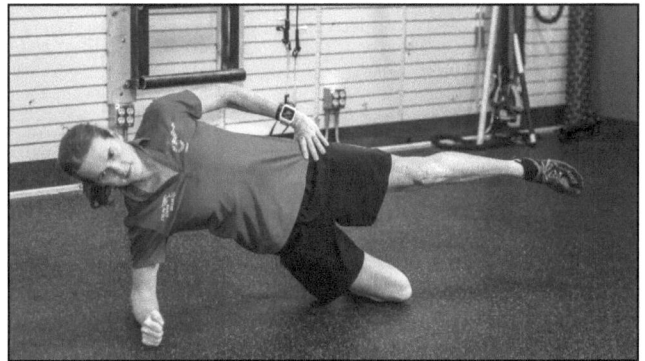

Tips and Progressions:

- This movement can be surprisingly challenging if you're doing it right. You can make it easier by allowing your top leg and foot to maintain contact with the floor. You can assist the hip lift by also pressing with that foot into the floor.

- To make it harder, use a light ankle weight, or place a lift bar parallel to your body with the end of it resting on the top leg. You will lift that end of the bar as you elevate that leg. You don't need much. A couple of pounds will make a big difference in the difficulty of the movement.

Half Get-Up

This is a fundamental movement that I include with some progression in almost all my programs. This is the level 1 progression, and the best one with which to start. Everyone should have the ability to easily and properly get up off the floor from a position of lying down, and this move will develop both the strength and motor patterns to do so. It will also develop a solid foundation to build on when progressing to more advanced variations of this move, such as adding the hip raise or performing it in half-kneeling or standing positions.

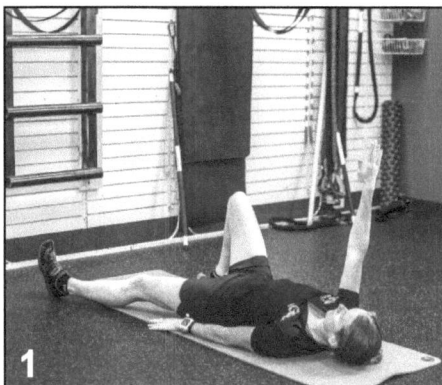

Primary Focus: Core

Secondary Focus: Hip flexor and arm

1. Lie on your back with one leg straight and the other bent. The arm on the bent-leg side should point straight up to the ceiling.

2. Start by lifting your shoulders off the ground as if you were doing a crunch, and continue ascending by pushing through the downed elbow. Keep your straight arm vertical and pointing at the ceiling the entire time.

3. Perform the desired amount of repetitions on one side. Rest, and then switch sides.

Starting Position   **Finishing Position**

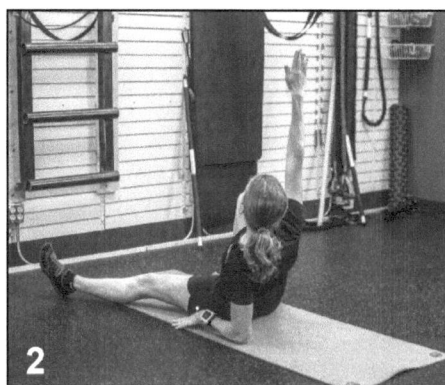

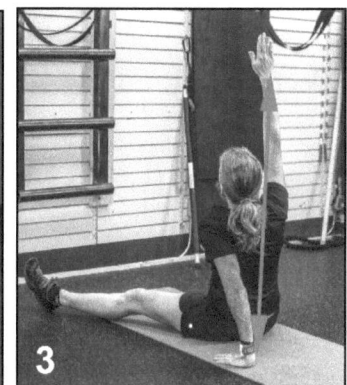

Note: Lift your chest and squeeze your shoulder blades together to create a straight line down your back from your fingers that are pointed up to your elbow that is on the floor.

Tips and Progressions:

- To make it harder, hold a weight in the hand that is reaching up. Keep it light; you don't need much to feel it. A light dumbbell, kettlebell, or even a can of soup or small sandbag will work. If you build to more than ten to fifteen reps, move on to the next advanced progression.

Bicycle Kicks

The hip-flexion movement (when the knee is pulled toward the chest) targets the core and hip flexors. Strengthening these can improve your gait, and benefit activities such as walking, running, stair climbing, and stepping over objects.

Primary Focus: Core

Secondary Focus: Hip flexors

Setup: Straps fully extended and approximately six inches off the ground.

1. Lie on your back with your feet in the cradles and your knees slightly bent.

2. Before you start the movement, make sure you engage your core (think about tightening your stomach muscles as if someone was going to poke you in the stomach).

3. Alternate pulling each knee toward your chest as you extend the opposite leg.

Starting Position	**Alternate Legs for the Finishing Position**

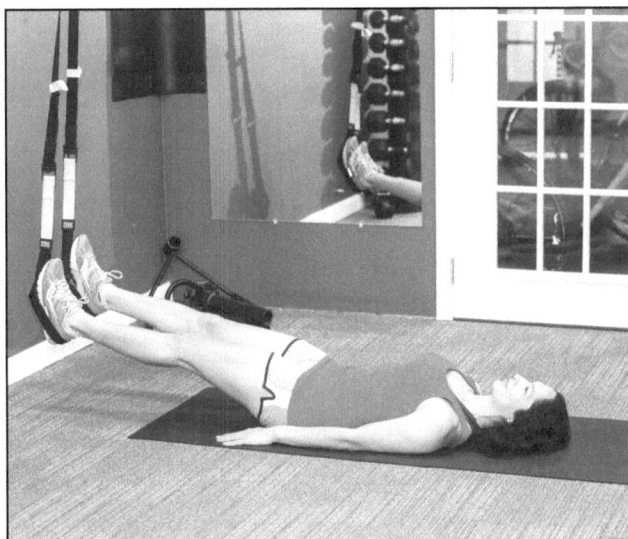

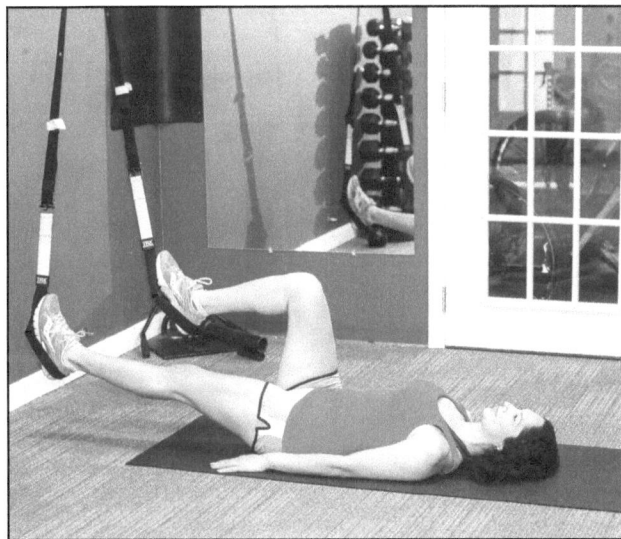

Tips and Progressions:

• The suspended bicycle kick is a great exercise for a beginner, and will help you learn to engage your hip flexors, which will result in better walking and running mechanics.

• Move out farther to make it harder. This will provide more resistance and require you to do more work to overcome the gravity pulling you back underneath.

• You don't need a suspended trainer to do this one, but having one helps the beginner master the movement by assisting with supporting some of the weight of the legs.

• You can progress this movement by lifting and holding your hips off the ground during the movement.

Crunch and Suspended Sit-Up

Starting Position

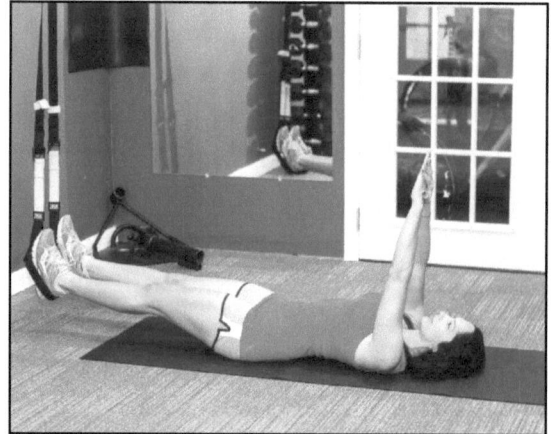

Develops all-around core and hip-flexor strength. This will give you a solid foundation that can better support the demands of all activities.

Primary Focus: Core

Secondary Focus: Hip flexors to assist the sit-up movement.

Setup: Straps fully extended and approximately six inches off the ground.

Crunch:

1. Lie on your back with your heels in the cradles, arms extended, and reach toward the ceiling.

2. Keep your arms vertical, and reach straight up toward the ceiling until your shoulder blades are off the ground.

3. Come back down, and as soon as you feel the floor with your upper back again, crunch back up to the top. This is a small but effective range of motion.

Crunch Finish

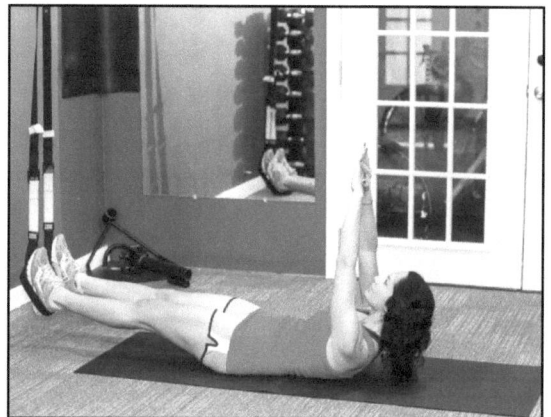

Sit-Up:

Instead of stopping to come back down when you feel your shoulder blades are no longer touching the floor, continue to ascend until your torso is vertical, keeping the arms extended upward toward the ceiling.

> **Note:** When doing the sit-up, strive to obtain full extension and reach for the ceiling at the top. That little extra move will do wonders in developing muscles that will support good posture.

Sit-Up Finish

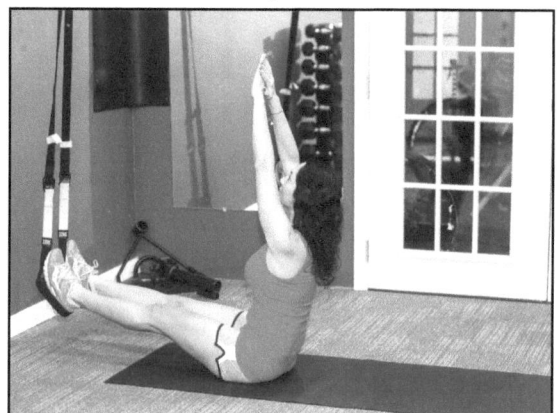

Tips and Progressions:

- Both exercises are effective. The crunch is also more suitable for a beginner or someone who has difficultly performing more than five sit-ups with good form. If you have difficulty with the sit-up at first, start with the crunch and progress to the sit-up later.

- Do one or the other. Don't get caught in "no-man's-land" – just going halfway up because that is as far as you can get. That is not the progression and usually results in bad form.

Hip Raise

Develops a solid foundation through the back side of the core, which includes your torso and hips.

Primary Focus: Hamstrings and hips.

Secondary Focus: Torso and lower back to help lift the hips and hold position.

Setup: Straps fully extended and approximately six inches off the ground.

1. Lie on your back with your feet in the cradles and your knees slightly bent. Your arms should be extended and at your sides on the mat.

2. Push your heels into the cradles to lift your hips off the floor. Focus on relaxed arms and pushing through the hips and heels.

3. Descend back down, keeping a stable position with your upper torso.

Starting Position   **Finishing Position**

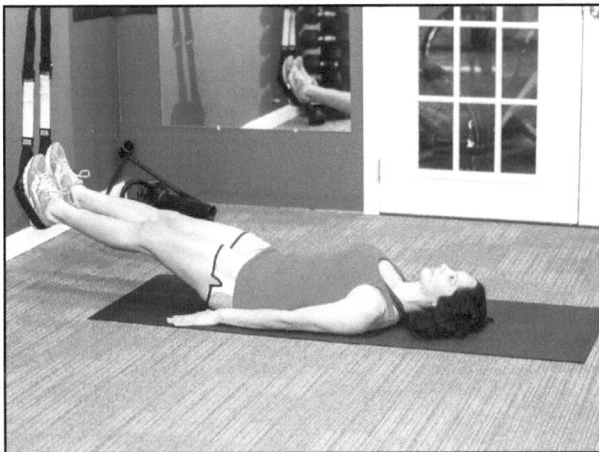

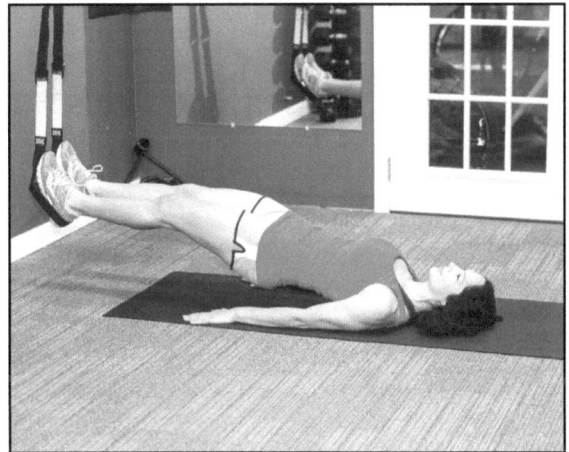

Tips and Progressions:

- Progress by adding more knee bend to your starting position, which will let you push your hips higher off the ground.

Half-Kneeling Rollout

The core is what drives the arm movement in this exercise. In addition, this half-kneeling position on one leg helps develop hip stability that is relevant to the single-leg-stance phase in walking and running.

Primary Focus: Core

Secondary Focus: Hips, arms, and back.

Setup: Straps fully extended.

1. Get on one knee and hold the straps in front of you. You will be supporting your weight on the downed knee and have the other leg right in front of you with the foot on the floor (you may use a folded-up towel, mat, or pad under the downed knee for comfort).

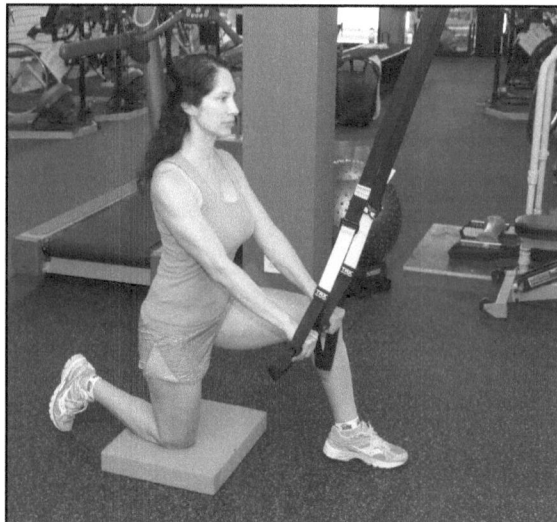

Note: Before you start the movement, make sure the muscles of the supporting hip are tight, and the hip is in line with your knee and torso. Squeeze the muscles in your butt to stabilize that hip.

2. Now push the straps away from you, and extend the torso and arms out in front and slightly to the side. Keep the back and torso flat.

3. Return to the starting position by pulling yourself back upright through your core. Do this by tightening your stomach muscles to drive the movement through the core and torso. Return to the upright position, and repeat for the desired number of repetitions.

4. Do a full set on one side. Switch sides and do a full set on the other side.

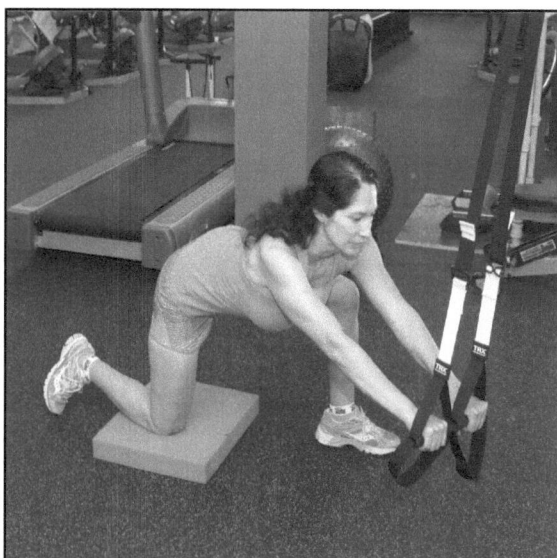

Tips and Progressions:

* The half-kneeling stance is a great position for developing hip stability because it requires the hip to work to stay stable without help from the knee and foot.

* To target stability more, keep a narrow stance by lining up the front foot with the back foot, which creates a narrow base of support.

* The farther out you extend, the harder the exercise becomes. Choose a distance that is appropriate for you.

Suspended Plank Intermediate and Advanced

This is a great all-purpose movement, as a strong core is beneficial to general strength for all activities as well as for good posture. It will build the strength to stabilize and create a solid center of mass to drive movement. A stronger, more stable midsection holds your body in alignment when lifting asymmetrical loads, such as a heavy suitcase, or when lifting or moving a piece of furniture.

Primary Focus: Core

Secondary Focus: Arms and shoulders to support your upper-body weight.

Setup: Straps fully extended and six inches off the ground.

1. Get on your hands and knees, facing forward and down so that your head is in alignment with your neck and spine, with your toes in the cradles.

2. Preload the core by tightening the muscles in your midsection, and straighten your legs to lift your knees off the ground. Your body should be straight like a table. Your elbows should be directly underneath your shoulders, and your head in line with your spine.

3. Time yourself, and hold until you feel fatigued.

Note: If you feel you can't hold your form, stop immediately and mark that as your time.

Tips and Progressions:

- If you're new to the plank exercise, start with your feet on the ground instead of in the straps. Progress to the straps after you feel you've mastered the traditional version of the plank.

- This exercise is all about form! Hips need to stay up, don't let the lower back sag, and keep shoulders soft and back flat (no rounding the back). Doing this one in front of a mirror will allow you to self-monitor your form.

- There is no need to hold this position for minutes at a time. Work up to holding it for forty-five to sixty seconds, and then progress by adding additional sets or progress to the suspended saw.

Starting Position

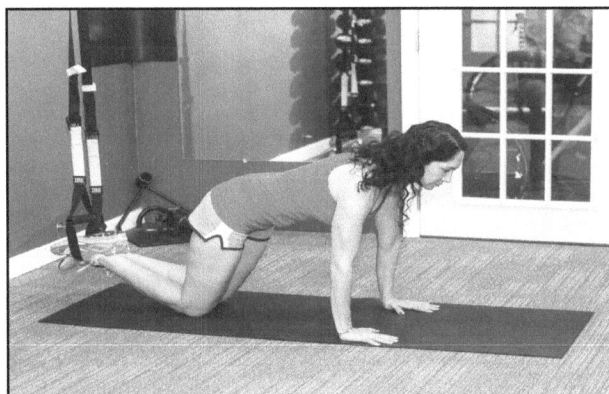

Finishing Position

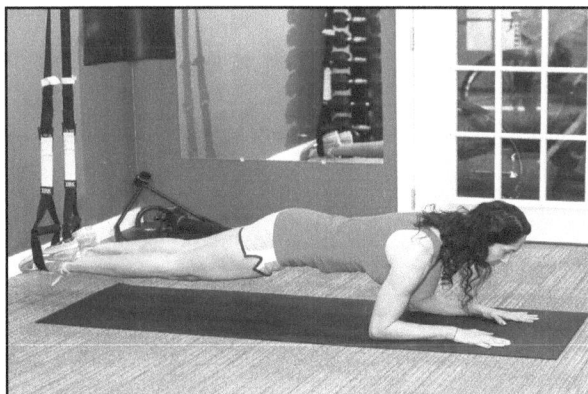

Pike Intermediate and Advanced

This is a challenging movement that will develop your overall dynamic core strength, as well as your ability to support and stabilize your body weight with your upper body while the lower body moves. This will translate into a solid foundation that will support all your activities and endeavors.

Primary Focus: Core and hip flexors.

Secondary Focus: Arms, which support and stabilize the upper body.

Setup: Straps fully extended and approximately six inches off the ground.

1. Face away from the suspended trainer on your hands and knees, with your toes in the cradles, right underneath the anchor. Your hands should be slightly wider than shoulder width, and your thumbs should be aligned with your chest.

2. To get in starting position, simply straighten your legs, which is going to lift your knees off the ground.

3. Pull your legs toward your chest by driving your hips upward toward the ceiling.

4. At the top of the movement, pause and slowly go back down to the starting position.

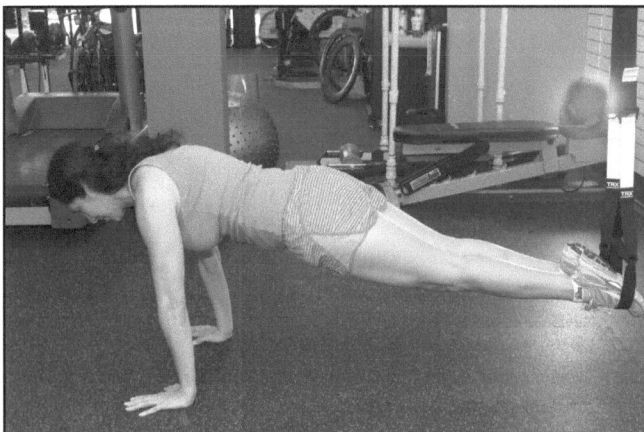

Note: Keep your core tight, and don't let your back or hips sag during this exercise.

Tips and Progressions:

- Starting farther out will be harder, and starting farther underneath the anchor point will be easier (refer to chapter 3).

- A common error is to allow your body to shift back too far, resulting in your hands being in front of you. Your hands should remain in line with your shoulders, and if you were to draw a line between them, this line would be directly under your chest (not your face).

Starting Position   **Finishing Position**

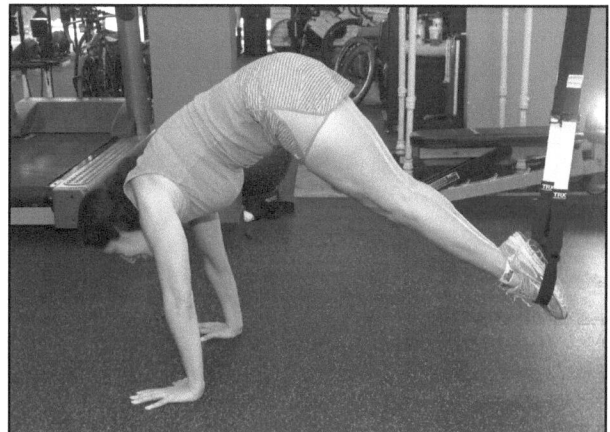

Suspended Side Plank Intermediate and Advanced

This move increases the power of your core, which drives rotational abilities and helps handle lifting and carrying uneven and asymmetrical loads. It will also help to develop good posture.

Primary Focus: Core, arms, and shoulders.

Secondary Focus: Lateral stabilizers in the hips to keep them up and in alignment during the exercise.

Setup: Straps fully extended and approximately six inches off the ground.

1. Start by lying sideways on the floor with your toes in the cradles. Your elbow should be directly underneath the shoulder, and the top leg should be forward.

2. Tighten the core and lift your hips off the floor, with your body weight supported by only the arm and shoulder and the feet in the cradles.

Note: If at any time you feel you're unable to maintain solid form as you fatigue or you feel pain in the shoulder, stop the set.

Tips and Progressions:

- You can self-spot this movement by placing your top hand on the floor to help stabilize.

- You can progress this movement by extending the top arm vertically toward the ceiling and adding a rotation. Do this by slowly reaching from the ceiling to the floor with the extended arm as you maintain the position.

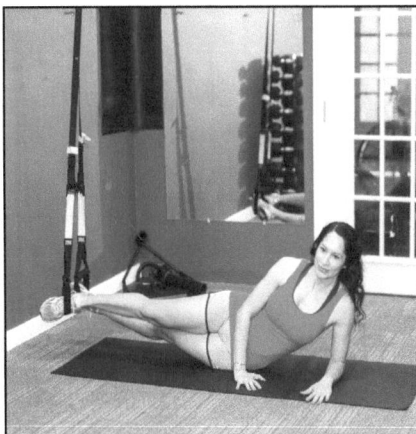

- Start with multiple short sets of ten to twenty seconds, and add time to your sets as you get stronger.

Starting Position   **Finishing Position**   **Finishing Position (self-spotting)**

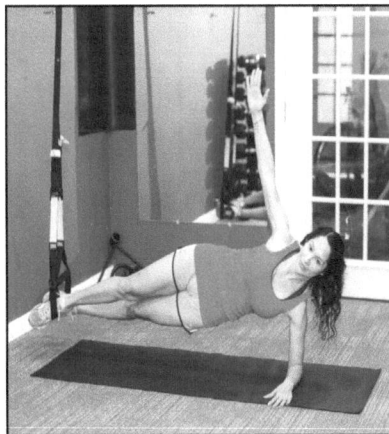

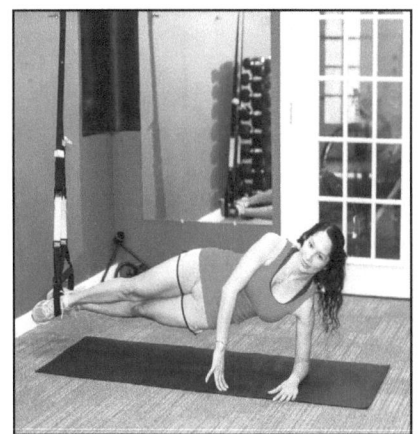

Mountain Climbers (Feet Suspended) Intermediate and Advanced

This is an excellent and challenging movement that trains the hip flexors, and deep core muscles to work together in a strong, powerful movement while the arms support your body weight.

Primary Focus: Core and hip flexors.

Secondary Focus: Arms and shoulders to support the upper body.

Setup: Straps fully extended and approximately six inches off the ground.

1. Face away from the suspended trainer on your hands and knees, with your toes in the cradles, right underneath the anchor. Your hands should be directly underneath your shoulders.

2. To get in starting position, simply straighten your legs, which is going to lift your knees off the ground.

3. Alternate bringing one knee to the chest and keeping the other leg extended.

Note: Keep your core tight, and don't let your back or hips sag during this exercise. Keep the hips level and your body straight like a board.

Tips and Progressions:

- Keep a solid position of the hips and torso. A common error of form occurs when allowing the hips to rotate or drop during the set. Stop the set if you feel you can no longer maintain good form.

- To make it harder, move your starting position farther out.

Starting Position

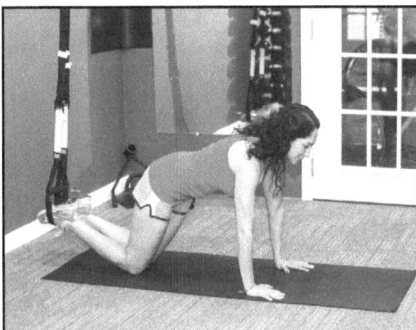

Finishing Position- alternate sides

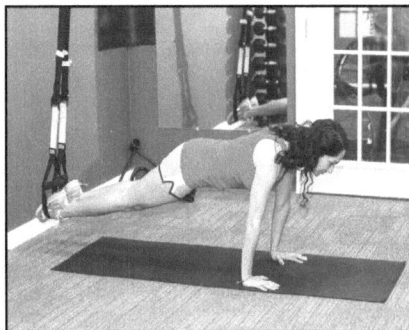

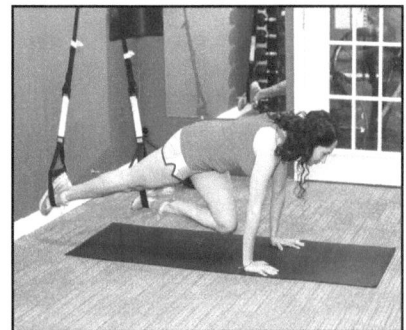

Tall Kneeling Rollout Intermediate and Advanced

This is a more advanced version of the half-kneeling rollout. The core drives the arm movement in both cases, but this version requires more strength because you don't have a foot forward to help support the resistance, as you extend out during the movement. Being able to hold your position with an extended body helps develop a strong and stable core and upper body.

Primary Focus: Core.

Secondary Focus: Arms and back.

Setup: Straps fully extended.

1. Face the suspended trainer, kneeling on both knees, torso upright, and holding the straps (place a pad, mat, or rolled-up towel under the knees for comfort).

2. Maintain good posture by making yourself tall, keeping shoulders relaxed, chest out, and looking forward. Tighten the core, lean forward, and extend the arms out in front of you.

3. Return to the start by pulling up with both your hips and core and bringing the arms back toward the body.

Note: It will get hard quickly as your body gets longer. Extend out to a position you can maintain with good form.

Tips and Progressions:

- Starting farther out will be harder, and starting farther underneath the anchor point will be easier (refer to chapter 3).

- Form is crucial! If you feel any pain in your lower back, don't go out as far, or skip this one.

Starting Position

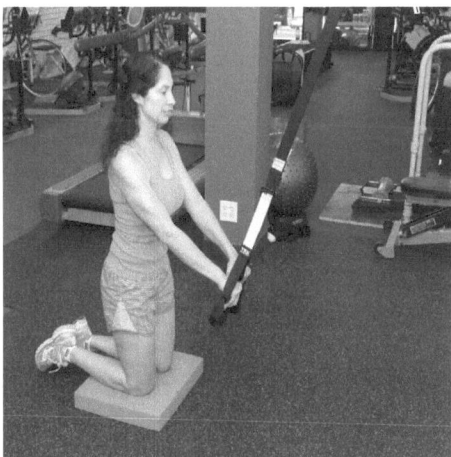

Finishing Position

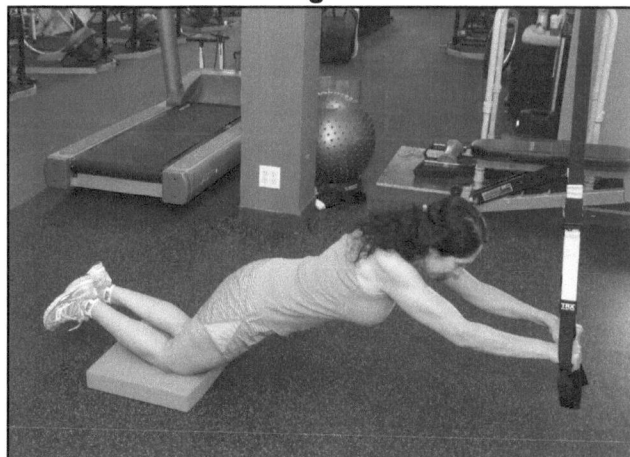

Atomic Crunches Intermediate and Advanced

Trains the hip flexors and deep core muscles to work together in a strong, powerful movement.

Primary Focus: Core and hip flexors.

Secondary Focus: Arms and shoulders, which support the upper body.

Setup: Straps fully extended and approximately six inches off the ground.

1. Face away from the suspended trainer on your hands and knees, with your toes in the cradles, right underneath the anchor. Your hands should be directly underneath your shoulders.

2. To start, straighten your legs, which is going to lift your knees off the ground. Keep a slight bend in the elbows, push the hips upward, and pull the knees toward the chest.

3. Finish with both knees bent and close to your chest, arms slightly bent and directly underneath your shoulders.

4. Extend the legs backward to return to the starting position.

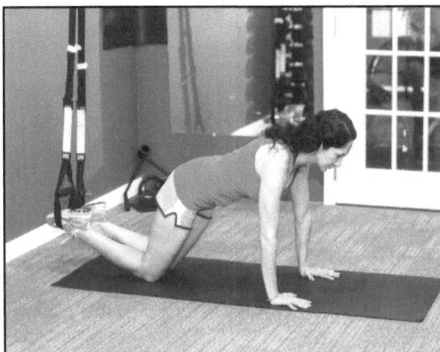

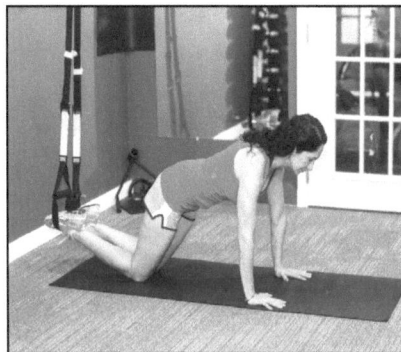

Note: Keep your core tight, and don't let your back or hips sag during this exercise.

Tips and Progressions:

- A degree of established core strength and maintenance of strong form is essential for this one.

- For some extra bang, alternate repetitions with the suspended floor push-up. For example, instead of 15 repetitions of atomic crunches, alternate between the two movements and perform 8 of each.

Starting Position   **Finishing Position**

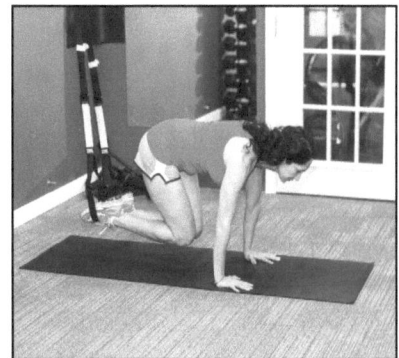

Suspended Saw Intermediate and Advanced

This movement requires extreme strength and stability to hold your body straight as a unit as you're moving in and out with your body. It increases in difficultly quickly as you move out, and you'll feel the position becoming much harder to maintain. This movement should only be done after a static suspended plank is mastered. It will continue to develop a strong, solid core to support all endeavors.

Primary Focus: Core.

Secondary Focus: Arms, which support the upper body.

Setup: Straps fully extended and approximately six inches off the ground.

1. Start on your hands and knees facing down, with your head in alignment with your neck and spine, and your toes in the cradles. Straighten your legs to bring your knees off the ground.

2. Now slowly move your body back while keeping it flat like a table. Your elbows should end up being in front of your shoulders at the farthest point. Move back until it's about as hard as you can handle while maintaining form.

3. Now slowly shift back to your starting position with your elbows under your shoulders. This movement can be done by time or repetitions.

Note: Your body should be straight like a table. Your elbows should be directly underneath your shoulders and your head in line with your spine. If you feel you can't hold your form, stop or reduce the distance you're moving forward and back.

Tips and Progressions:

- Master the standard and then the suspended plank before progressing to this version.

- You will not need to move very far out to feel the difficulty increase.

- Form is crucial! If you feel any pain in your lower back, avoid this exercise, or go back to doing just a regular or suspended plank.

Starting Position

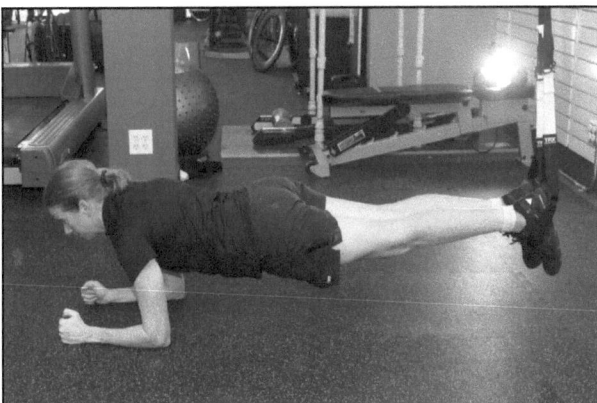

Finishing Position

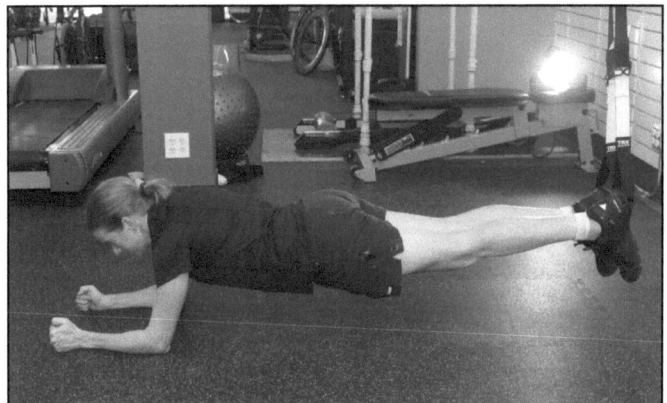

Plank with Arms Suspended Intermediate and Advanced

This position requires extreme strength and stability to hold your core while your arms are suspended.

Primary Focus: Core.

Secondary Focus: Arms, which support and stabilize the upper body.

Setup: Straps fully extended and approximately six inches off the ground.

1. Start on your hands and knees facing inward. Place your hands through the foot cradles, and allow your forearms to rest on the straps while supporting your upper body.

2. Slowing shift your body weight forward over your forearms until you feel tension in your core.

3. Hold for target amount of time.

Note: I recommend doing this movement from your knees, and I think you'll find that position plenty challenging if you shift your body weight forward enough during the movement. Doing it from your toes puts a lot of strain on the lower back and tends to shift the focus of the exercise from the area of the core we want to target.

Tips and Progressions:

- Form is crucial! If you feel any pain in your lower back, avoid this exercise or go back to doing just a regular or suspended plank.

Side View

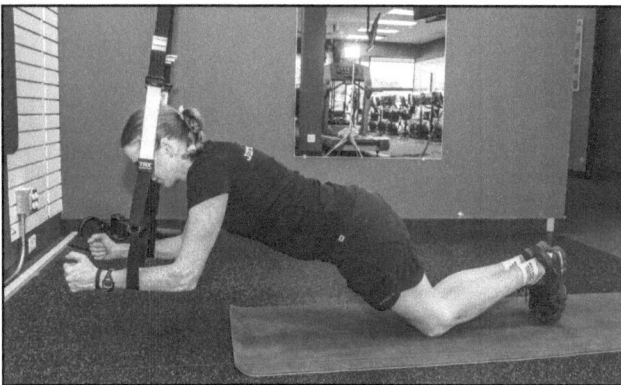

Rear View

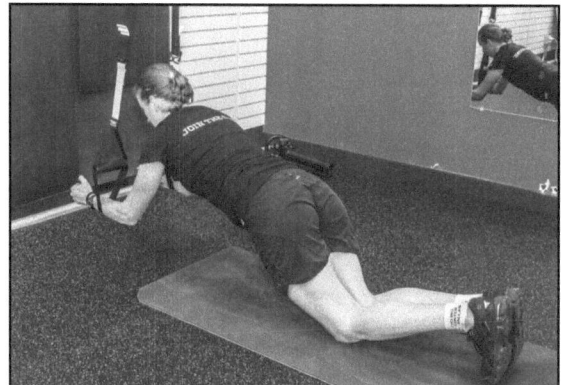

Suspended Straight-Arm Plank Intermediate and Advanced

This movement requires extreme strength and stability in your core and torso as well as your arms and shoulders, in particular, the core and upper-body strength that drives all movement and supports strong posture.

Primary Focus: Core, arms, and shoulders.

Secondary Focus: Legs and hips, which must work to maintain the straight body position from the torso to the feet.

Setup: Straps fully extended and approximately six inches off the ground.

1. Start on your hands and knees facing away from the suspended trainer, with your toes in the foot cradles. Your hands should be slightly wider than your shoulders and in line with your chest.

2. Straighten your legs to go into the position. You will now be supporting your upper body with your arms and lower body through your feet in the cradles.

3. Hold for the target amount of time.

Note: Keep your body straight like a board from head to toe, and keep your head position in line with your spine (eyes looking just in front of you).

Tips and Progressions:

• You can do the same position with your feet on the floor. Progress to the feet in cradles when you're ready.

• Form is crucial! If you feel any pain in your lower back, avoid this exercise or go back to an alternate version.

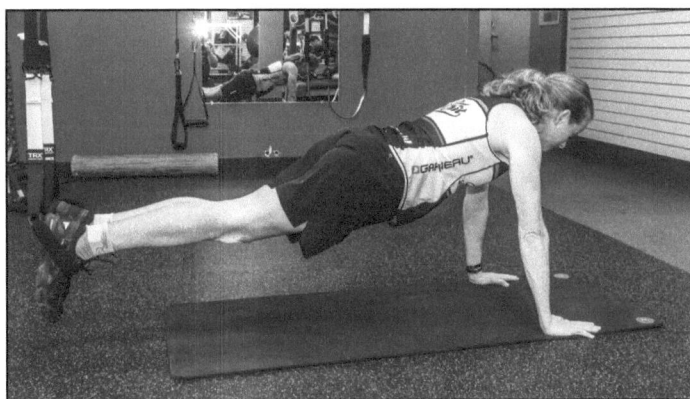

Side View   **Side/Front View**

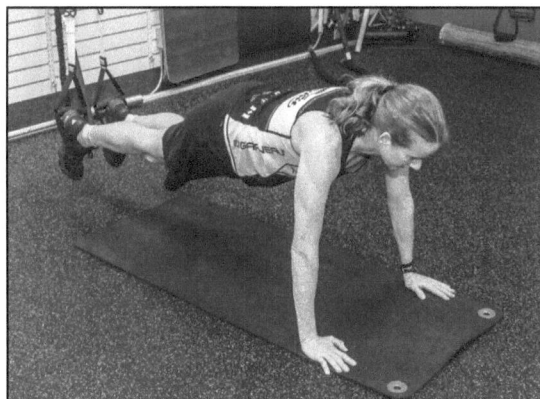

Upper-Body Movements

Push-Up Variations

I have included several variations of this movement. The variation from your knees is the least difficult one, but that does not necessarily mean it's easy. Try it out and see how you do. If you can do at least four to six solid push-ups, but not more than fifteen to twenty, that's probably a good place to start. If that version is too hard, stick to the suspended trainer version (hands suspended) where you can further unload the weight you're lifting. When that version gets to be too easy, continue to challenge yourself with more advanced progressions.

There are also additional variations not shown here. For example, the spider push-up on the suspended trainer can also be done on its own.

Primary Focus: Chest and shoulders

Secondary Focus: Core

Start the push-up from the straight-arm plank position. If you are not quite ready to do full or modified pushups, work on increasing the time you can hold this position. Working on this will develop the upper body and core strength and stability that you need to able to progress to push-ups when you are ready.

Modified from your knees: Make sure you keep your body weight over your arms.

Traditional from your feet: Keep your body straight like a board and no sagging hips.

Plank to push-up: Transition from a plank position on your elbows to a straight-arm plank position and then back again. Make sure to keep your body straight and hips down and level during the transition. Also, change the arm you lead with halfway through your set, or perform a set leading with each arm to keep things balanced.

Power Push-Up: Explode up from the bottom. Catch some air! You can do these from your knees or from your feet.

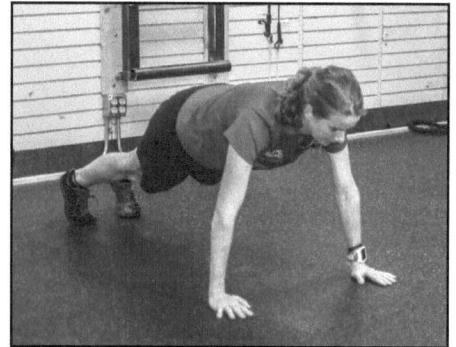

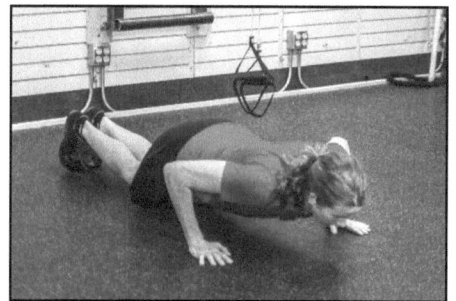

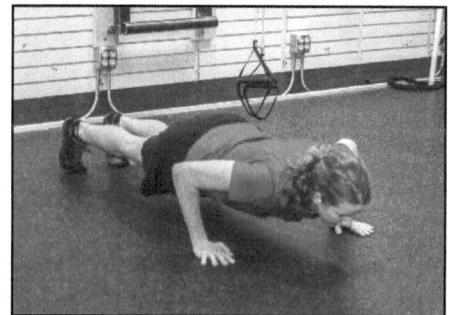

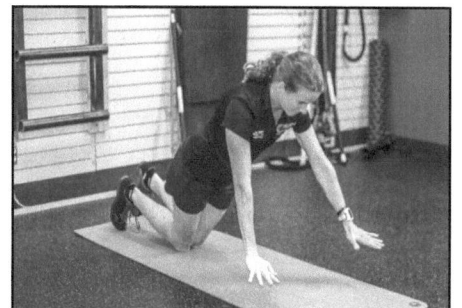

Note: *Still want more? Add a weight vest, or do the spider push-up (p. 202), which can be performed with or without a suspended trainer.*

Push-Up (Hands Suspended)

This is an all-purpose pushing movement that increases both strength and stability of the upper body and core.

Primary Focus: Chest and shoulders.

Secondary Focus: Arms, which assist the movement, and core muscles, which stabilize the position.

Setup: Straps fully extended.

1. Face outward, holding the straps with a shoulder-width stance.

2. Step back and lean forward into the straps with the arms straight. Get a board-straight body position from your head to feet, that you will maintain through the movement.

3. Allow your arms to bend, and lower your body until your elbows reach ninety degrees and are aligned with your shoulders. Don't let your elbows get behind your shoulders.

Push yourself back up to the straight-arm position, exhaling as you do so, and maintain a tight core and straight body from head to feet.

Note: Keep your arms up at shoulder level as you descend. Make sure you're keeping your core tight and body straight (don't allow the hips to sag) throughout the movement.

Tips and Progressions:

* To make it harder, step back to load more of your body weight onto the straps. To make it easier, step forward to load more of your body weight onto your feet.

* To focus on improving balance and stability during this exercise, narrow your foot position or progress to standing on one foot only. Both will narrow your base of support, giving you less stability and making you work harder to balance during the movement.

Starting Position

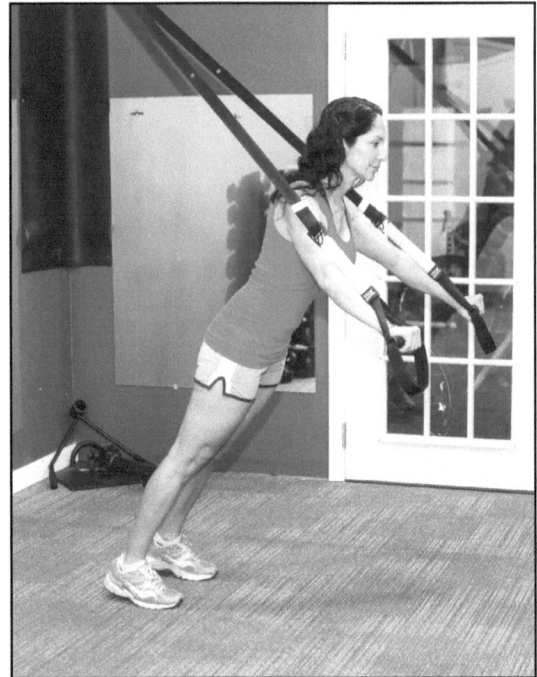

Finishing Position

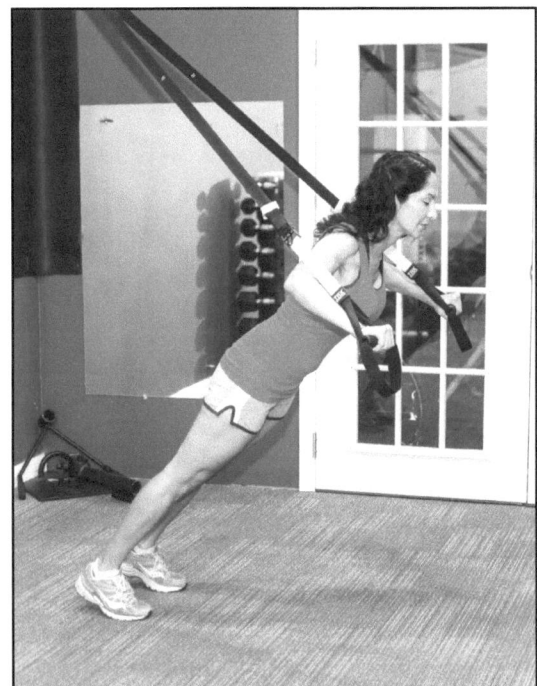

Row

An all-around movement that targets the large muscle groups in your back. It can improve posture by strengthening the muscles that pull your shoulders back. This move is especially great for those who spend extended amounts of time at a desk, computer, or behind the wheel.

Primary Focus: Back and arms.

Secondary Focus: Back of the shoulders as well as core and hips, which are used to stabilize and maintain body position.

Setup: Straps shortened to mid-length.

1. Face toward the anchor point, holding the straps with a shoulder-width stance. Now step forward, lean back, and straighten your arms.

2. Pull yourself up until your elbows are bent and at your side, exhaling as you pull yourself up. Keep a solid core and straight body position from your head to feet and your head aligned with the spine.

3. When you get to the top, lower yourself back down by allowing the arms to straighten out again until you are back in the starting position.

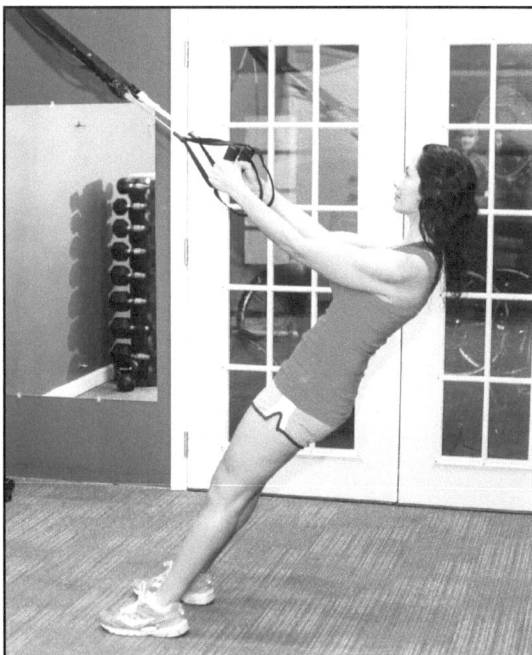

Tips and Progressions:

* To make it harder, step forward and place your feet farther underneath the anchor. This will increase your lean, putting more body weight on the straps, which is more weight you'll have to lift.

* Those at a more advanced level could try starting farther underneath to make it harder. As fatigue sets in, step back to take some of the weight off, which will allow you to do a few additional reps per set.

Starting Position   **Finishing Position**

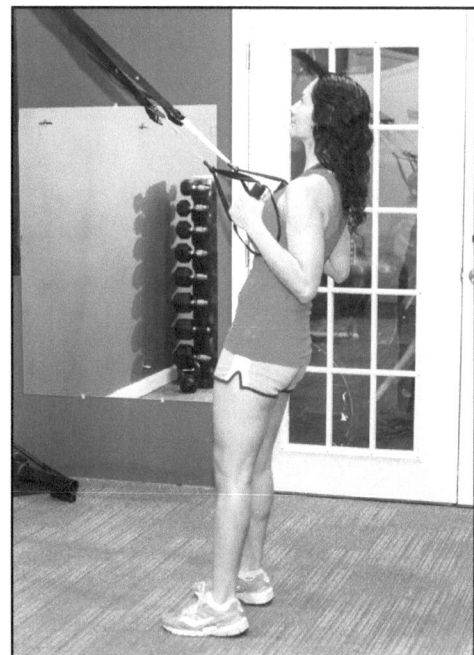

Triceps Extension

Starting Position

This one targets the underside of the arm, and that's where you should feel it. You will also feel this in your core as you maintain your position during the movement. You are basically doing a triceps press and a plank at the same time.

Primary Focus: Triceps.

Secondary Focus: Core.

Setup: Straps fully extended.

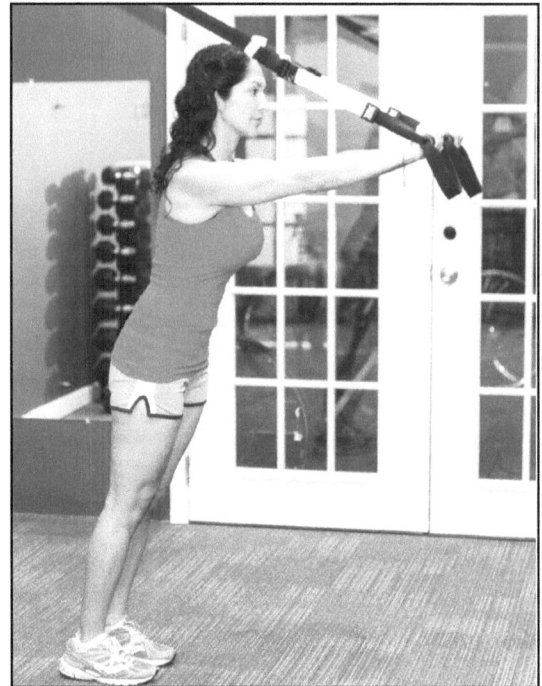

1. Face outward, holding the straps with your arms straight in front of you and parallel with the ground.

2. Start the movement by allowing your elbows to bend and your body to descend toward your hands.

3. Allow your body to come toward your hands until the tops of your hands are close to your forehead. Always maintain your tight core and a body straight like a board.

Finishing Position

4. Return to the starting position by straightening the arms and pushing the body back up and away from the hands.

    Note: Keep the elbows in and up! Your upper arm from your elbow to shoulder should remain parallel with the ground as your elbows bend.

Tips and Progressions:

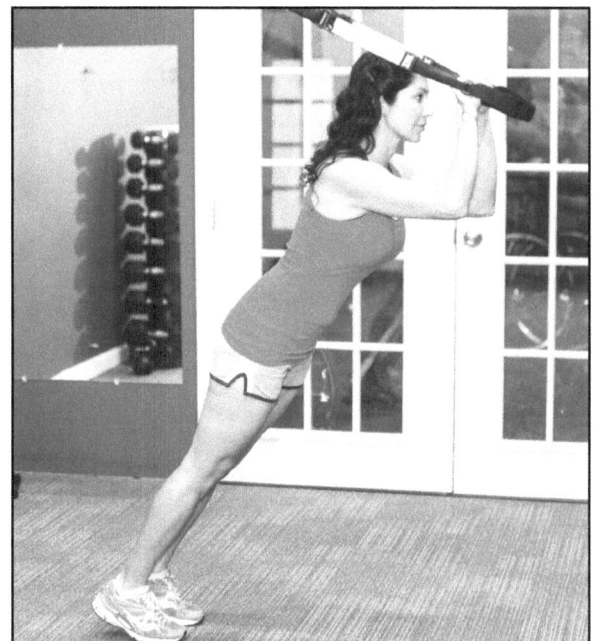

- Step back and increase your body angle for more resistance; step forward for less resistance.

- Focus on your elbow and arm position during this movement, and fully extend the arms on each repetition. Give the triceps an extra squeeze at the end of the range of movement to really stress them.

- The most common mistake in form for this movement is to allow the elbows to drop or flare out. Keep them high and tight. They should point straight ahead at all times.

Bicep Curl

This movement works more than just your biceps. Stabilizing the core and upper part of the torso during the movement is equally important. The increased strength and stability of your core while the arms pull the body is what makes this version of a bicep curl more functional than the traditional version.

Primary Focus: Biceps and forearms.

Secondary Focus: Core, which stabilizes your body to stay in a straight line during the movement.

Setup: Straps fully extended.

1. Face inward, holding the straps, and lean back with arms fully extended and parallel to the ground.

2. Start the movement by bringing your palms toward your forehead while keeping the elbows up and the rest of your body as straight as a board. Continue to pull until your elbows are bent at about a ninety-degree angle and the palms of your hands are at your forehead.

3. At that point allow the arms to extend back to the starting position.

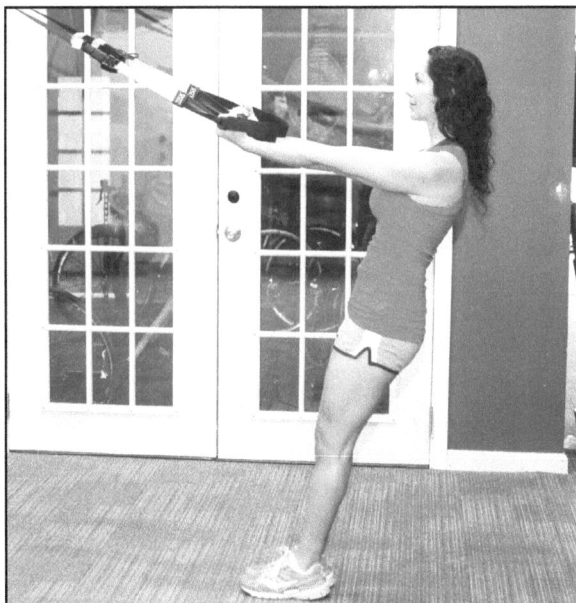

Note: Keep your elbows up throughout the movement!

Tips and Progressions:

- Step underneath the straps and increase your body lean for more resistance. Step back for less.

- Keep your shoulders down and relaxed, chest out, and shoulder blades down and back throughout the movement. This will help you to maintain a strong connection in your shoulders and upper torso.

Starting Position

Finishing Position

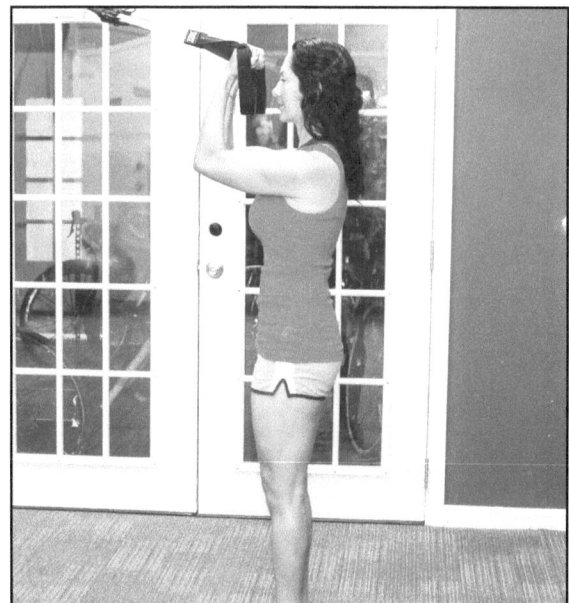

Fly

This movement helps to develop a strong and stable upper body to support the demand of all activities. You should feel it in the front of the shoulders, and in your chest and core.

Primary Focus: Chest and shoulders.

Secondary Focus: Core, which stabilizes your position.

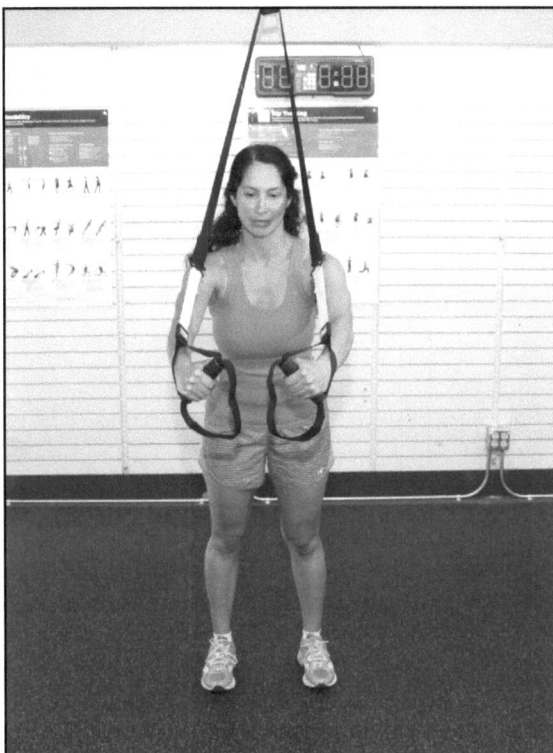

Setup: Straps fully extended.

1. Face out, and hold the straps with your arms extended out in front of you. Maintain a slight bend in your elbow.

2. Allow your arms to open up and go from right in front of you to extended out to the side. Your body will come forward as your arms go back. Stop when they are in line with your shoulders.

3. Come back to the top of the movement by bringing your arms back together in front of you as if you were hugging a barrel.

Tips and Progressions:

- Your body will lean forward as you go down into the movement, but remember to keep it straight from your feet to your head.

- Don't shrug. Relax the shoulders and keep them down by pulling your shoulder blades down toward your butt.

Starting Position   **Finishing Position**

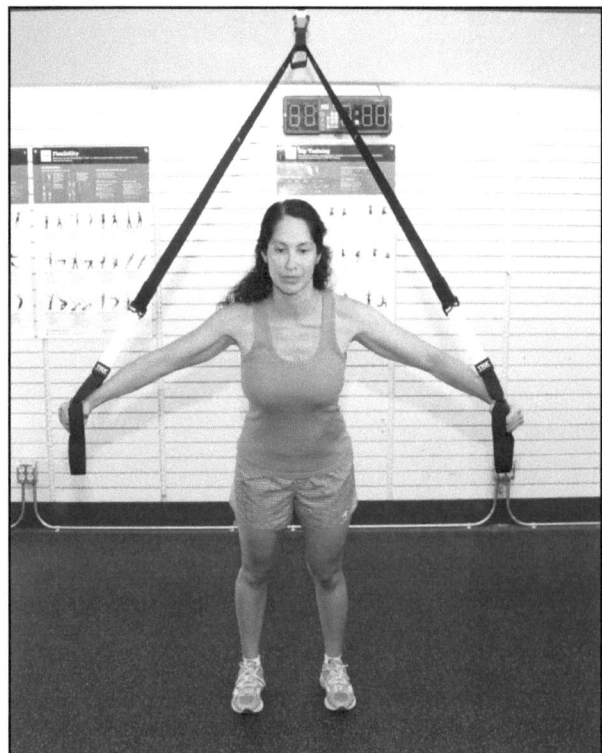

Reverse Fly

This move targets muscles needed for good posture. It's also known as the posterior deltoid. You may have seen the big weight machines in the fitness centers that target this area. This version is better (and requires less equipment) because you're learning to move and stabilize your body instead of sitting down and moving a plate behind you.

Primary Focus: Upper back and the rear part of the shoulders.

Secondary Focus: Core and lower back to stabilize your body position.

Setup: Straps fully extended.

1. Face the anchor with your arms extended and together in front of you with a slight backward lean. Place your feet in an offset stance with one foot in front and the other foot placed behind you.

2. Keeping the arms straight, open them up, and extend out from your shoulders. This will bring your body forward.

3. Bring the arms back together to the front, holding good form as you do so.

Note: Keep your abs engaged, and do not allow your back to arch as you bring the arms back. This is especially important to remember as you fatigue during the set!

Tips and Progressions:

- This is a great exercise to train the core to maintain proper alignment while the upper body moves against resistance.

- Those of you who spend a lot of time at a desk or behind the wheel during your day will really benefit from this one because it will strengthen the back muscles that pull the shoulders back to help maintain good posture.

Starting Position **Finishing Position**

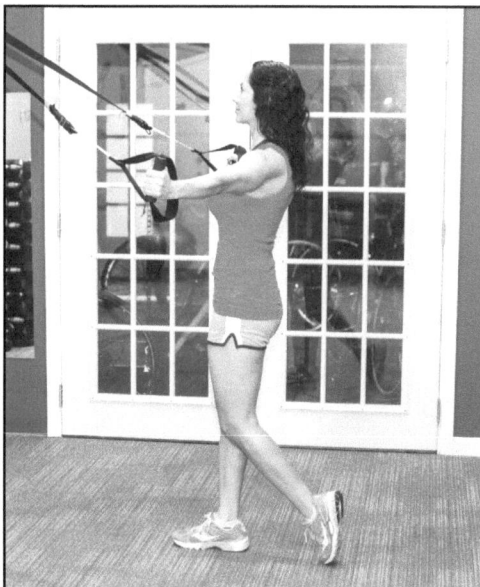

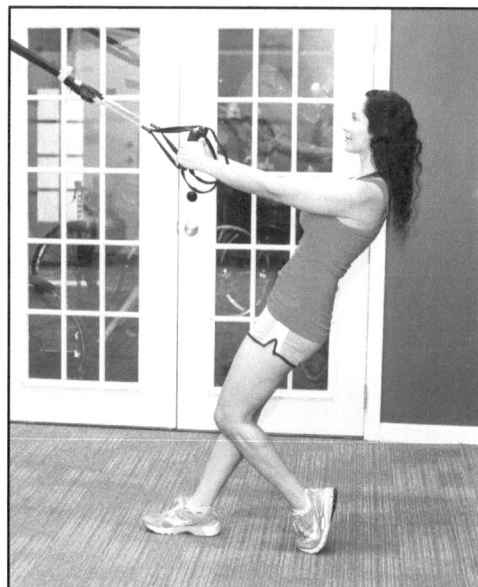

Single-Arm Row

A rowing movement with a twist—literally. You are pulling, which strengthens the back muscles, and you are also generating rotational forces through your core.

Primary Focus: Back and arms.

Secondary Focus: Core, to rotate the body and maintain position.

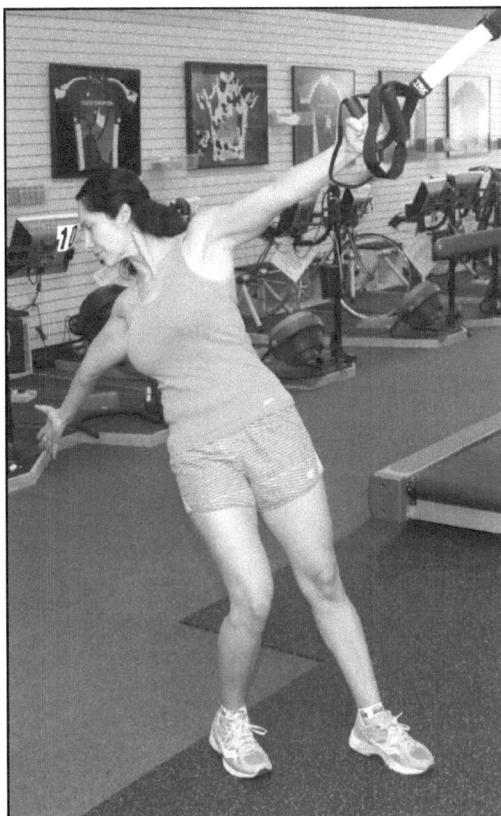

Setup: Straps mid-length and single-handle mode.

1. Face inward, and hold the single handle with one hand. Get into an offset foot stance by stepping back with the foot opposite the hand that is holding the handle.

2. Allow the arm holding the handle to extend, and reach for the floor behind you with the free hand. Allow your weight to shift a bit to your back foot if needed.

3. When you get to the bottom of the movement, pull yourself back up, and finish the rotation by reaching forward with the free hand toward the strap.

Tips and Progressions:

- To make it easier, get into a wider offset stance, or position yourself more upright so more of your weight is being supported by your legs.

- Although you will rotate your torso and hips, still maintain good posture, and keep your body straight like a board.

Starting Position　　　　　　　**Finishing Position**

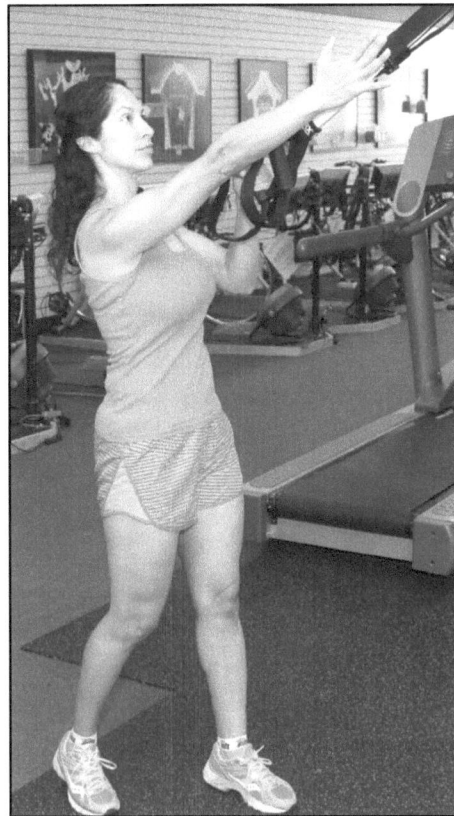

Back Extension

Since this movement targets the entire back side of the torso and core, it helps develop good posture and a stronger, more injury-resistant torso.

Primary Focus: Back and rear shoulders.

Secondary Focus: Hips, in the standing variation.

Setup: Straps fully extended.

1. Stand and face toward the anchor, holding the handles.

2. Allow your hips to hinge, and push your butt back behind you while keeping your arms straight.

3. At the bottom of the movement, extend your arms up over your head as you bring your hips back underneath you to straighten your body again.

Note: Maintain a strong connection with your shoulders. Think about pulling the shoulder blades in and down toward your pockets.

Tips and Progressions:

• Performing a seated version will take the hips out of the movement and target the lower and upper back only.

• Make sure to extend the arms through the full range of motion overhead.

Starting Position

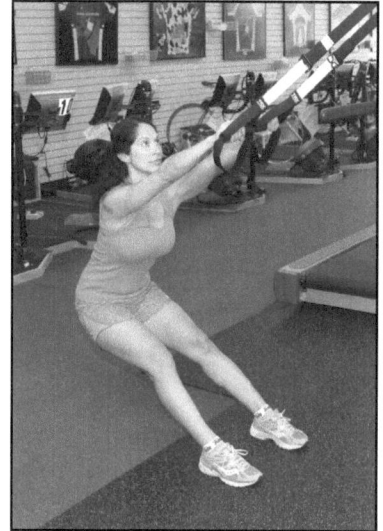

Finishing Position

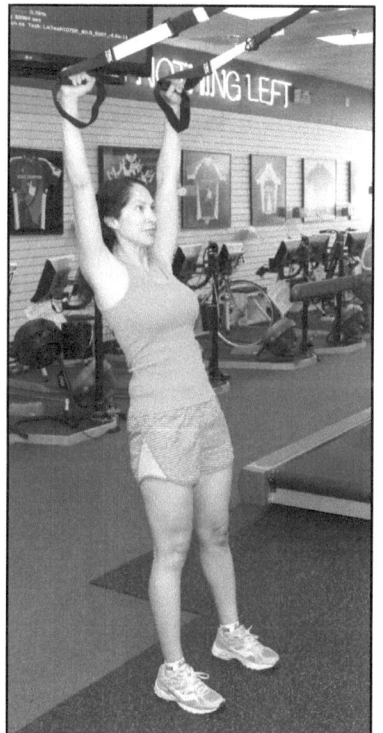

Seated Version

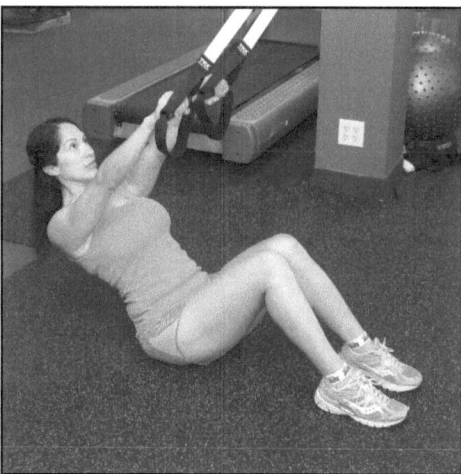

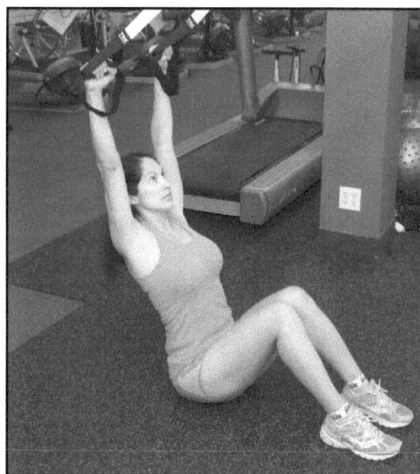

Assisted Pull-Up

This is a pull-up that allows you to assist and self-spot by pushing a portion of your body weight with your legs. A great all-purpose pulling movement that makes pull-ups accessible to a variety of strength levels.

Primary Focus: Back and arms.

Secondary Focus: Rear shoulders, core to maintain posture, legs to help spot.

Setup: Straps super-shortened, which will allow you more room underneath to perform this movement.

Starting Position

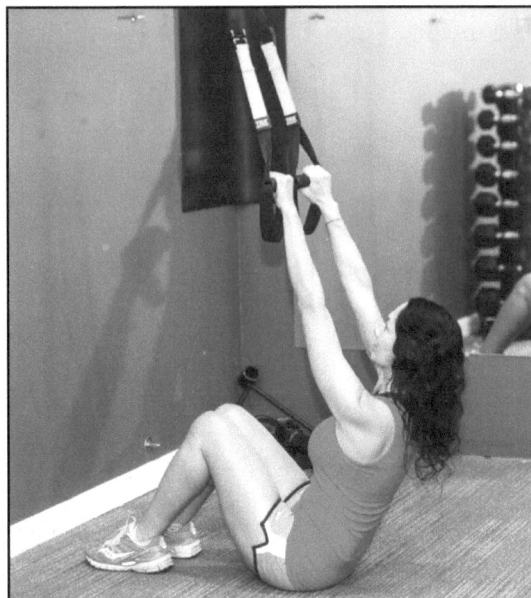

1. Start by sitting on the floor directly underneath the suspended trainer, holding the handles, with your knees bent.

2. Pull yourself straight up from the floor and up until your chin is level with your hands. Think about pulling yourself over an imaginary bar.

3. Hold your position at the top for a second with good form and then come back down in a slow, controlled movement.

Note: Use your legs to spot you as much as you need to but as little as you must. Perform as much of the work as you can by pulling yourself up with your arms.

Tips and Progressions:

Finishing Position

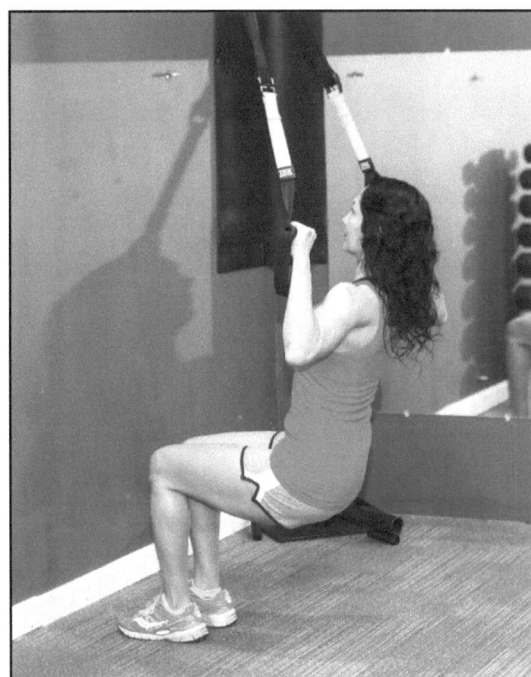

- Keep the elbows out wide, shoulders back, and chest out as you're pulling yourself up.

- A variation would be to use a chin-up grip, which is a narrow, reversed grip where the arms and elbows remain closer to the body and the palms face toward you.

Golf Rotation

This movement is a great one for loosening and warming up the upper torso and arms. It's also excellent for increasing shoulder and upper-torso mobility for those who are lacking it, and for improved posture in all activities. The rotation and reach will also open up the front of the body and improve strength in the muscles in the upper back.

Primary Focus: Upper back and shoulders.

Secondary Focus: Core to stabilize your body position.

Setup: Straps fully extended.

1. Face the anchor, hold the straps, and get into a shoulder-width stance.

2. Keep one arm in place and reach up and slightly behind you with the other arm, rotating your torso and looking in the same direction.

3. Hold for one to three seconds on each side. Alternate sides.

Tips and Progressions:

- Those of you who spend a lot of time at a desk or behind the wheel during your day will really benefit from this movement, because it will increase the strength as well as the mobility of your upper torso.

Starting Position

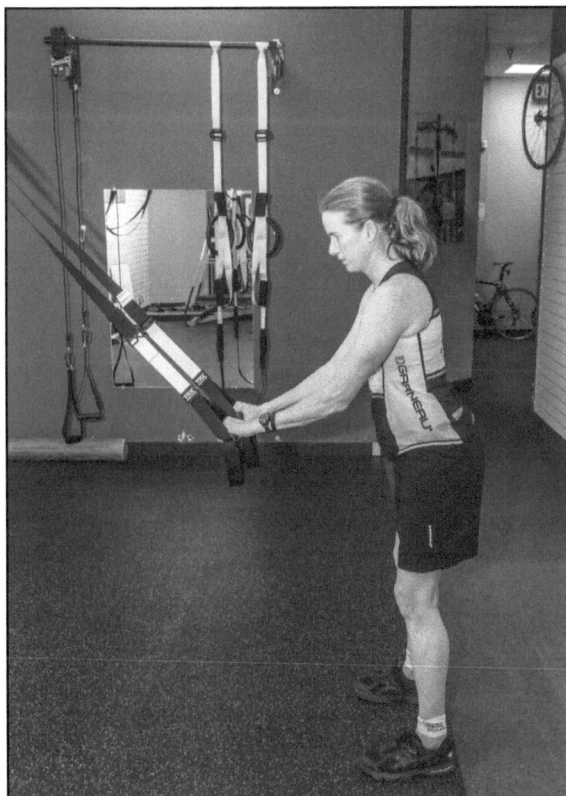

Finishing Position

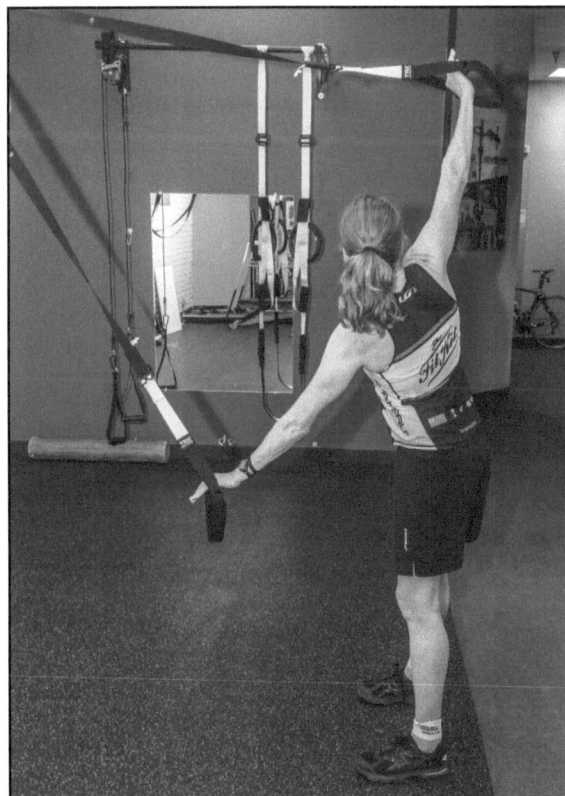

Wall Slide

An excellent movement for increasing shoulder and upper-torso mobility, strength in the upper back, and improved posture in all activities.

Primary Focus: Upper back and shoulders.

Secondary Focus: Core to stabilize your body position.

Setup: Straps fully extended.

1. Face the anchor with your arms up, elbows bent and at shoulder level, and the backs of your hands pressed into the foot cradles.

2. As you continue to press your hands back into the foot cradles, extend your arms upward until they are completely straightened.

Note: Keep your abs engaged, and do not allow your back to arch as you bring the arms back. This is especially important to remember as you fatigue during the set!

Tips and Progressions:

- If your hands tend to migrate in front of your body as you press them overhead, you might have some limited mobility in the upper spine and/or shoulder area. Work on this one by working through the range of motion as much as you can. Also consider adding the thoracic spine stretch (pp. 68, 70) in the flexibility section to your program as well.

- Those of you who spend a lot of time at a desk or behind the wheel during your day will really benefit from this one because it will increase the strength as well as the mobility of your upper torso.

Starting Position   **Finishing Position**

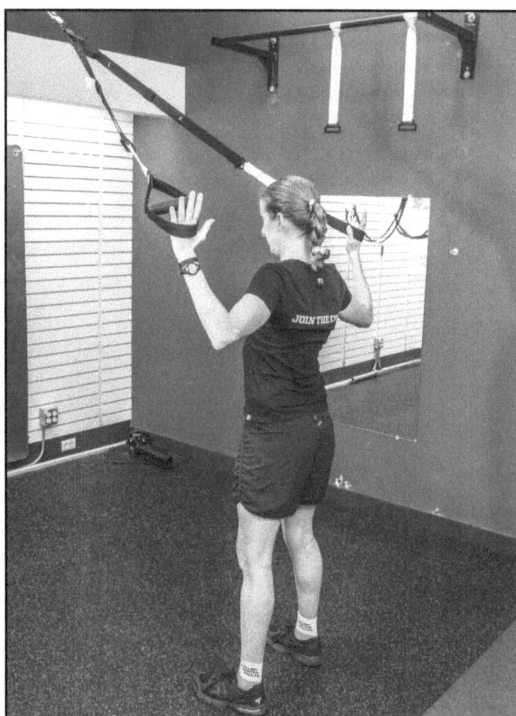

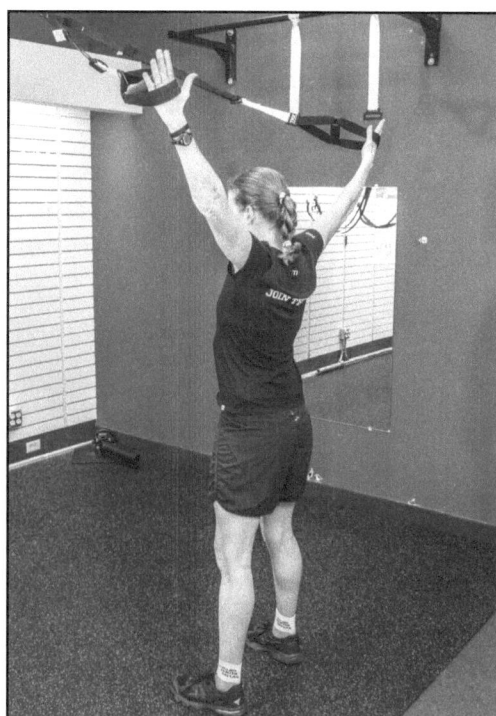

Inverted Row Intermediate and Advanced

This movement develops upper body pulling strength. Great for developing your back muscles and overall posture in all activities. The inverted version puts you directly under the straps and requires more strength than the suspended rows that can be found earlier in the library.

Primary Focus: Back and biceps.

Secondary Focus: Core, which holds proper alignment of the torso.

Setup: Straps mid-length.

1. Face inward, and lower yourself all the way under the anchor with your arms straight. Your knees will be bent, and your torso will be flat like a table, parallel to the ground.

2. Pull your torso up to the handles until your elbows are bent at your side.

3. Lower yourself back down, keeping the straight body position and with control of the descent.

Tips and Progressions:

- What is shown in the pictures is a narrow row. A variation of this movement is a wide row, where elbow and hand position is wide and in line with the shoulder (think about an inverted push-up position).

- You may also make it harder with external resistance such as a weight vest, or elevating your feet on a flat bench or platform.

Starting Position

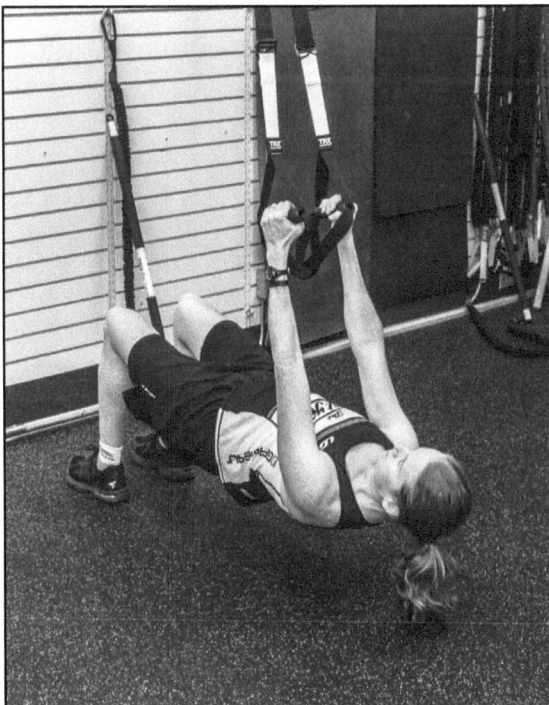

Finishing Position

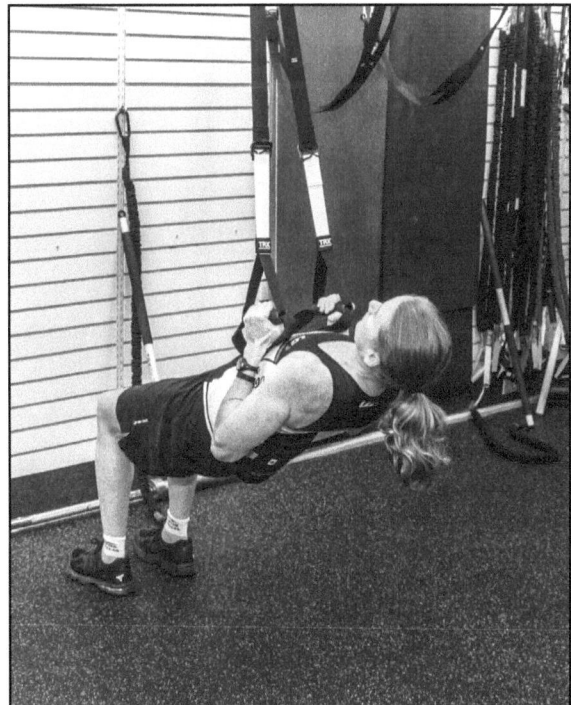

Suspended Push-Up from Floor Intermediate and Advanced

A great all-purpose pushing exercise. This version of the pushing movement requires torso and upper-body strength as well as proper timing of the stabilizer muscles to maintain a straight body.

Primary Focus: Chest and arms.

Secondary Focus: Core.

Setup: Straps fully extended and approximately six to twelve inches off the ground.

1. Face away from the suspended trainer on your hands and knees with your toes in the cradles, right underneath the anchor. Your hands should be slightly wider than shoulder width, and your thumbs should be aligned with your chest.

2. Start by straightening your legs, which will lift your knees off the ground. Keep your body straight, and go down until your elbows bend to approximately a ninety-degree angle.

3. At the bottom, push through the floor to raise your body back up to the starting position as one unit.

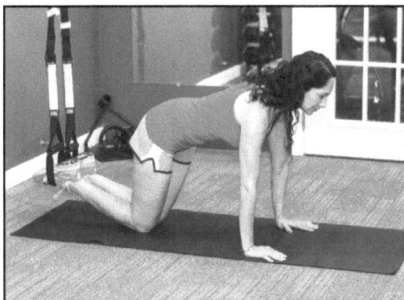

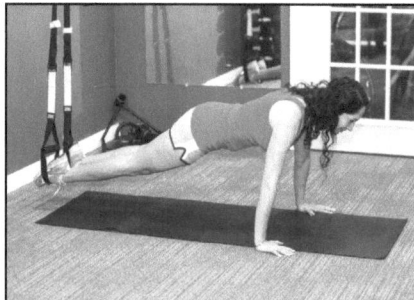

Note: Keep your core tight, and don't let your back or hips sag during this exercise.

Tips and Progressions:

*   Keep the hands in line with the chest. The imaginary line between your hands should be directly under your chest (not your face).

*   The instability of the suspended trainer will add to the difficulty level of the traditional push-up. Because of this, holding your core position should be the primary focus during the movement.

*   This version of a push-up should not be attempted until you can perform several full traditional push-ups first. Become proficient with the traditional push-up by performing push-ups on your knees and progressing to full traditional push-ups. Advance to suspending your feet at that point.

Resting Position	**Starting Position**	**Finishing Position**

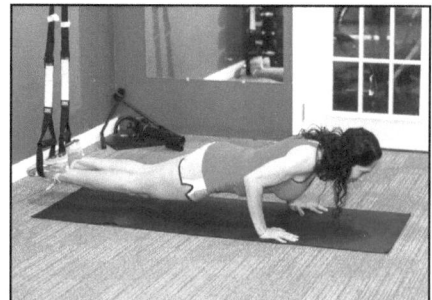

Swim Pull Intermediate and Advanced

This movement mimics the pull of the freestyle swim stroke. It will help develop the muscles that drive the arm down as well as the core.

Primary Focus: Back and arms.

Secondary Focus: Core, which stabilizes the torso and drives the arm movement.

Setup: Straps fully extended.

1. Start with an offset stance that will allow for some weight shifting during the movement. Lean back and find a starting position that will provide the amount of resistance you want.

2. Keeping your body and your arms straight, push your arms down to your sides, which will bring your body forward and vertical. Make sure the arms stay extended and straight.

3. Repeat by lowering yourself back down in a controlled descent.

Note: Keep your shoulders back and shoulder blades actively retracted in and down toward your pockets.

Tips and Progressions:

- The offset stance will allow you to shift your weight forward and back over your feet during the movement to provide a more constant resistance through the arms as you pull your body up to the top of the movement.

- Once at the top of the movement, finish it by giving your triceps a squeeze and straightening the elbow all the way. If you've ever done the swim-stroke drill where you flick the water after you finish the pull through, this last small movement is very similar.

Starting Position   **Finishing Position**

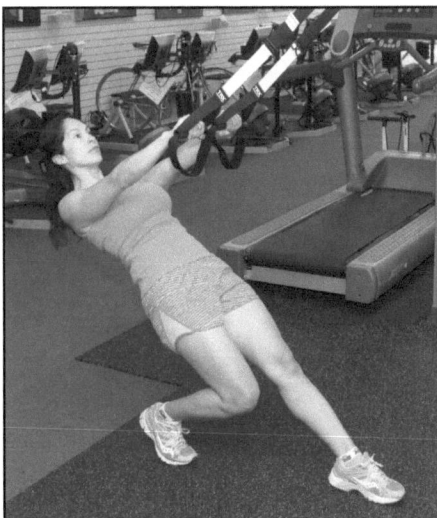

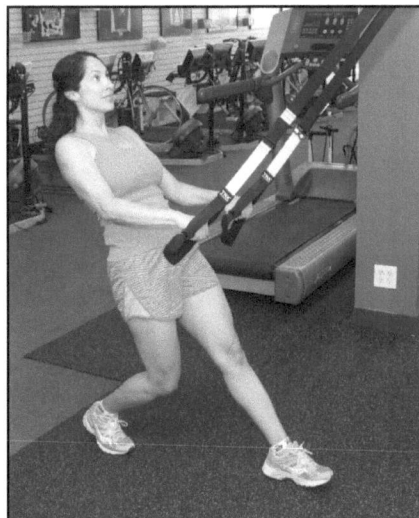

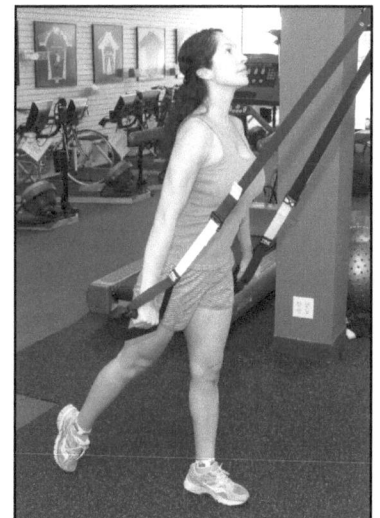

Assisted Dip Intermediate and Advanced

An advanced all-purpose upper body pushing movement that develops upper body strength, as well as a strong core alignment, strength, and stability, which benefits all disciplines and all aspects of training.

Primary Focus: Shoulders and arms.

Secondary Focus: The assisting leg and the core, which holds proper alignment of the torso.

Setup: Straps mid-length.

1. Start by facing away from the anchor, holding the straps so that they are positioned behind you and on the inside of your arms. Your palms will be facing inward to your sides.

2. Lower yourself down by allowing the elbows to bend back behind you. Keep good posture with an upright torso, shoulders back (no shrugging). Use your legs to assist as much as you need to and as little as you must.

3. Descend until you have roughly a ninety-degree bend in the elbow, and then push yourself back up.

Note: This is a self-spotting exercise, and you will use your legs to help support your body weight if needed. You may partially support yourself with one leg or both legs, depending on your level of ability.

Tips and Progressions:

- A common error of form with this movement is letting your elbows flare out. Keep them in and tight to your side.

- To make it harder, use only one leg, or extend both legs in front of you while keeping your torso vertical. This results in having to lift more of your body weight.

Starting Position

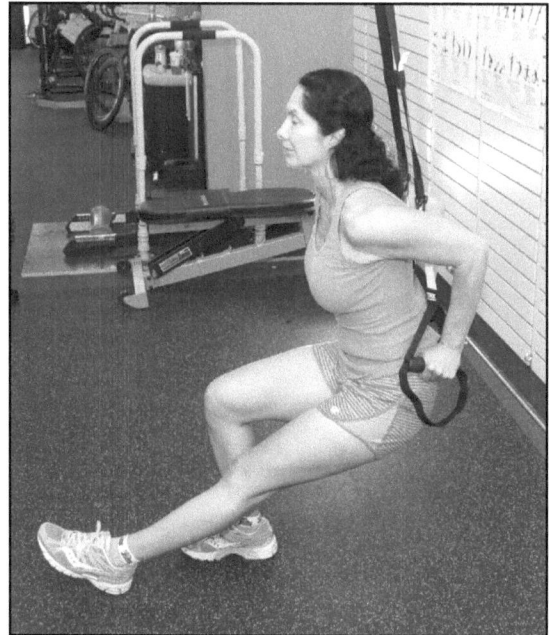

Finishing Position

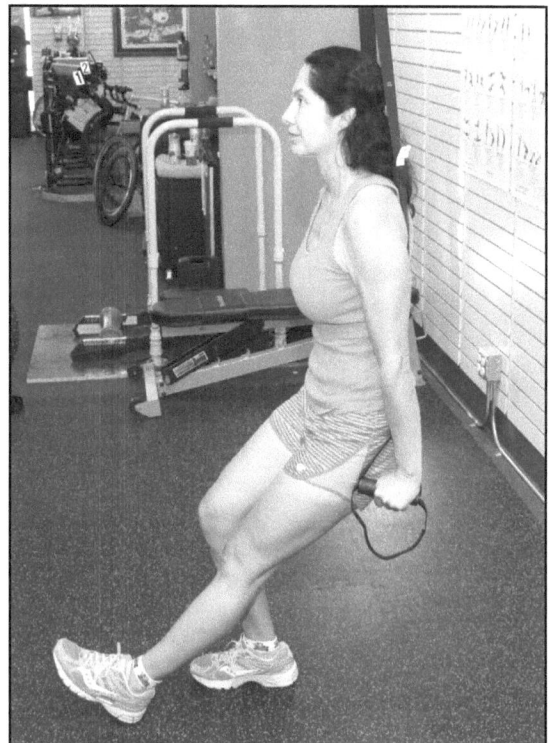

Chin-Ups and Hangs

Pull-ups and chin-ups are hard. That's why you don't often see people doing them. The more body weight you have, the more difficult they are, for obvious reasons. As they do require a bar on which to pull up, it's not technically body weight only, but I wanted to include it and share a variation that may help more people be able to include this one in their program. Even if you find you can't do one pull-up, read on and consider trying one of the hang positions, which will work the same muscles.

Primary Focus: Back, biceps, and core.

Variations and Progressions:

Starting Position   **Finishing Position**

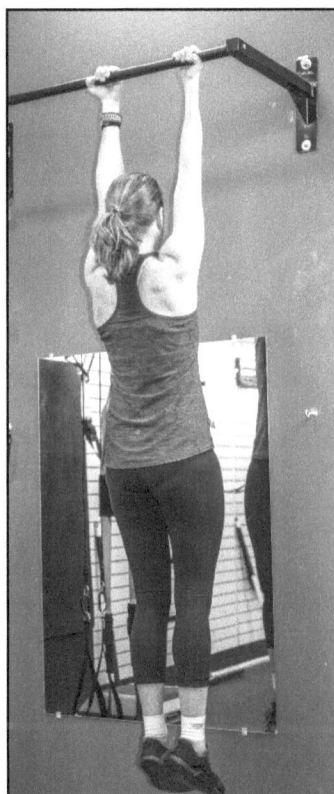

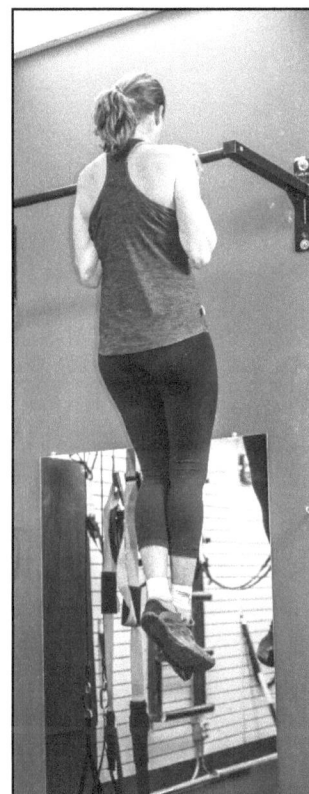

1. **Arm Hangs.** Use a narrow and underhand grip on the bar. Hang at the top of the movement, and then when you have had enough, hang at the bottom of the movement. Work on increasing the duration you can do this. By working both ends of the movement, you will eventually develop the strength to pull yourself up a few times, and you can build from there.

2. **Full Chin-Ups.** Note the starting position. Jumping up to the top of the bar is not part of it. Neither is swinging your body in any way to generate momentum. Keep your torso tight and still, and make your muscles do the work.

Keep good form. Don't let your shoulders disconnect on the bottom. Prevent this by pulling your shoulder blades down to your pockets, especially at the bottom of the movement. Don't forget to breathe!

Want more? Add a weight vest, or switch to a pull-up using a wide overhand grip.

Chin-ups are performed with an underhand narrow grip as shown. Pull-ups are performed with an overhand wide grip. Pull-ups with the overhand wide grip tend to be even harder because the lever between your body and your hands on the bar is longer.

Lower-Body Movements

Basic Squat

The Squat develops strength in the legs and hips. Mastering the squat movement will teach and reinforce proper squatting form, and give you a solid base for more advanced exercises that combine the squat with other movements.

Primary Focus: Legs.

Secondary Focus: Core and upper torso, which are responsible for maintaining good posture

Setup: Straps fully extended to mid-length.

1. Face the anchor, holding the straps with a shoulder-width stance.

2. Keep the arms relaxed and shoulders back, and drop your hips down toward the floor as if you were sitting on a bench behind you. Maintain good posture through your upper body, and keep your shoulders back and relaxed.

3. When you reach the bottom, push yourself back up through your legs and hips while keeping your weight centered over your feet (not on your heels or toes), exhaling as you do so.

Note: Knees should be directly over the feet during the squat.

Tips and Progressions:

- This is a great exercise if you're a beginner to learn the proper squat while receiving some balance assistance from the suspended trainer. If you're more advanced, it works well as part of a warm-up circuit.

- The depth of the squat you descend to depends on your fitness level and the comfort level of the movement. If you are just starting out or have any knee or hip issues, a shallow squat is OK.

Starting Position   **Finishing Position**

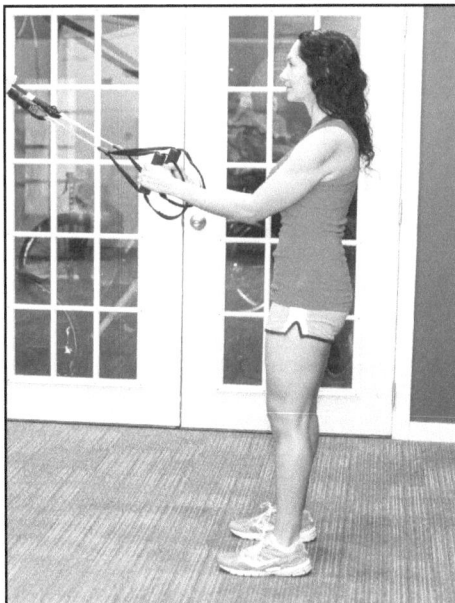

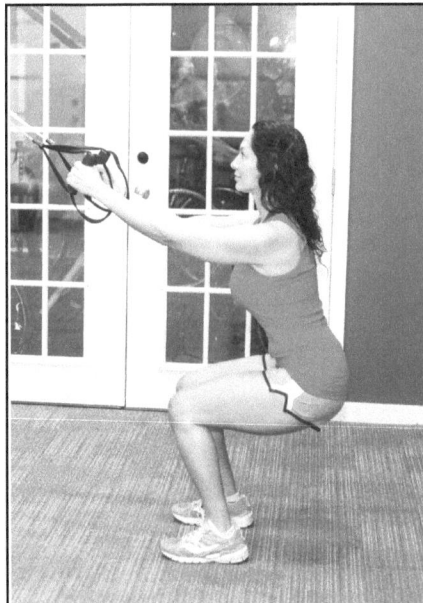

Split Squat

This movement develops strength and balance control in the legs and hips. This movement pattern of the legs and hips working together, although they're in opposing positions, is important for overall good movement abilities. It's also highly transferable to walk and run gait mechanics.

Primary Focus: Front and back of the legs as well as the hips.

Secondary Focus: Posture and stability of torso and hips to maintain good form.

Setup: Straps fully extended or shortened to mid-length.

1. Face the anchor and hold the straps in front of you. Take a large step behind you with one leg while keeping the other leg where it is.

2. Begin the movement by dropping the back knee down toward the floor as low as you are comfortable doing. The knee of the front foot should stay directly over that foot as it bends.

3. Return to the starting position by pushing through the toes of your back foot and the front foot.

Note: Throughout the movement, keep your arms relaxed, shoulders back, and torso upright.

Tips and Progressions:

- If you're at a beginner level, it's OK to not go down as far. As you get more comfortable doing this exercise, you can progress to go deeper.

- Widening your feet will make you more stable. Narrowing your feet will challenge your balance more. Find a stance that is challenging but allows you to perform the movement with good technique.

- This movement can be progressed by doing it without holding the straps or by holding additional weight (dumbbells or a medicine ball) at your side or in front of you.

Starting Position   Finishing Position

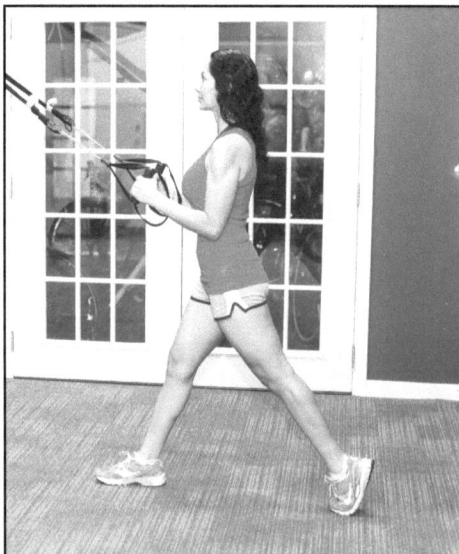

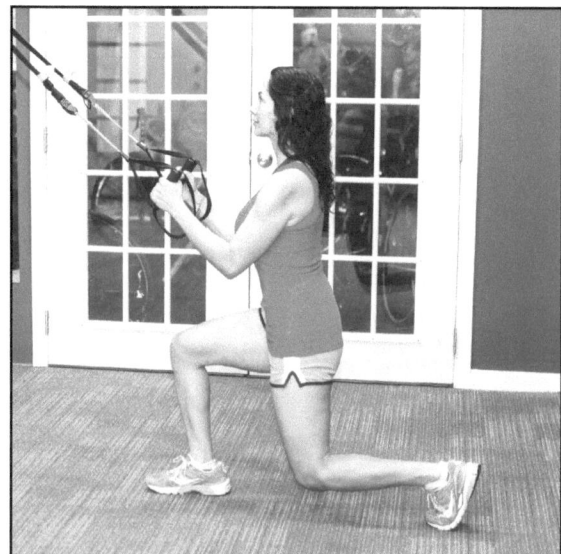

Reverse Lunge

This is a great exercise for your single-leg strength and stability because of the requirement of decelerating, stabilizing, and then pushing your body weight forward with one leg at a time. Training the muscles to not only be strong in a single-leg stance, but also to be stable is a critical component in strong gait mechanics.

Primary Focus: Hip and legs.

Secondary Focus: Stabilizer muscles in legs and hips.

Setup: Straps fully extended or shortened to mid-length.

1. Face the anchor, holding the straps with a shoulder-width stance.

2. Take a big step back with one foot, and immediately drop the back knee straight down to the floor. Descend to a depth that challenges you.

3. From there, ascend by pushing up through the front leg and bringing the back leg back to the starting position.

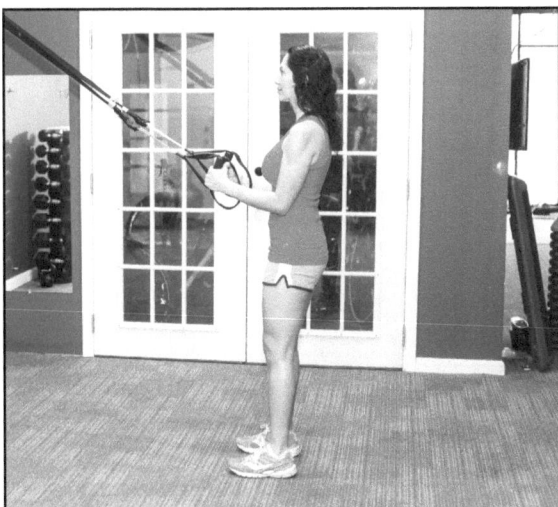

4. Repeat all repetitions on the one leg, recover, and then perform a set on the other leg.

Note: Keep your torso upright (don't bend forward).

Tips and Progressions:

- The front leg is the one you want to be working. Focus on pushing through that leg to return to the starting position from the bottom.

- Focus on keeping the knee right over the midfoot as you descend and ascend. If you feel wobbly or your knees tend to cave inward, don't descend as far down, and focus on improving the stability of the supporting leg before progressing.

- Progress this one by doing it freestanding, without holding the straps. Progress even further by holding additional weight (dumbbells or medicine ball) at your side or in front of you.

Starting Position   **Finishing Position**

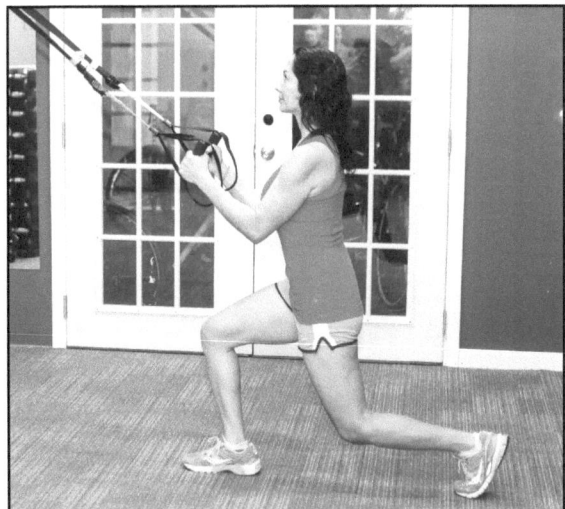

Calf Raise

This is a great exercise to support walking, riding, climbing, and jumping activities. It will also help in developing muscle definition in your calves.

Primary Focus: Calves.

Secondary Focus: Core (hold your plank to maintain your body alignment).

Setup: Straps fully extended.

1. Face away from the anchor with the straps underneath your arms.

2. Place the handles between your thumbs and index fingers, and with bent elbows, lean forward so the straps are supporting a portion of your weight. It's OK if your heels come off the ground. Keep your body straight like a board.

3. Drop your heels down to the floor (you will probably feel a slight stretch in the calves) and then push all the way back up on your toes.

Tips and Progressions:

- Increase the speed of the movement to make it harder, and give the calf muscles a good squeeze at the top of the movement.

- For a progression, just use one leg and either self-spot with the other leg or hold it off the ground completely.

Starting Position   **Finishing Position**

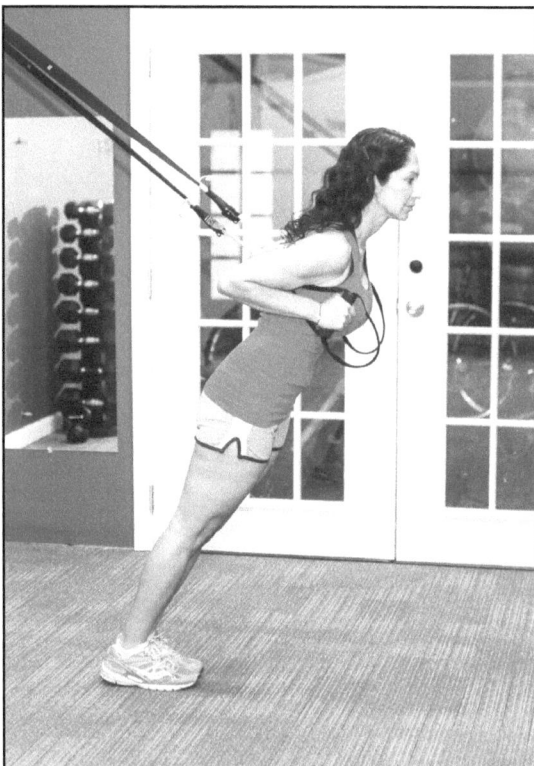

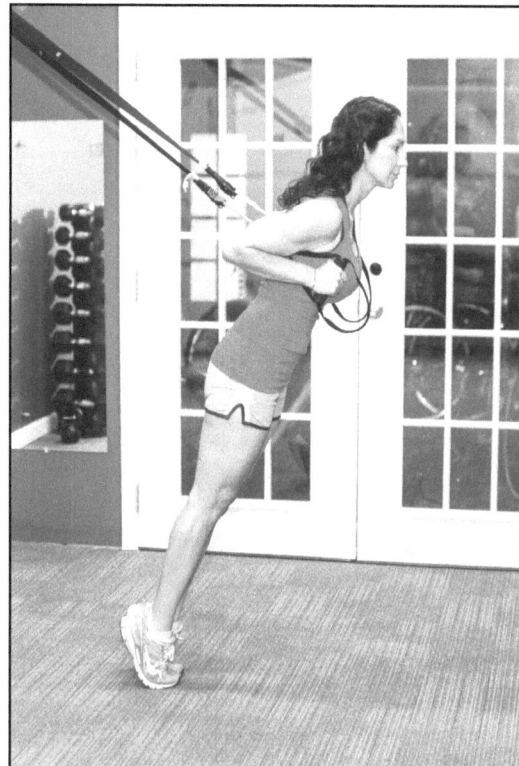

Hip Hinge

This movement will train the muscles to maintain stability while supporting the body on one leg. Walking and running require the stance leg to support and stabilize all your body weight while the rest of the body moves. A lack of stability in your single-leg stance can cause compensations and harmful forces in the knee and hip as well as poor balance.

Primary Focus: Legs and hips.

Secondary Focus: Core and stabilizers of the legs to maintain a proper single-leg stance.

Setup: Straps fully extended.

1. Face the anchor, holding the straps with your arms extended in front of you.

2. Lift one leg and extend it behind you while bending forward from the waist and pushing your arms out in front of you.

Note: Think about hinging at the hip, and keep your back flat like a board as you reach forward with your arms. The supporting leg should stay extended with a slight bend in the knee. Do not lock out the knee.

3. At the bottom of the movement, your body should be as straight as possible from your arms to your extended foot. Think about making a flat table out of your arms, torso, and leg. Focus on maintaining a strong, stable position with the supporting leg, with the knee directly over the foot and hips aligned.

4. Return to the starting position with both feet on the ground again.

Tips and Progressions:

*   If you feel wobbly or are losing your balance, don't go as far down into the movement until you can get it under control. Start again slowly, only going down to the point where you feel it challenges your balance, and then come back up.

*   If you're feeling comfortable with this exercise, try preforming consecutive repetitions without allowing the extended leg to touch the ground.

Starting Position   **Finishing Position**

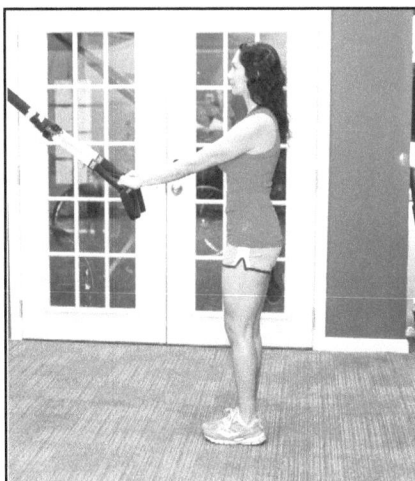

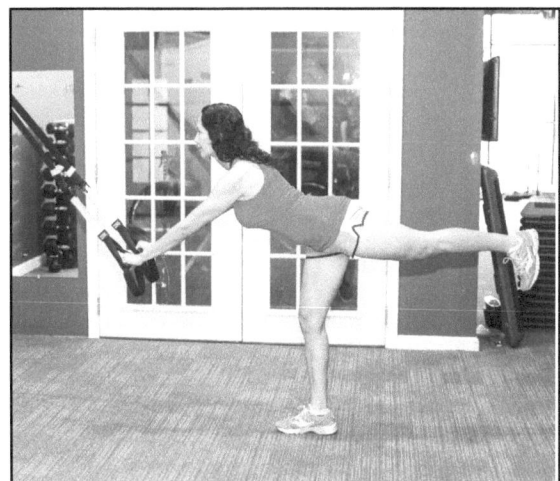

Hamstring Curl

This movement will develop hamstring power and strength. This is especially relevant to having a strong and snappy heel kick during running, as well as being able to step over objects. Elevating your hips during this movement also strengthens the back side of the core.

Primary Focus: Hamstrings.

Secondary Focus: Backside of the core and hips to lift the hips.

Setup: Straps fully extended and approximately six to twelve inches off the ground.

1. Lie on your back with your feet in the cradles of the straps and your knees slightly bent.

2. Keeping just a slight bend in the knees, push through your heels and raise your hips.

3. Keep them elevated and pull your heels toward your butt. Extend your legs back out, keeping the hips raised. Repeat.

Tips and Progressions:

*   This exercise can also be done as a combination with the hip raise. Instead of keeping your hips elevated, just lower them back down and then lift them back up between each hamstring curl.

*   This movement is harder than it looks. But if you still want more, move your position farther out from underneath the anchor point (see chapter 3 on adjusting resistance levels). You'll be working against gravity more and will have to overcome more resistance to pull your heels to your butt.

Starting Position

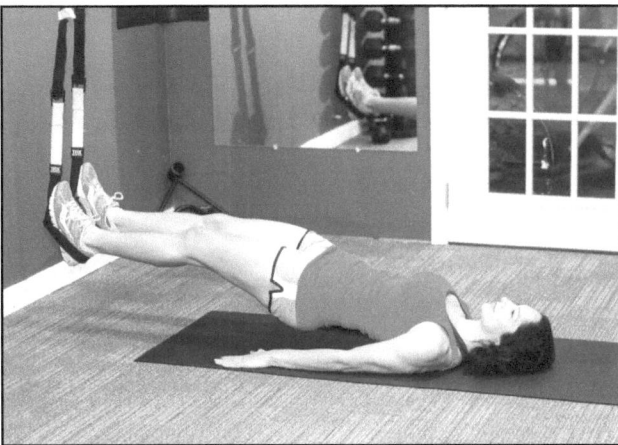

Finishing Position

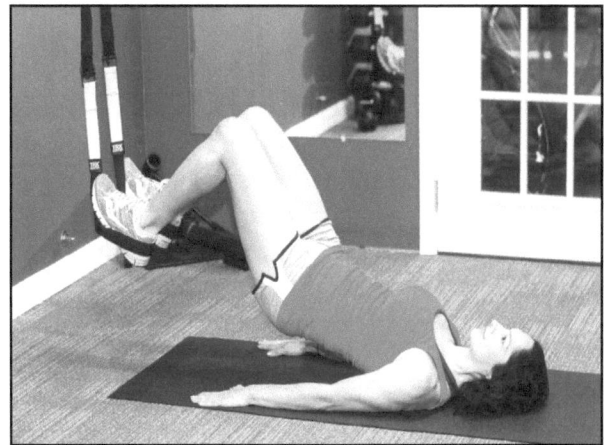

Front Squat

The squat is an all-purpose movement that will strengthen the legs and hips. It develops strong hip and leg extension. This move can also progress to the front squats with the jump, which is a great exercise for developing explosive power as well.

Primary Focus: Front and back of the legs as well as the hips.

Secondary Focus: Calves.

Setup: Straps fully extended.

Starting Position

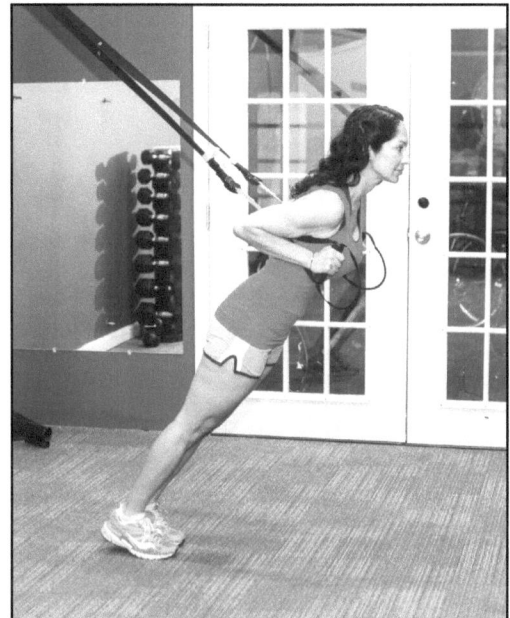

1. Start by facing away from the anchor with the straps underneath your arms. Place the handles between your thumbs and index fingers with your elbows bent and at your side.

2. Lean into the straps so they're supporting a portion of your weight (think about making chicken wings with your arm and elbow position). It's OK if your heels come off the ground when you're leaning forward, but your body should stay in a straight line. You should feel like you're just hanging on the straps at this point.

3. Allow your knees to bend and your hips to descend back and down behind you toward the floor, following along the angle of your lean.

Finishing Position

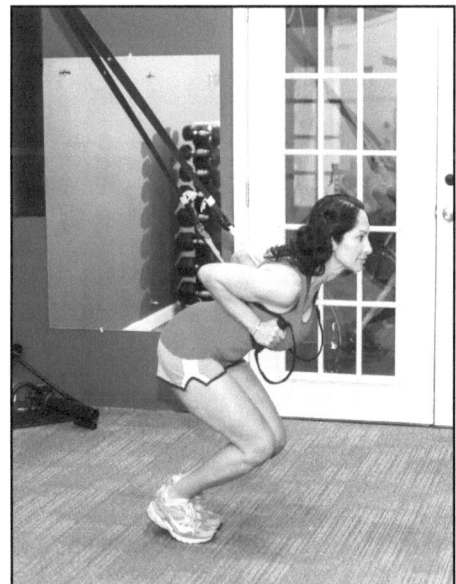

4. At the bottom of the movement, make sure you still have good posture and a tight core, and push back up, exhaling as you do so.

Note: Maintain your torso position (don't bend over at the waist), and look straight ahead (not at the floor).

Tips and Progressions:

- Start slowly and increase the speed of the movement as you become more comfortable.

- Add a calf raise at the top of the movement for more bang.

- Progress to a hop. It can either be a single small hop, leaving and landing in the same spot, or a double hop that lands you about an inch forward, followed immediately by a second hop that lands you back the same inch. The impact will develop explosive power, is great for your bones, and will burn more calories.

Crossover Lunge

This movement requires you to stabilize and decelerate through a single leg, before the transition to pushing off again. This will develop the ability to maintain alignment of the hip, knee, and ankle in the single-leg stance. A lot of soft tissue tears occur because the hip and knee can't keep the alignment needed under stress during sudden changes of direction, or quick stops and starts (common in tennis, basketball, and soccer). This movement strengthens the components that protect the knees when those types of stresses are placed on them.

Primary Focus: Legs and hips.

Secondary Focus: Lateral stabilizers of the legs and hips to stabilize the knees and hips.

Setup: Straps shortened to mid-length.

Starting Position

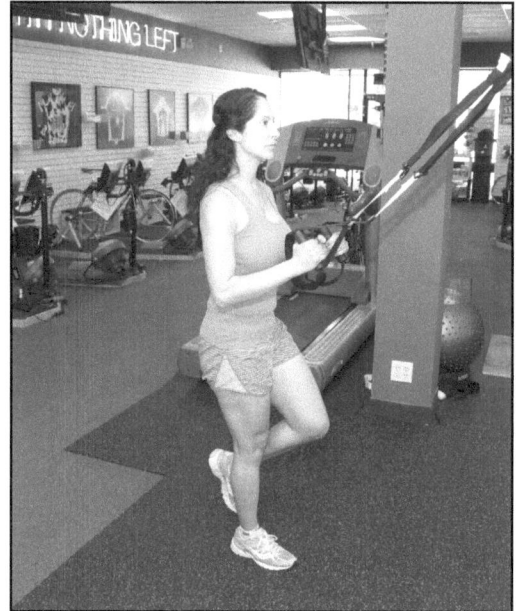

1. Face the anchor, holding the straps.

2. Lift one leg, cross it behind the supporting leg, and dip down toward the ground by allowing your hips and knees to bend.

3. When you get to the bottom of the movement, push yourself back up through the supporting leg until you are upright again.

Note: Make sure you keep the knee over the foot on the leg you're pushing back up with. Your hips should drop straight down to the floor. Don't use your arms to pull yourself up; instead push yourself back up through your supporting leg.

Finishing Position

Tips and Progressions:

- You may touch the ground with the back leg that crosses over if you need to.

- Don't lean back on the straps to make it easier. Make your supporting leg do the work of pushing you back up to the top.

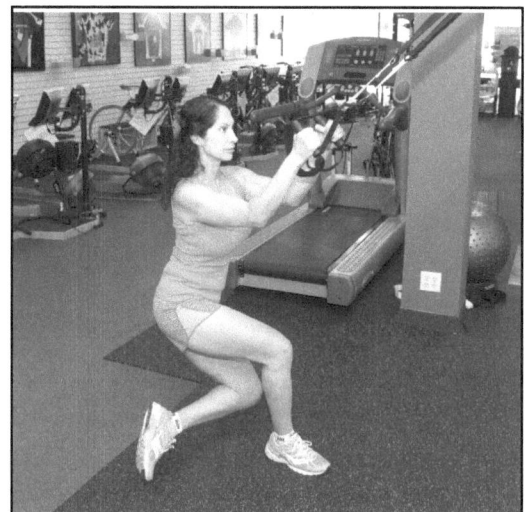

Hip Abduction

This is an excellent movement for strengthening hip stabilizers, which are extremely important in maintaining strong gait mechanics. You may have seen people whose hips drop when they walk. "Model walk" is actually an informal name for when this happens. If the hip stabilizers are weak, they can't maintain the hip alignment when you're on one leg during your gait. This causes the opposite hip of the supporting leg to drop with every step. This movement, along with other single-leg movements, will help keep strong gait mechanics.

Primary Focus: Lateral muscles of the hips.

Secondary Focus: Hamstrings and lower back.

Setup: Straps fully extended and approximately six inches off the ground.

1. Start by lying down with your heels in the cradles directly below the anchor point. Your arms should be at your side, palms down on the floor. Push through the heels to lift the hips off the ground.

2. Now, keep the hips up off the ground and extend the legs out to the side. Go as far out to the side as you can while keeping proper form. At that point bring them back to the middle and your feet back together.

3. Repeat for the targeted number of repetitions.

Tips and Progressions:

- Don't allow the knees to cave in; keep them in a straight line with your hips and feet.

- Don't allow the back to arch up.

- The arms may provide some leverage, but keep good posture, with shoulders relaxed and shoulder blades pulled tight toward your butt.

Starting Position

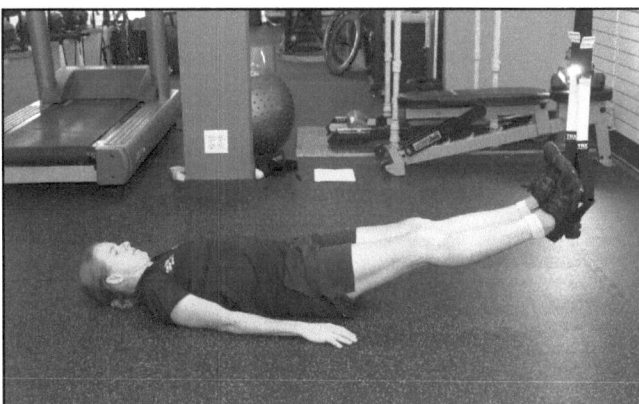

Finishing Position

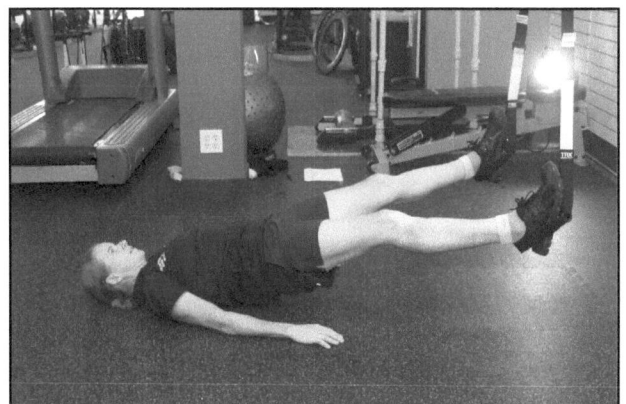

Sprinter Starts

This is one of my favorite movements because it improves strength, stability, and power, all with one movement. It's easy to modify and progress. It's also a fun exercise. It will help develop a strong leg extension that is required for forward propulsion, and pushing up inclines. It also improves stability and balance because you're pushing through one leg while simultaneously controlling your body hanging on the straps.

Primary Focus: Legs and hips.

Secondary Focus: Calves and hip flexors.

Setup: Straps fully extended.

1. Face away with the straps underneath your arms. Place the handles between your thumbs and index fingers, and with your elbows bent and at your side, lean forward into the straps.

2. Go down into the movement by taking a large step back with one leg, allowing the front leg to bend.

3. Come back to the starting position by pushing back up through the front leg, and then finish the movement by driving the knee of what was the back leg up and toward your chest (like a person sprinting from the starting blocks).

4. Repeat all repetitions on one side, rest, and then switch legs.

Note: Think about making chicken wings with your arm and elbow position. It's OK if your heels come off the ground when you're leaning forward, but your body should stay straight like a board.

Tips and Progressions:

- Keep good torso position and your head and eyes looking forward during the movement. This will help maintain good alignment and posture.

- Start slowly and increase the speed of the movement when you feel comfortable with it.

- To progress this exercise, add a hop to it. This can be either a single small hop, leaving and landing in the same spot, or a short double hop (think about putting a piece of tape down and hopping over it and back quickly at the top of each repetition).

Starting Position   **Finishing Position**

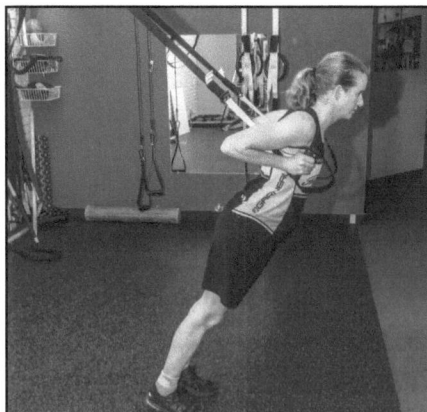

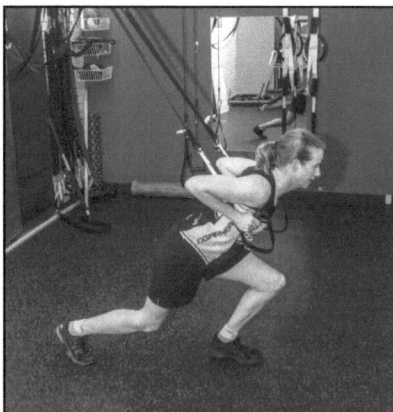

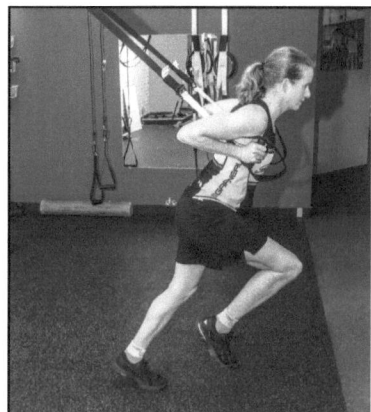

Jump Squat

This exercise will develop explosive power of the hips and legs. It will train your muscles to be able to fire more of the larger muscle fibers more quickly. The impact is good for your bones, and catching air is fun!

Primary Focus: Legs and hips.

Secondary Focus: Power.

Setup: Straps fully extended.

1. Facing the anchor, hold the straps, and stand with your feet a little wider than shoulder width.

2. Keep the arms relaxed and shoulders back, and squat down toward the floor.

3. When you reach the bottom, immediately power back up through the hips and legs, and jump as high as you are able.

Note: Maintain good posture through your upper body, and keep your shoulders back and relaxed. Keep your weight over your feet when going into and coming out of the squat. Your knees should be directly over your feet, **not** out in front of them.

Tips and Progressions:

- You should master both the comfort and technique of the squat movement before adding the jump.

- Make sure you maintain correct form. Common form errors are caving the knees in, bending forward too far at the waist, and leaning back on the straps to make it easier. Keep your knees in line with your feet and your weight over your legs and feet.

- This movement can be progressed by doing it freestanding, holding weight, or wearing a weight vest.

Starting Position   **Finishing Position**

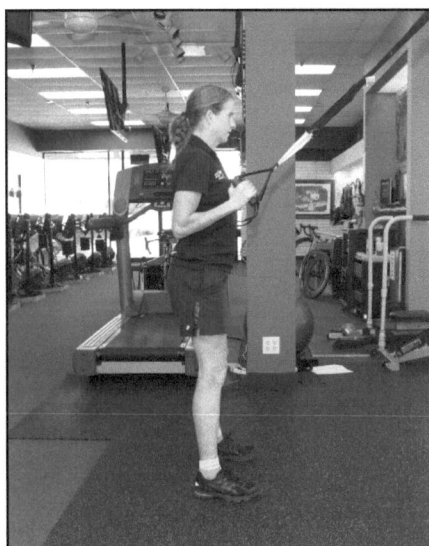

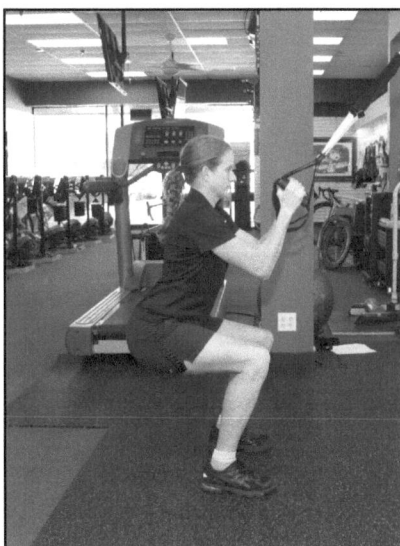

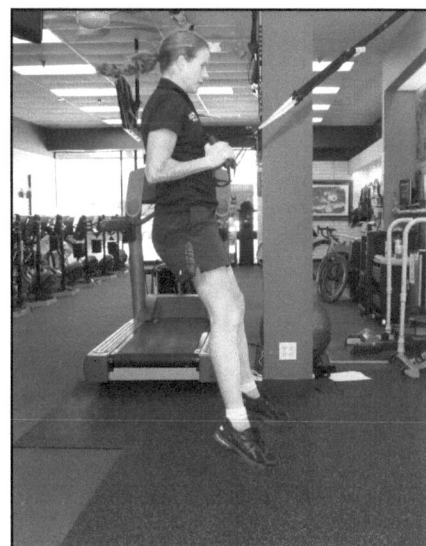

Skaters

This movement develops leg and hip strength and power. It also develops stability, and the ability to control and decelerate your body weight while keeping your ankle, knee, and hip aligned. It's a fun movement where you can catch some air and increase the distance you jump from side to side as you get stronger and more fit.

Primary Focus: Legs and hips.

Secondary Focus: Cardio.

Setup: Straps fully extended.

1. Face the anchor, holding the straps. Step out to the side with one leg, and drop down into a lateral lunge movement.

2. Power back up through that leg, pushing yourself to the opposite side, stepping down on the opposite leg and allowing yourself to descend toward the floor on that leg. As you descend on the supporting leg, cross the unsupported leg behind you, and reach even farther out to the side of you with it.

3. Push back up through the supporting leg and repeat.

Note: Keep the knee aligned straight over the foot of the supporting leg! Make sure your knee stays right over and in line with your foot as you are controlling your deceleration and then pushing off.

Tips and Progressions:

- Master the crossover lunge before doing skaters.

- Start slowly, and only step out to the side as much as you are comfortable with. As you get proficient with this one, increase the distance you step out to the side.

- To make it even harder, add a jump to it. Spring yourself up from the side to catch some air in the middle before landing on the other side.

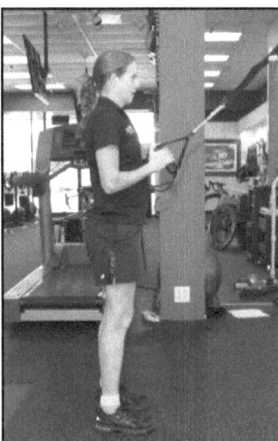

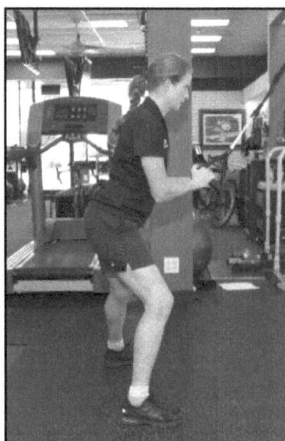

Starting Position   **Finishing Positions Alternating Sides**

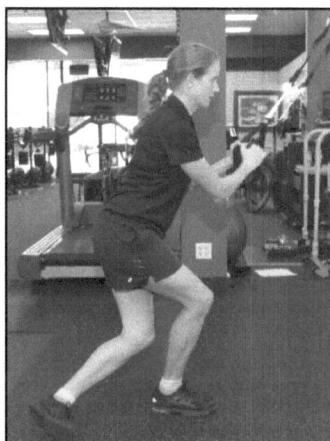

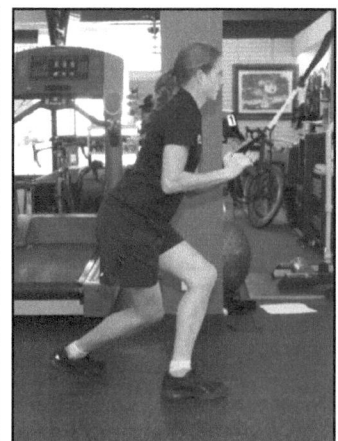

Lateral Hip Hinge

This movement is similar to the standard hip hinge, but is a little more challenging because the lateral resistance will pull you off balance even more. This variation will put an increased amount of lateral stress on the body that the supporting leg and core will be required to work against.

Primary Focus: Legs and hips.

Secondary Focus: Core and stabilizers of the legs to maintain a proper single-leg stance alignment.

Setup: Straps fully extended.

Starting Position

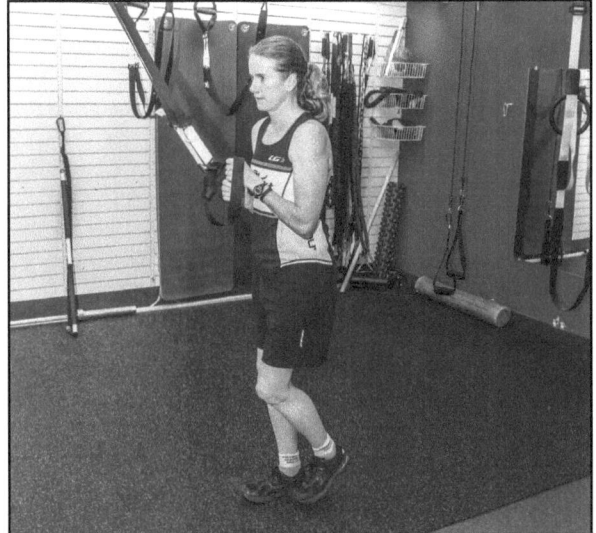

1. Face sideways, holding the straps in front of you.

2. Lift one leg and extend it behind you while bending forward from the waist and pushing your arms out in front of you.

3. At the bottom of the movement, your body should be as straight as possible from your arms to your extended foot. Make a flat table out of your arms, torso, and leg. Focus on maintaining a strong, stable position with the supporting leg, with the knee directly over the foot and hips aligned.

4. Return to the starting position with both feet on the ground again.

Note: Think about hinging at the hip, and keep your back flat like a board as you reach forward with your arms. The supporting leg should stay extended, with a slight bend in the knee. Do not lock out the knee.

Finishing Position

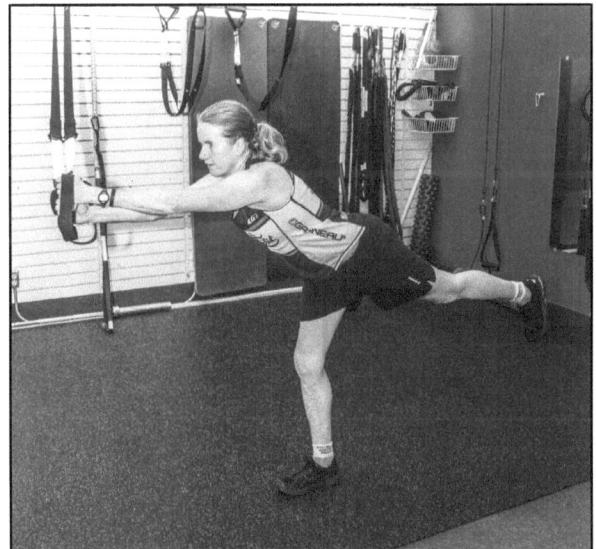

Tips and Progressions:

- If you feel wobbly or are losing your balance, reduce the range of motion until you can get it under control. Start again slowly, only go down until the point where you feel it challenges your balance, then come back up.

- Start by allowing your trailing leg to touch the ground in between repetitions to help stabilize you. If are feeling comfortable with this one, do it without touching in between.

- You don't need much lateral tension to increase the difficultly level. Find the amount that challenges you while still allowing you to perform the movement correctly by slightly adjusting your position closer to or farther from the anchor.

Swim Starts

In addition to extending the push leg, you will also be simultaneously extending the free leg back behind you. This gives the glutes a nice extra kick during the movement. Good for developing strength and stability in the hips, legs, and calves.

Primary Focus: Legs and hips.

Secondary Focus: Calves, glutes, and lower back.

Setup: Straps fully extended.

1. Face away with the straps underneath your arms. Place the handles between your thumbs and index fingers, and with your elbows bent and at your side, lean forward into the straps.

2. Go into the movement by taking a large step back with one leg, allowing the front leg to bend.

3. Come back to the starting position by pushing back up through the front leg while extending the back leg behind you as if you're trying to reach and touch the wall behind you.

4. Repeat all repetitions on one side, rest, then switch legs.

Note: Think about making "chicken wings" with your arm and elbow position. It's OK if your heels come off the ground when you are leaning forward, but your body should stay straight like a board.

Tips and Progressions:

- Keep good torso position and head and eyes looking forward during the movement. This will help maintain good alignment and posture.

- Start slowly and increase the speed of the movement when you feel comfortable with it.

- Give the back leg an extra squeeze when it's in the fully extended position.

Starting Position   **Finishing Position**

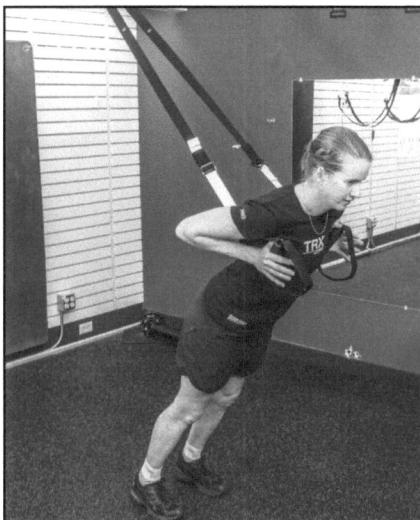

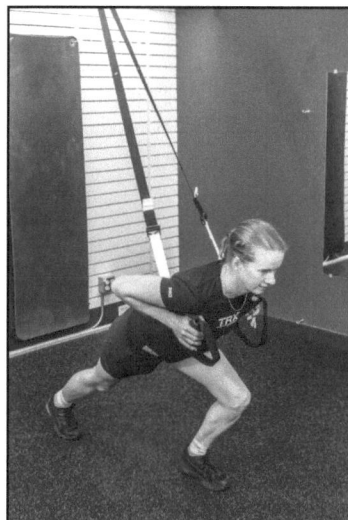

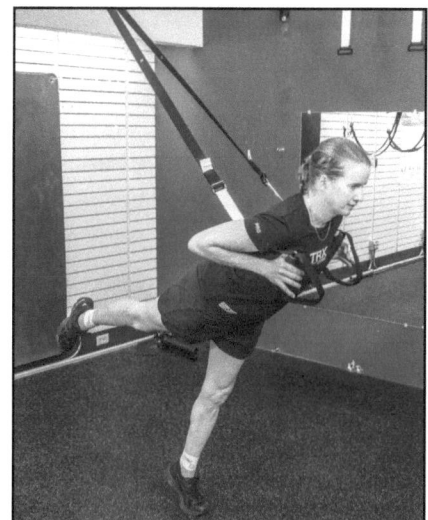

Suspended Reverse Lunge Intermediate and Advanced

This is a reverse lunge with the foot of the non-working leg suspended in both cradles. This takes away the support of the ground at the bottom of the movement, and adds a degree of instability. This exercise will help both strengthen and stabilize the leg and hip muscles all the way from the feet to the hips. It will also be a balance challenge for most of you. Hold a dowel, bar, or hiking pole to help with balance if you need to, until you can master the balance through the whole movement.

Primary Focus: Legs and hips.

Secondary Focus: Stabilizer muscles of the legs and hips.

Setup: Straps fully extended and approximately six inches off the ground.

1. Start by facing away from the anchor with the toes of one foot in both cradles of the suspended trainer. Keep a slight bend in the knee of the leg that is now supporting all of your weight.

2. Drop down into the movement by pushing back with the foot that is in the cradle, allowing the front leg to bend and your hips to drop down toward the floor.

3. Return to the starting position by stepping back up through the front leg, and bringing the back leg back in line with the front leg. Perform a set of consecutive repetitions on one side, then repeat on the other side.

Note: The work is to be performed by the supporting leg. Minimize the weight you're putting on the strap of the suspended leg to the extent you are able.

Tips and Progressions:

- Make sure you have mastered the reverse lunge before progressing to the suspended variation.

- Add some hip flexor work by pulling the knee of the leg that's in the cradle all the way up instead of just in line with the other leg.

Starting Position

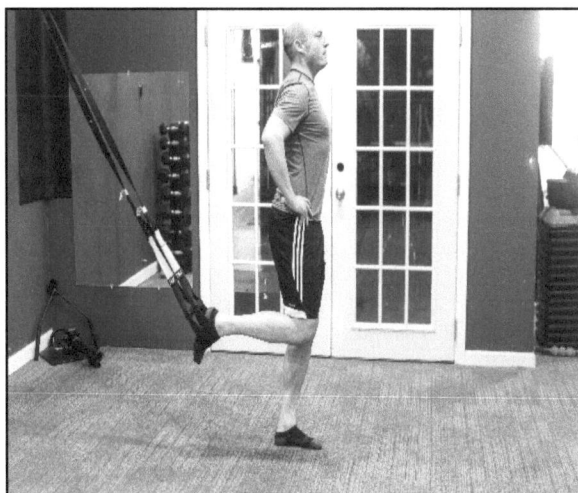

Finishing Position

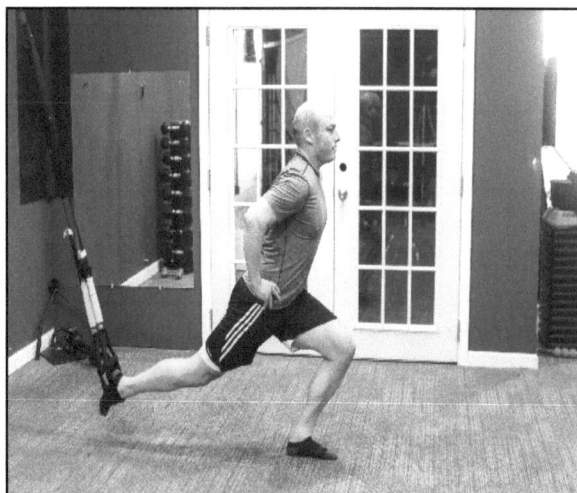

Suspended Lateral Lunge Intermediate and Advanced

A form of a single-leg squat with some hip adduction for the inner thigh.

Primary Focus: Legs and hips.

Secondary Focus: Inner thighs, which help pull the suspended leg back toward the body.

Setup: Straps fully extended.

1. Stand on one leg to the side of the suspended trainer, with the other leg in both cradles.

2. Keeping the arms relaxed and shoulders back, push the suspended leg out to the side and descend on the stance leg toward the floor. Go down as low as you are comfortable, maintaining good form and posture with the upper body.

3. When you get to the bottom, push back up through the stance leg, and bring the suspended leg back to the center by engaging the muscles in the inner thighs.

Tips and Progressions:

- Start with a shallow lunge, and progress by increasing the depth of the lunge as you get stronger. Hold onto a pole or dowel if needed to help with stability, but try to wean yourself off of it as you improve.

- This one challenges both strength and stability. Additional weight can be added by holding a ball or dumbbell either in front or in one hand at your side. In most cases, however, this is not needed. Make sure you have mastered the movement before progressing with added weight.

Starting Position

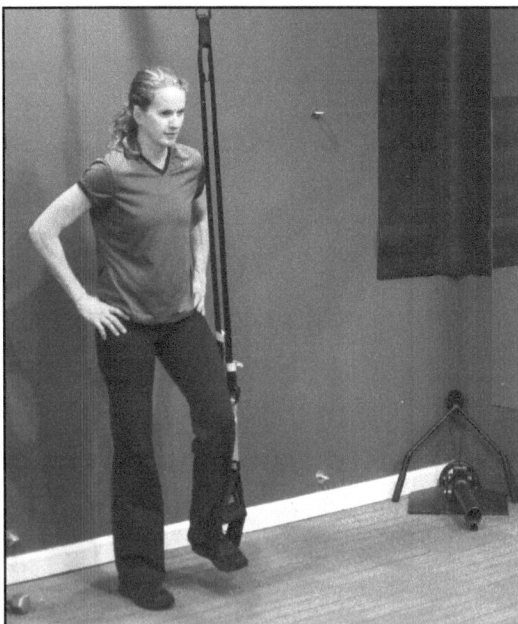

Finishing Position

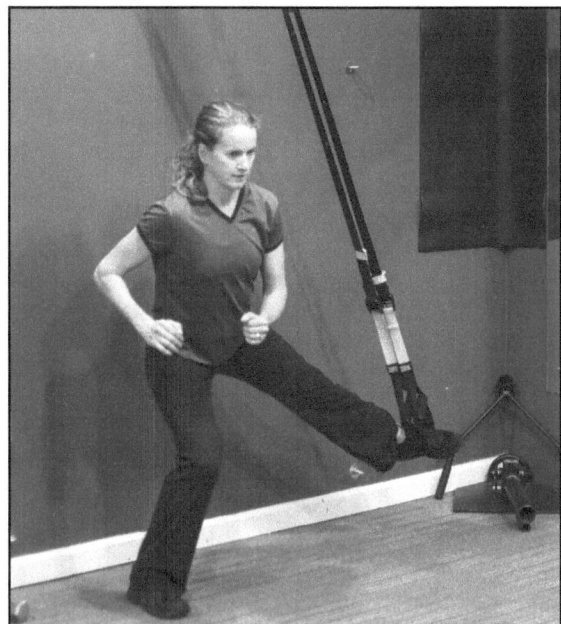

Suspended Power Lunge Intermediate and Advanced

An explosive movement that will increase strength and power of the hips and legs. The legs and hips must stay aligned while absorbing impact, decelerating body mass, and then producing explosive power to push the body back up—all with just one leg. The impact and high force generated are great for bone health.

Primary Focus: Hips and legs.

Secondary Focus: Hip flexor of the suspended leg, which drives the knee forward.

Setup: Straps fully extended and approximately six inches off the ground.

1. Face away from the anchor on one leg, with the foot of the other leg suspended in both cradles.

2. Drop down into the movement by pushing back with the foot that's in the cradle, allowing the front leg to bend and your hips to drop down toward the floor.

3. Now, when you get to the bottom, power back up with as much acceleration as you can produce. Push through the front leg as you pull the suspended knee back in line with the supporting knee. The result should be a hop or jump off the ground.

Note: Always keep a slight bend in the knee of the leg that is supporting all of your weight. Make sure you don't lock out your knee.

Tips and Progressions:

*   Master the suspended lunge movement before attempting the suspended power lunge.

*   Don't rush it. Make sure to control the landing, and maintain good form on the way back down.

*   Make sure the knee stays over the foot, and your torso stays straight up and down.

Starting Position   **Finishing Position**

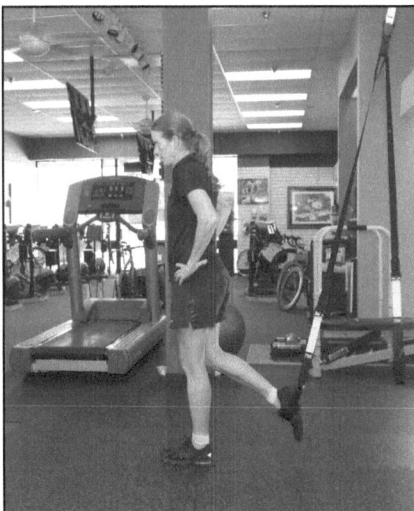

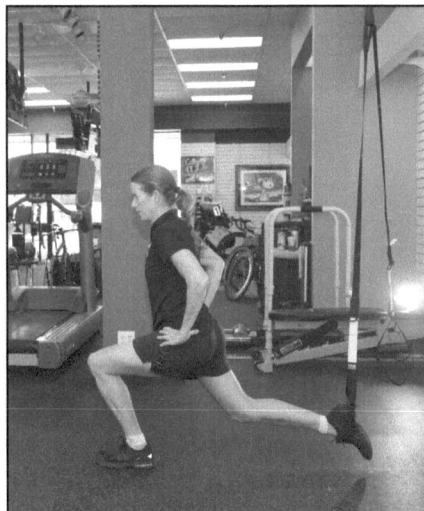

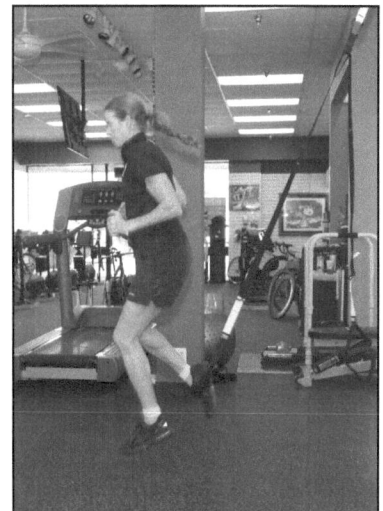

Single-Leg Squat Intermediate and Advanced

You may have heard of the pistol squat. This is a version of it. You will need optimal strength and stability to descend into the lowest version of this movement. The good news is that using the straps will help you maintain form as you progress and increase the depth to which you can descend to.

Primary Focus: Legs and hips.

Secondary Focus: Stabilizer muscles of the hips and legs to hold the alignment of the ankle, knee, and hip.

Setup: Straps mid-length.

1. Facing the anchor point, hold the end of each strap in each hand, and assume a shoulder-width, or slightly wider stance.

2. Keep the arms relaxed and shoulders back, lift up one leg, and support your body weight with your other leg.

3. Descend toward the floor using only the supporting leg. Keep an upright torso and good posture.

4. At the bottom, push yourself back up through the supporting leg, exhaling as you rise.

Note: Make sure you maintain good form throughout the movement, with the shoulders back, core engaged, and head in line with the spine and torso (don't look down during the movement).

Tips and Progressions:

• Use the straps for balance, but don't lean back on them too much. Use your legs.

• Start with a shallow squat. As you get stronger, descend further.

• Descending to the bottom of the range of motion is also known as the pistol squat, and can be done with or without a suspended trainer.

Starting Position

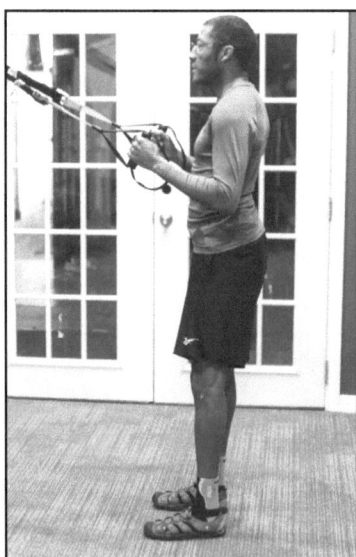

Finishing Position

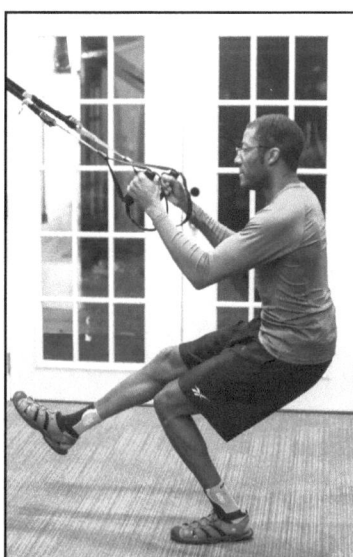

Split-Squat Jumps Intermediate and Advanced

This movement is great for hip and leg strength. It will get your heart pumping, and help improve and maintain bone density too!

Primary Focus: Legs and hips.

Secondary Focus: Cardio.

Setup: Straps fully extended.

1. Face the anchor, hold the straps, and assume a long split-stride position, with one leg forward and the other behind you.

2. Keep the arms relaxed and shoulders back, and drop the back knee down to the floor.

3. When you reach the bottom, immediately power back up through the hips and legs, jump as high as you are able, and quickly switch legs while you're in the air. When you land, the leg that was behind you is now in front, and vice versa.

Note: Maintain good posture through your upper body, and keep your shoulders back and relaxed. Your jump should be straight up, and you should land in the same spot with the legs reversed.

Tips and Progressions:

- Make sure you maintain correct form. Common errors of form include: knees caving in or coming too far over the toes, or bending forward too far at the waist. Keep your knees in line with your feet and your weight over your legs and feet.

- Make sure you've mastered proper technique of the split-stance squat before adding the jump to this movement.

- This movement can be progressed by doing it freestanding, holding weight, or wearing a weight vest.

Starting Position　　　　　　　　　　　　　　　　　　　　**Finishing Position**

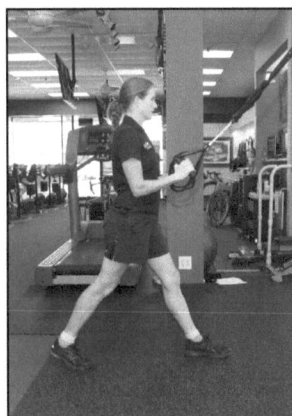

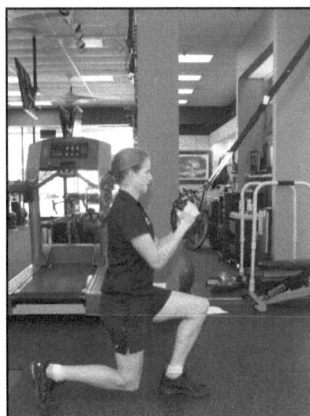

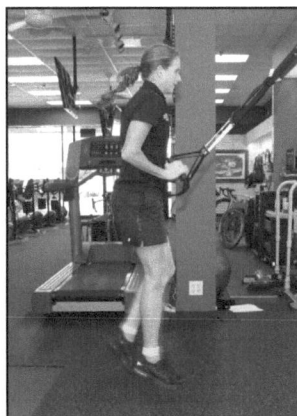

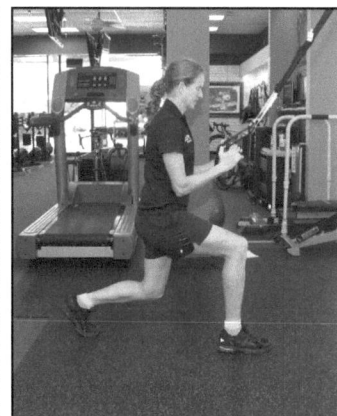

Whole-Body Movements

Forward Lunge with Fly

A good total-body foundation movement to teach the core to stabilize and assist movement of the upper and lower body simultaneously.

Primary Focus: Legs and chest.

Secondary Focus: Core and shoulders.

Setup: Straps fully extended.

1. Facing away, hold the straps in front of you with your arms extended.

2. Take a big step forward with one foot, and drop the back knee down toward the floor to go down into the lunge. At the same time, allow the arms to open up and move from the front to the side. They should stay parallel with the floor and extend straight out from your shoulders at the end of the movement.

3. To come back up, tighten your core, push back up through the front leg, and squeeze the muscles in your chest to bring your arms back together in front of you.

Tips and Progressions:

- The emphasis can be shifted from the upper body to the lower body, depending on which you push with more to get back up to the top of the movement.

- This movement uses a lot of muscles at the same time, and requires multiple larger muscle groups to work together.

Starting Position

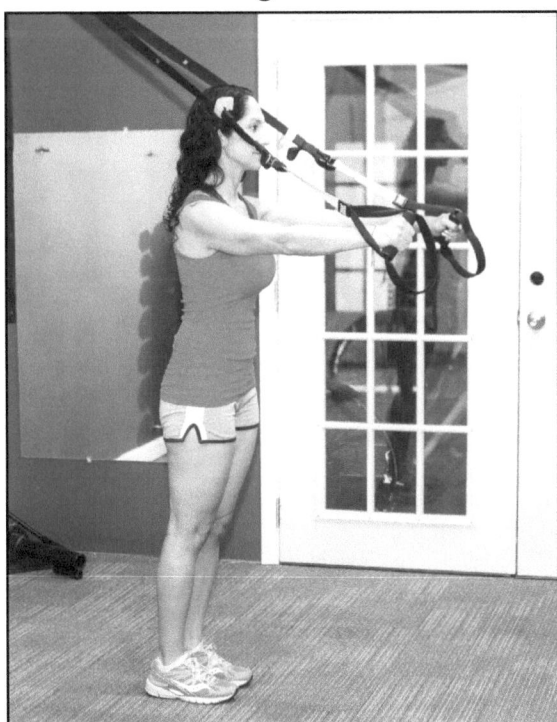

Finishing Position

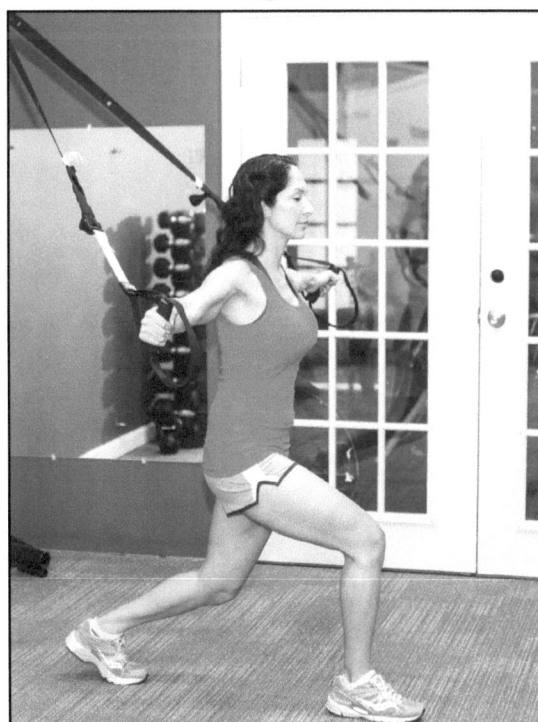

Squat Press

This is a great full-body exercise that will challenge those at a beginner-to-intermediate level. It can also serve as a functional warm-up, or part of a circuit program for more advanced levels. It will provide some dynamic flexibility for those with tight shoulders and chest muscles.

Primary Focus: Legs and hips.

Secondary Focus: Shoulders, to push the arms overhead.

Setup: Straps fully extended.

1. Face away from the anchor with a handle in each hand and the straps on the outside of your arms. Assume a slight forward lean.

2. Start the movement by dropping your hips to the floor behind you. Stay straight up and down as much as possible with your upper torso.

3. From the bottom of the movement, tighten your core and push back up with your legs and hips, exhaling as you do so. As you push back up, press your arms overhead.

4. Your finishing position should be full extension of both your arms and legs, leaning slightly forward.

Note: At the lowest part of the movement, you should be on the balls of your feet and have a slight forward lean, elbows bent, and the handles in line with your shoulders.

Tips and Progressions:

- Try hard to obtain the full extension at the top of the movement. Think about squeezing your arms to your ears and reaching toward the sky.

- Keep the hands as close to being directly overhead as possible at the time of the movement. Don't let them finish too far in front of your body.

Starting Position   **Finishing Position**

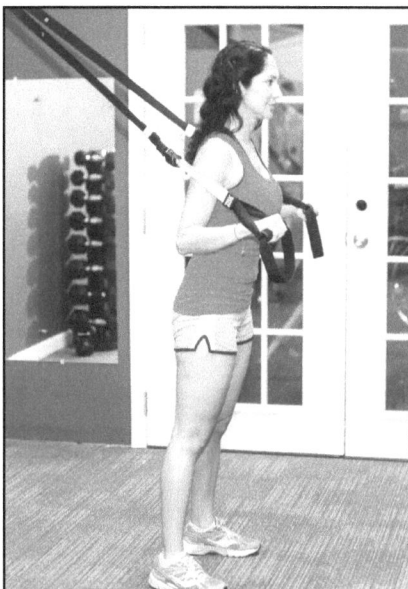

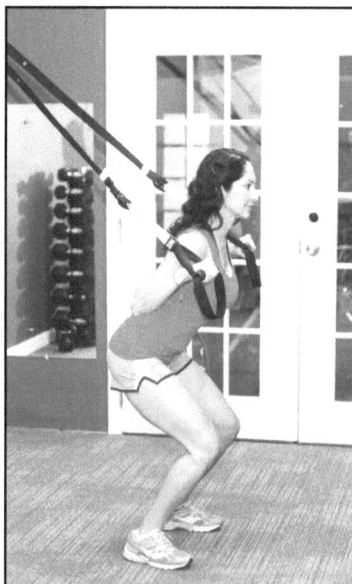

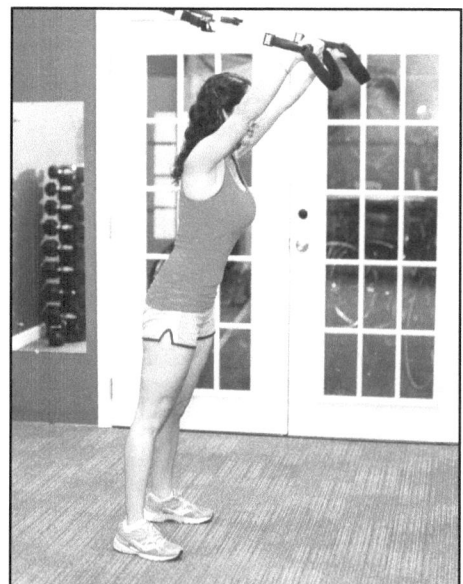

Squat Row

This is an all-purpose foundational movement that reinforces squat form, while also targeting the chain of muscles in the back and torso that are responsible for good posture. This exercise will challenge those at a beginner-to-intermediate level, and can serve as a functional warm-up or part of a circuit program for more advanced levels

Primary Focus: Legs and back.

Secondary Focus: Torso and core.

Setup: Straps shortened to mid-length.

1. Facing the anchor, hold the straps with a shoulder-width stance. Lean back slightly.

2. Sit down into the squat by dropping your hips down toward the floor. When you get to the bottom, your arms should be straight and extended in front of you.

3. Push yourself back up with your legs while simultaneously pulling your upper body toward the straps. Your finish position should be standing tall with your elbows bent at your side.

Tips and Progressions:

- Those who spend a lot of time at a desk or behind the wheel would benefit from combining the squat press (p. 190), which will help open up the chest and shoulders, with the squat row, which targets the large and small posture muscles.

Starting Position   **Finishing Position**

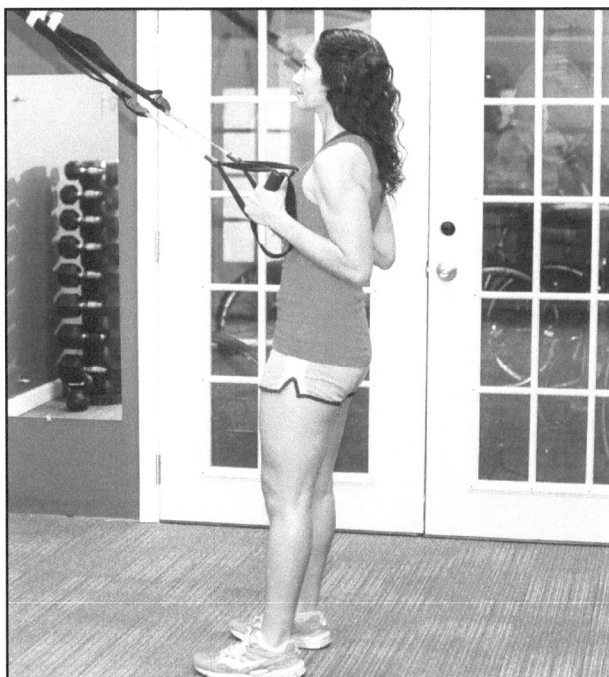

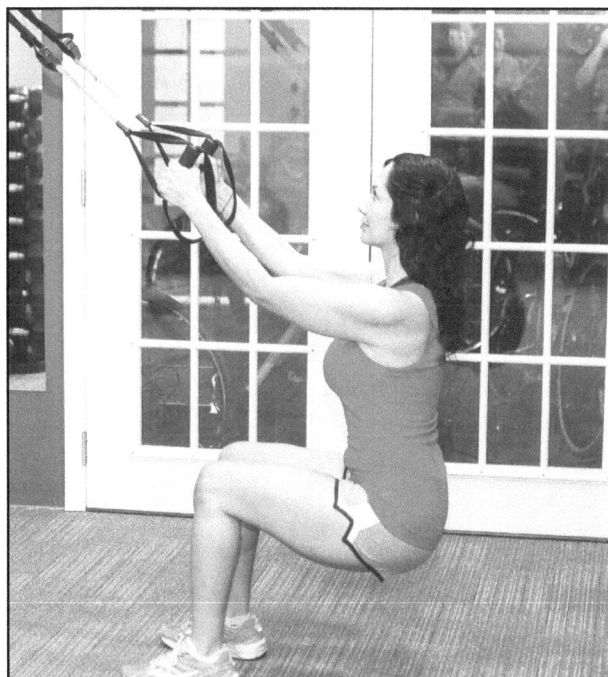

Squat to Reverse Fly

These two movements performed together will result in working many muscle groups at the same time. The reverse fly movement will help your posture, and adding the squat at the same time will get the entire chain of muscles in your back and torso working together.

Primary Focus: Rear shoulders and legs.

Secondary Focus: Back and torso, which stabilizes your position.

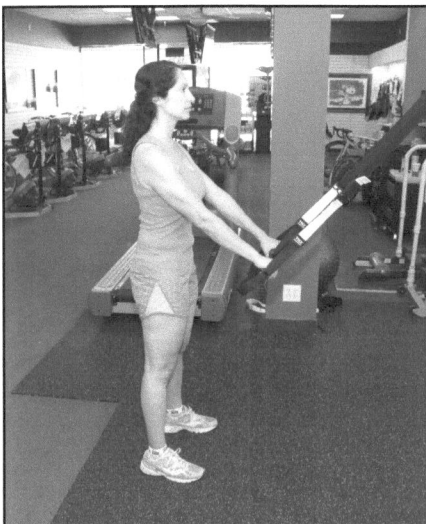

Setup: Straps fully extended.

1. Facing the anchor, with a slightly wider than shoulder-width stance, hold the straps with your arms extended in front of you.

2. While keeping your arms straight, sit down into the squat. Go down as low as you feel comfortable with.

3. At the bottom, push back up, and when you get close to the top of the movement, immediately move your arms out to the side until they are in line with your shoulders.

Tips and Progressions:

- Get into an amount of lean that will load the desired amount of weight onto the reserve fly movement. You will still be leaning back to some extent during the squat, but that's OK.

- Keep the movement controlled, and don't use momentum to swing you back up from the squat. Make your legs and hips do the work.

- This move is a terrific addition to a workout if you are short on time, or looking to add a cardio component to get your heart rate up and burn more calories in less time.

Starting Position   **Finishing Position**

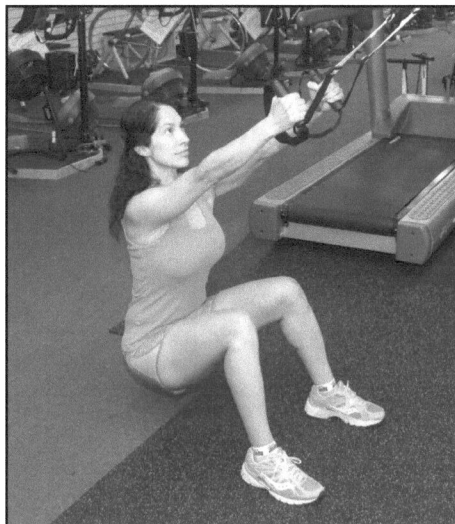

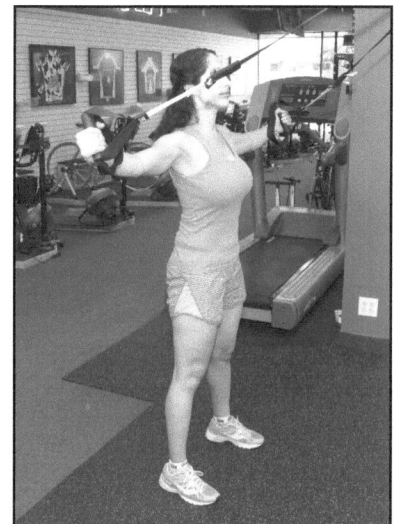

Run in Place

A great high-knee drill for runners and walkers that will help improve knee lift, forward lean, and stride turnover. It will also get your heart pumping and blood moving.

Primary Focus: Legs and hip flexors.

Secondary Focus: Calves and core as well as cardio.

Setup: Straps fully extended.

1. Face away with the straps underneath your arms. Lean forward into the straps. It's OK if your heels come off the ground when you are leaning forward, but your body should stay straight like a board.

2. Start by essentially jogging in place with small but frequent steps while maintaining forward lean.

3. Increase both the speed of your foot turnover and how high you are lifting your knees as you get comfortable with the movement.

Tips and Progressions:

• Keep good torso position and your head and eyes looking forward during the movement. This will help maintain good alignment and posture.

• You adjust the intensity level by both how fast you are running, as well as how high you are lifting your knees.

• Adds a great cardio component to a routine.

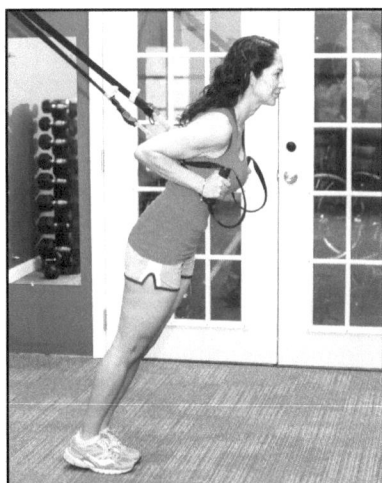

Starting Position   **Finishing Positions with Alternating Sides**

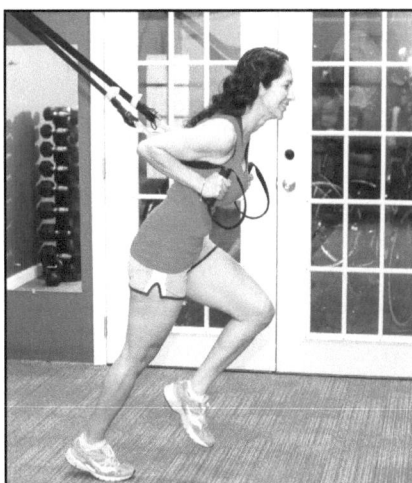

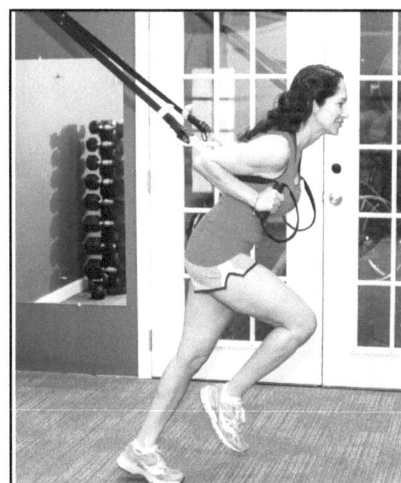

Streamline Squat

A good movement for both hip strength and upper body posture. It challenges the mobility and strength of the muscles in the upper torso and shoulders, while the lower body is moving.

Primary Focus: Legs, upper torso.

Secondary Focus: Core and lower back, to hold the arm overhead position during the squat.

Setup: Straps fully extended, handles in single-handle mode.

Starting Position

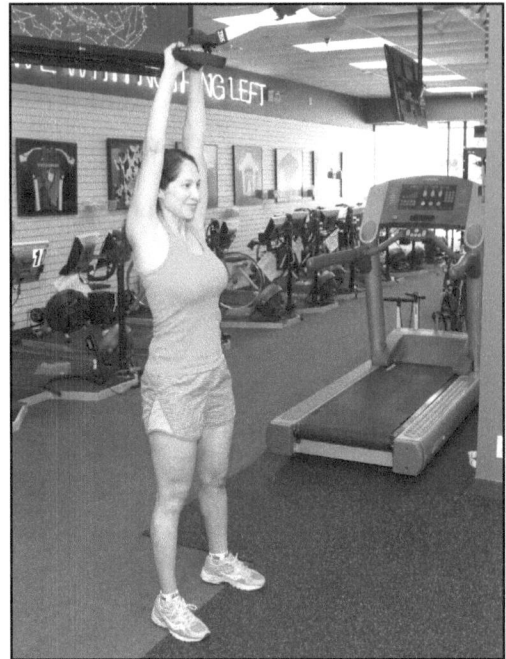

1. Face the anchor with a shoulder-width stance, holding one handle with both hands.

2. Extend your arms with the handle straight up over your head. Squeeze the arms together as if you are streamlining yourself in the pool while swimming or diving.

3. Hold this upper-body position, and then sit your hips down into a squat. Keep your arms extended and straight over your head while maintaining an upright torso. Go down as low as you feel comfortable with.

4. When you get to the lowest point in your squat, push yourself back up with your legs and hips, exhaling as you do so.

Note: Keep the muscles in your back and shoulders working to keep your arms overhead the whole time.

Finishing Position

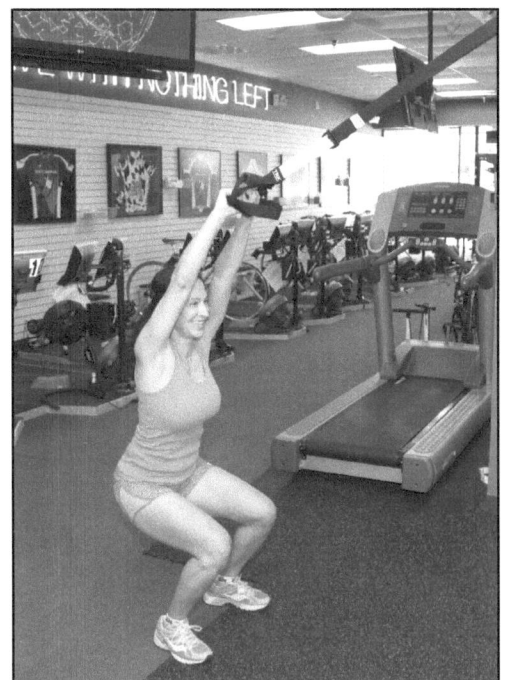

Tips and Progressions:

- Proper execution of this movement requires optimal mobility and strength of the hips, legs, and upper body. Those who are tight in the shoulders and upper torso have difficultly performing this movement. If this sounds like you, limit your squat to a shallow depth, and add some rotational stretches to help give you more range of motion.

- The depth of the squat also depends on your fitness level and comfort level. If you're just starting out or have any knee or hip issues, begin with a shallower squat. Squat deeper as you are able.

Ski Jumps Plyometric

This movement works to develop explosive power and quickness. The impact created by hopping will also help develop and maintain strong bones.

Primary Focus: Legs and calves.

Secondary Focus: Cardio—this one will get your heart pumping.

Setup: Straps fully extended.

1. Face inward with a shoulder-width stance, holding one strap in each hand.

2. Keeping your feet close to each other, perform side-to-side hops over the center line.

3. Adjust the level of intensity by increasing the speed of the hops, increasing the lateral distance of the jumps, or both. Maintain good posture throughout the set.

Tips and Progressions:

* You can mark your center line with tape to give you a visual aid or just use an imaginary one.

* Progress to jumping farther out to each side or higher up as you get more fit.

* Use either repetitions (e.g., set of 20 hops), or time (e.g., set of thirty seconds) to structure this exercise into your routine.

Starting Position

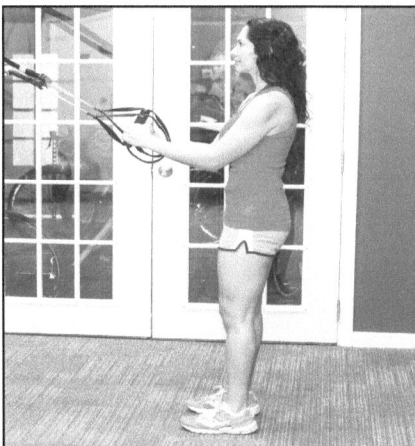

Finishing Positions/Alternate Sides

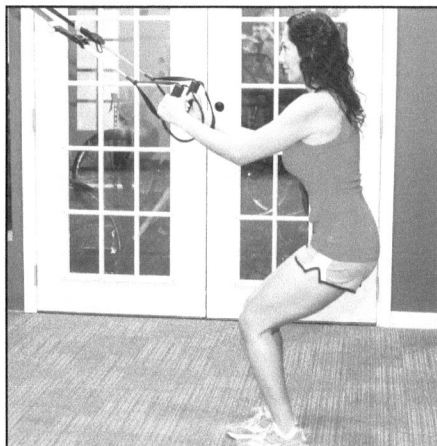

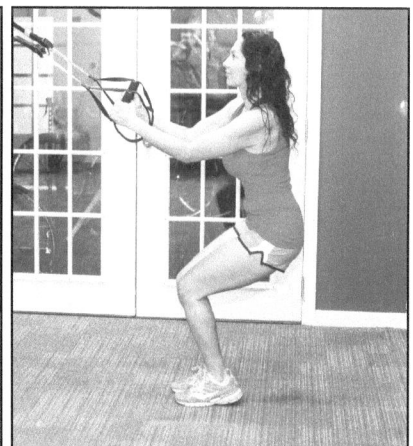

Mountain Climbers (Hands Suspended)

This will increase the strength and stability of the core, single-leg stance, and upward drive of the knee. Great for posture and overall mechanics of walking and running. The supporting (non-moving) leg learns to remain in proper alignment as the knee is driven upward in the opposite leg. The core is working to maintain the body in a static position as this is happening. The movement benefits both parts of the stride. One leg is working on strength and mobility of the hip, and the other is working on stability of the single-leg stance.

Primary Focus: Legs and hips.

Secondary Focus: Cardio.

Setup: Straps fully extended.

1. Facing away, get into a forward lean with your arms fully extended and supporting you on the straps. Your body should be leaning but straight like a board.

2. Maintaining your straight body, drive the knee of one leg upward toward your chest, while maintaining the alignment of the supporting leg.

3. Bring the leg back down to return to the start position, and switch legs. Alternate legs as if you are marching.

Note: Find the amount of lean that is most appropriate for you.

Tips and Progressions:

- To make this one harder, step back and increase the lean. To make it easier, step forward to decrease the lean.

- This one is about maintaining proper alignment as you alternate legs. Pay attention to possible asymmetries in your body. Do you feel one side is easier? If so, reduce the lean until both sides can be worked with proper form. Progress at the level of the weakest area.

Starting Position	**Finishing Position/Alternate Sides**

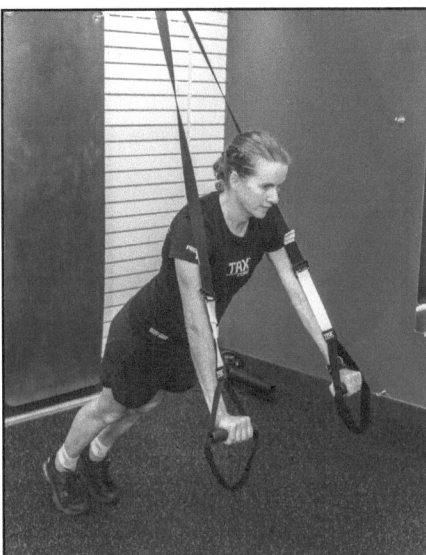

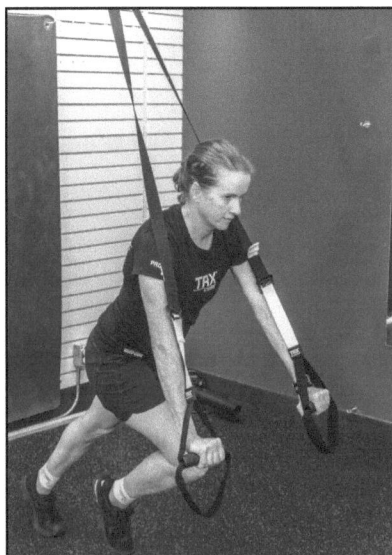

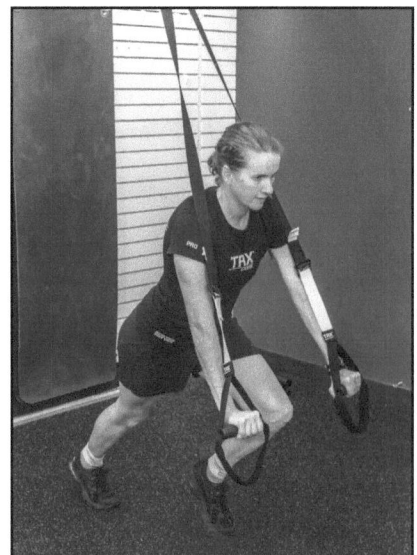

Suspended Get-Up

This is a great all-purpose, foundational movement that combines three movements into one exercise. It will get your heart rate up as well, and if you're short on time, it will give you a lot of bang for your buck!

Primary Focus: Legs, back, and arms.

Secondary Focus: Core.

Setup: Straps fully extended.

1. Sit on the floor facing in and holding the straps. The straps should have tension on them at this point. Extend one leg straight in front of you with the other leg bent at the knee.

2. Start the movement by pushing through the hip of the bent leg while simultaneously pulling yourself with your arms. Keep good posture (shoulders back, head looking forward) while making the ascent.

3. When you reach the top, your feet will be together. Immediately continue into a triceps press down, straightening the arms until they are fully extended and at your side.

4. To descend back to the starting position on the floor, simply perform the movement in reverse. Perform consecutive repetitions on one side, then switch legs.

Tips and Progressions:

- This is an excellent full-body movement that requires aspects of stability, strength, and mobility. It will get your heart pumping and burn tons of calories as well!

- This movement combines a single-leg squat, row, and triceps extension movement all in one.

- Start this one by performing the reps slowly, and master the form. Progress by performing more reps consecutively, and add a little speed. Don't cut range of motion short at either end. Make sure you finish the movement.

Starting Position   **Finishing Position**

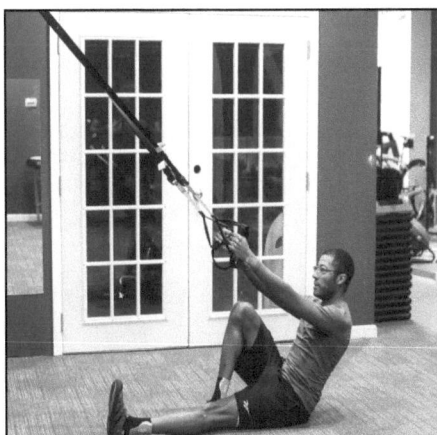

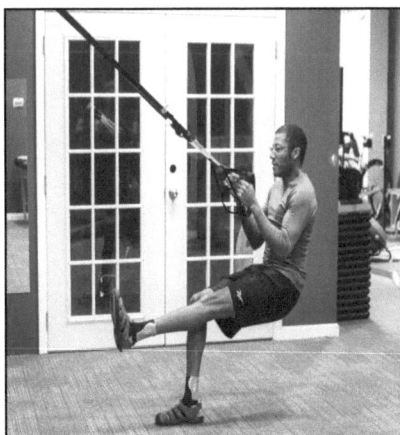

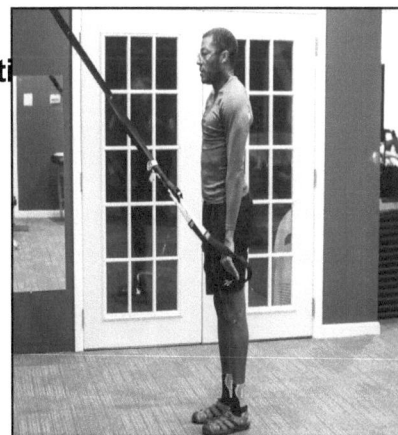

Overhead Squat Intermediate and Advanced

This is a challenging movement that requires optimum strength, stability, and mobility throughout the ankles, hips, torso, and shoulders. This movement develops and maintains a strong and solid movement foundation that will support all demands of strength and endurance training and activity.

Primary Focus: Legs, hips, upper torso.

Secondary Focus: Arms, to keep the straps overhead.

Setup: Straps fully extended.

Starting Position

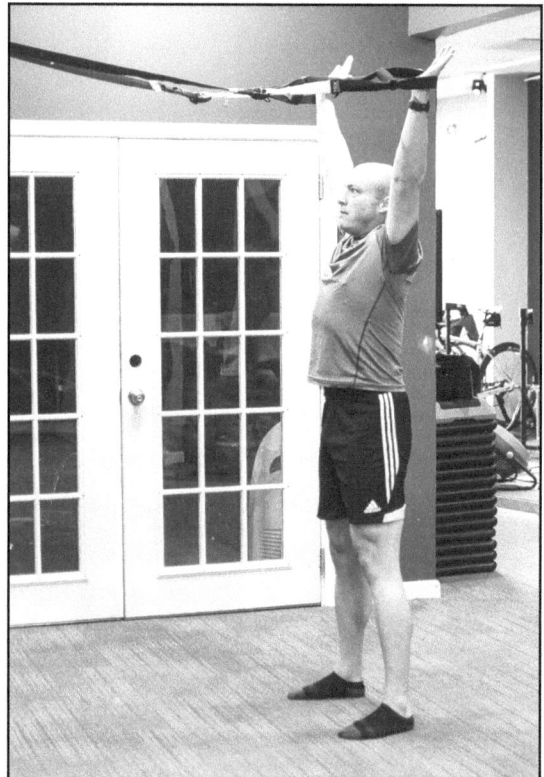

1. Facing the anchor, with a shoulder-width stance. Place your hands in the straps with your fingers extended, the backs of your hands pressing into the foot cradles, and arms extended straight above your head.

2. Drop your hips down into your squat while keeping your arms extended straight above your head, applying light pressure on the straps with the back of your hands. Descend below parallel if able to do so while maintaining form.

3. Immediately stand back up by pushing though the legs and hips while maintaining the arms overhead.

Note: Keep your torso vertical and knees and hands directly over your feet during the squat. Your arms should not come forward, and your knees should not extend in front of your toes.

Finishing Position

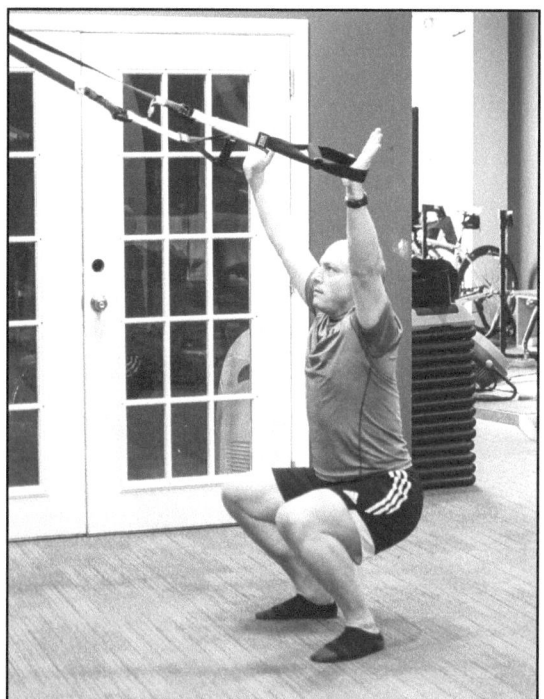

Tips and Progressions:

- Inadequate mobility or stability in any area of your body may prevent you from achieving ideal form in this movement. If this sounds like you, focus on some flexibility work of both upper and lower body, and work on the squat and the overhead arm extension separately until you get to a point you can successfully maintain form.

- If you experience knee, hip, or shoulder pain during this movement, stop immediately.

Squat-Press Jump Plyometric

This is a full-body explosive movement that will develop strength and power in the large muscles of the legs and hips. It will train the muscles how to fire more fibers faster. This will increase the ability to generate more power in cycling, running, and all other active endeavors. The impact and high force of the jump is great for developing strong bones.

Primary Focus: Legs and hips.

Secondary Focus: Cardio.

Setup: Straps mid-length to fully extended.

1. Facing away, holding the straps at shoulder level with a shoulder-width stance.

2. Drop your hips and descend into a squat, keeping your arms in the same position.

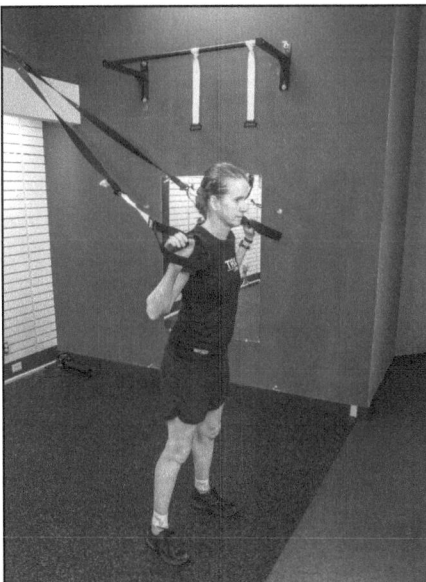

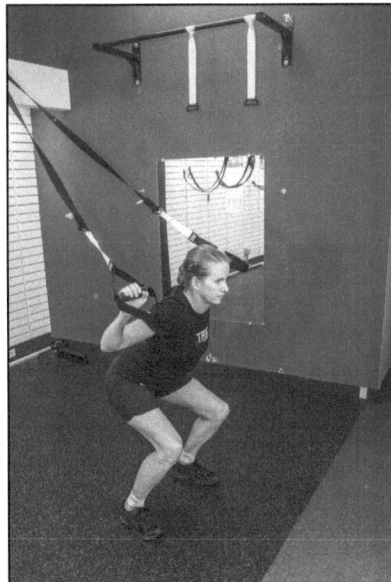

3. When you reach the bottom, explode upward while simultaneously pressing your arms up.

Tips and Progressions:

- Descending lower into the squat will increase the range of motion and increase the difficulty.

- Catch some air. Try to get as far off the ground as possible.

- Keep the transition time as short as possible. As you reach the bottom of the movement, explode back up as quickly as possible.

Starting Position   **Finishing Position**

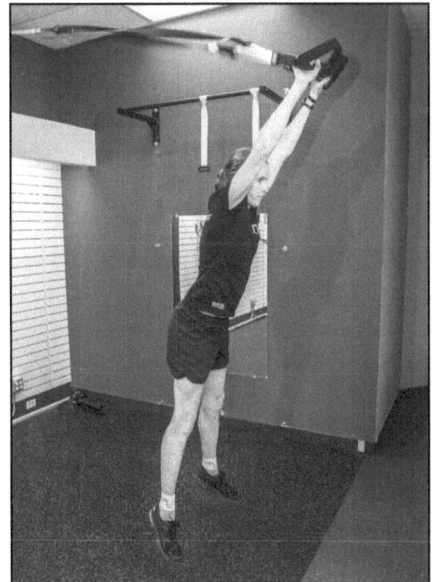

Burpee Intermediate and Advanced

This is a challenging, all-purpose movement that works the entire body.

Primary Focus: Legs, core, and upper body.

Secondary Focus: Cardio.

No equipment needed

1. From a standing position, bend down until your hands are on the floor.

2. Kick both legs out behind you until you are in a straight-arm plank position.

3. Immediately pull your legs back up underneath you at the same time in a strong movement.

4. Push off the ground with your hands, and stand up through your legs to return to the starting position. Repeat for targeted repetitions or time.

Note: Don't cut the range of motion short on either end. Extend the legs all the way out, and return to a vertical standing position each time.

Tips and Progressions:

- To progress the movement, add a push-up at the bottom, a squat jump on top, or both!

Starting and Finishing Position

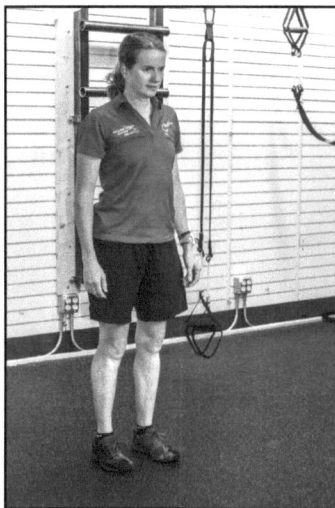

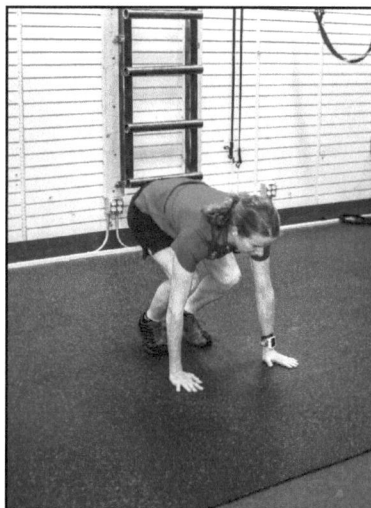

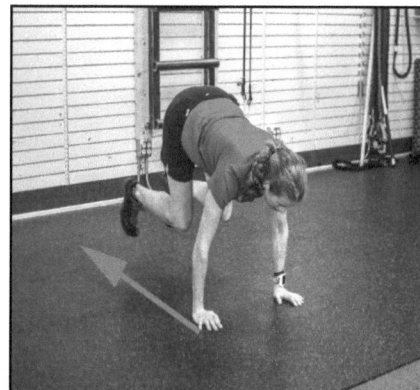

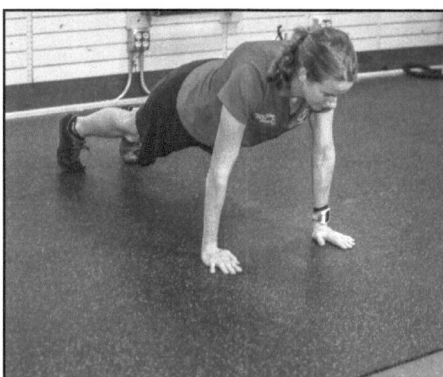

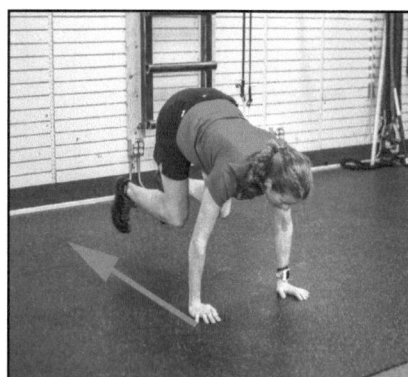

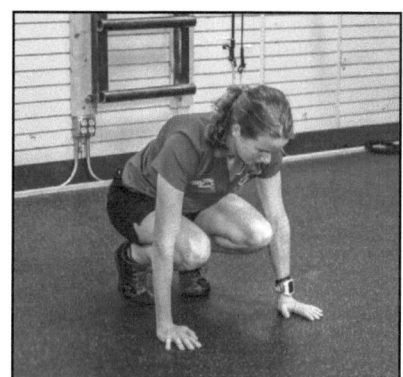

Suspended Burpee Intermediate and Advanced

This movement gives you a lot of bang for your buck. It's a challenging total-body movement that requires all-purpose strength, stability, and mobility.

Primary Focus: Supporting leg and arms.

Secondary Focus: Everything. The transition between the standing and floor position works the entire movement chain.

Setup: Straps fully extended and approximately six inches off the ground.

1. Start by facing outward, standing on one leg with your other foot suspended in both cradles.

2. To start the movement, push the suspended leg back behind you as you lower your upper body to the ground until your hands are on the ground in front of you. At this point, your supporting leg will still be underneath you with the knee bent.

3. Extend the bent leg behind you until that foot is next to the suspended foot. Your arms are now supporting your upper torso (as if you were going to do a push-up). Your body should be straight like a board.

4. To get back up, drive the unsuspended knee forward and back underneath you while keeping the suspended leg extended behind you. Now stand back up by returning your torso to upright as you push back through the front leg.

Tips and Progressions:

- This exercise is about quality, not quantity. Use time or repetitions as a target goal for your sets, but don't get sloppy. If you feel you're losing your perfect form because of fatigue, stop.

- Want even more? Add a push-up movement to the bottom of each repetition.

Starting Position

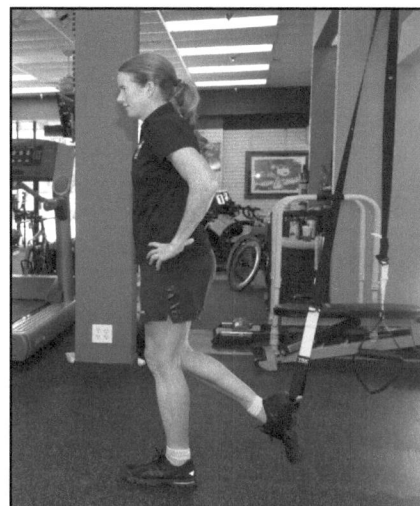

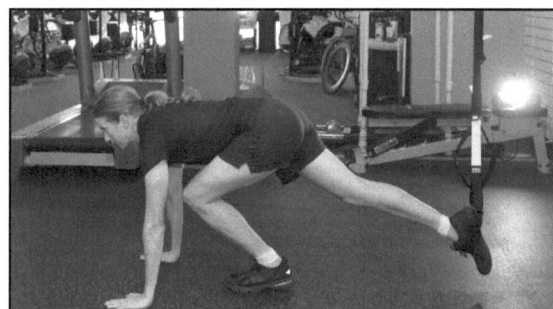

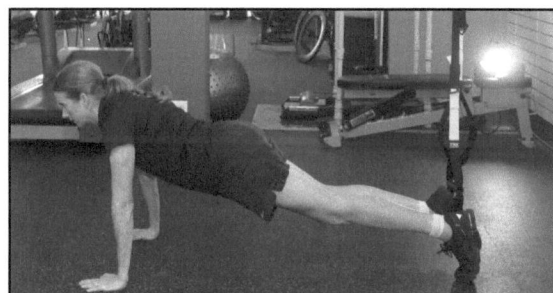

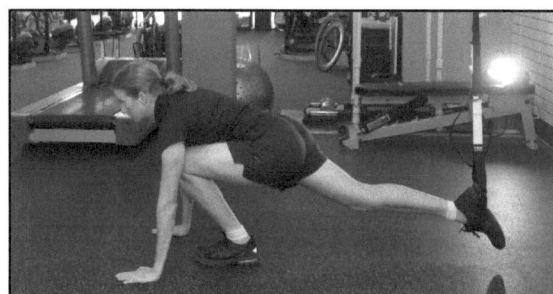

Finishing Position (see starting position)

Spider-Man Push-Up Intermediate and Advanced

This is a great upper-body and core movement that also requires hip mobility and strength. The simultaneous extension of one leg, and hip flexion of the opposing leg, develops strength and a movement pattern that is relevant to the run stride. The upper-body pushing and core stabilizing will develop strength that will drive a strong swim stroke and hold a proper body position through fatigue and adverse elements.

Primary Focus: Arms and core.

Secondary Focus: Legs and hips.

Setup: Straps fully extended and approximately six inches off the ground.

1. Start on your hands and knees facing away from the straps with the toes of one foot in both cradles. Your hands should be a little wider than shoulder width, but at the same level as your shoulders.

2. Straighten both legs and push them back so you're supported by only your arms in front and the suspended leg. The free leg should still align with the suspended leg.

3. Now, go down into the push-up movement while at the same time pulling the knee of the free leg up toward your chest. Keep your body straight and in alignment as you do this leg movement.

4. Go down until your elbows are at least bent to ninety degrees, and then push back up as you extend the free leg back and move it back and in line with the suspended leg.

Tips and Progressions:

- Keep your form! Don't sacrifice form for repetitions. Think quality over quantity.

- Keep the suspended leg actively extended to help maintain alignment. You'll feel the muscles in the front of the leg working hard to hold your position.

Starting Position   **Finishing Position**

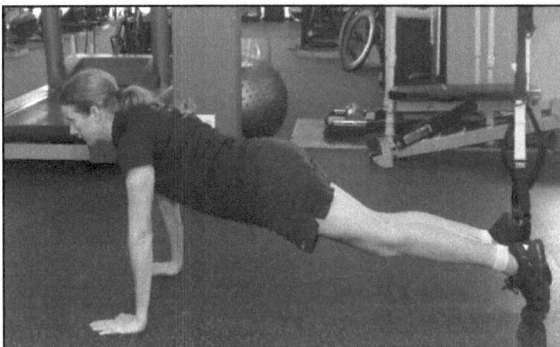

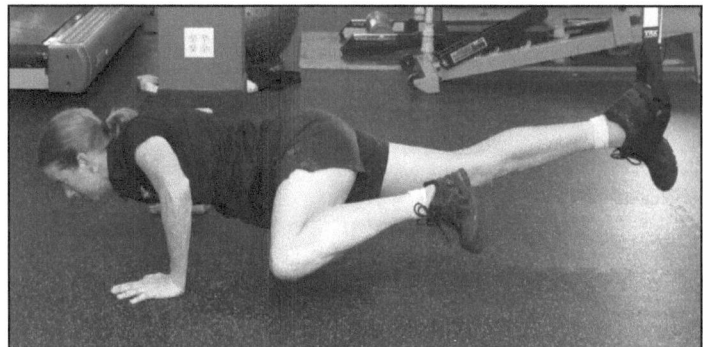

Shrimp Kick Intermediate and Advanced

This movement requires extreme strength and stability through the core and legs as well as strength and mobility of the hips. Core mechanics in all movements will benefit from the elevated level of core stability and hip mobility that this movement will build.

Primary Focus: Core and arms.

Secondary Focus: Legs and hip flexors.

Setup: Straps fully extended and approximately six inches off the ground.

1. Start on your hands and knees facing away from the straps, with just one foot in both cradles, leaving the other foot unsupported.

2. To start the movement, get into a fully suspended position by straightening both legs.

3. With a strong, solid movement, pull the unsupported leg underneath and across the body toward the opposite arm, and then back to the starting position. Repeat all repetitions on one side, then switch sides.

Note: At this point you, will have removed your knee support on the ground and are only connected with your arms on the ground and one leg in the cradle behind you. Stabilize through the core and arms as if you were going to perform a push-up.

Tips and Progressions:

- Keep the hands in line with the chest during the movement. The imaginary line between your hands should be directly under your chest (not your face).

- Focus on stabilizing your midsection, and don't allow the core to rotate as you pull the knee up and under your body.

- Build up to this one with some planks (p. 126) and then atomic crunches (p. 140) or pikes (p. 136). This movement requires a solid foundation of core strength, stability, and hip mobility.

Starting Position

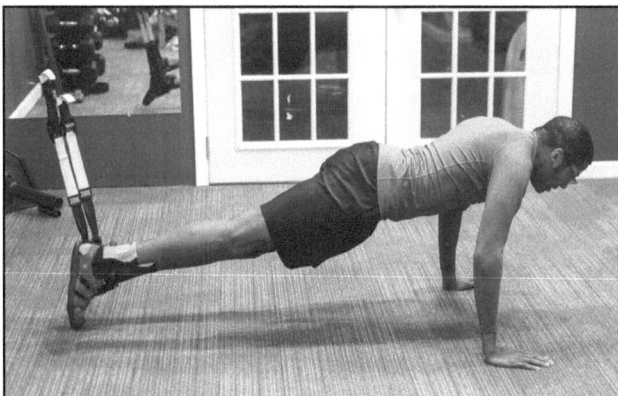

Finishing Position

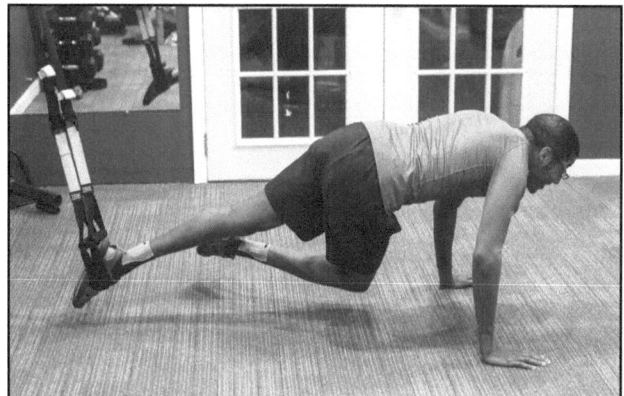

Bear Crawl Intermediate and Advanced

This is a great full-body and core movement.

Primary Focus: Core and the front of the upper body.

Secondary Focus: Hip flexors.

No equipment needed

1. Start in a straight-arm plank position.

2. In one movement bring one arm forward in front of you, along with the opposite leg and foot.

3. Repeat the same thing on the other side, bringing your body forward over your hands and legs as you go.

4. Perform for a targeted amount of repetitions for each side, time, or distance.

Note: Keep a straight body, aiming to get your advancing knee close to the trailing arm each time.

Tips and Progressions:

- To increase the challenge, increase time or distance or reverse the movement and go backward. Going forward and backward also works if you have a limited amount of space with which to work.

Starting and Finishing Position

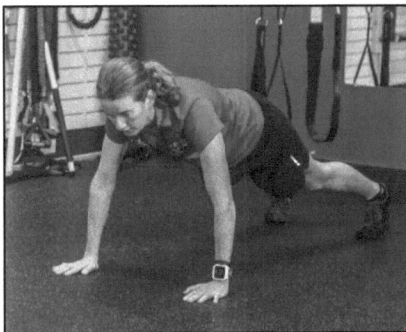

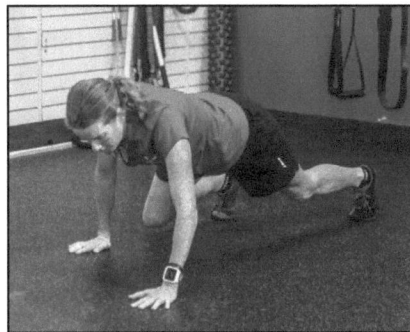

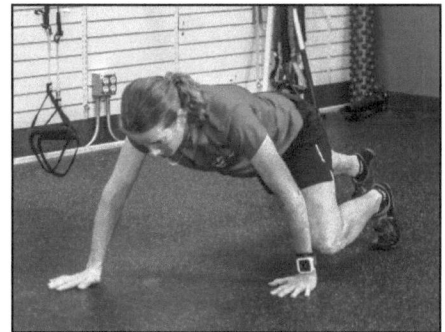

Full Get-Up Intermediate and Advanced

This is a fundamental movement that requires maximum mobility, stability, and strength through the entire chain of the body. Make sure you have mastered the half get-up (p. 130) before progressing to this one! Also, I suggest adding one progression step at a time. For example, if you're doing well with the half get-up (and have even added some weight), add the hip raise. Master that for a few workouts, and then go to half-kneeling. Going to the full get-up does not need to be the end goal. Do the progression that is most appropriate for you based on your level and abilities.

Primary Focus: Core and full body.

Secondary Focus: Cardio.

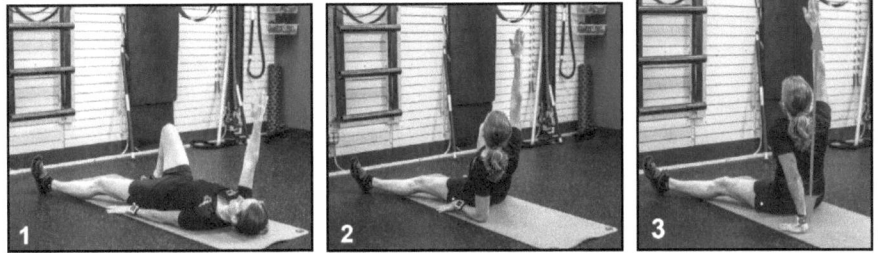

Half Get-Up

1. Lie on your back with one leg straight and the other bent. Point the arm on the bent-leg side straight up to the ceiling.

2. Start by lifting your shoulders off the ground as if you were doing a crunch, and continue ascending by pushing through the downed elbow. Keep your straight arm vertical and pointing at the ceiling the entire time!

3. Perform the desired amount of repetitions on one side. Rest, and then switch sides.

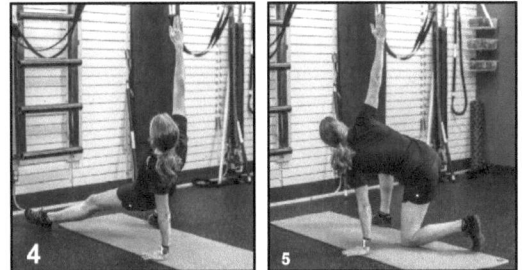

Full Get-Up

1. When you get to the top of the half get-up, push through your arm and both legs to bring your hips off the ground and in line with the rest of your body

2. From this position, bring your extended leg back underneath you so you're now positioned on that knee. That knee should now be close to your grounded hand. Continue to keep your other hand pointed straight up.

3. Only at this point, allow your grounded hand to come off the ground as you bring your torso upright and vertical over your hips.

4. Push through the front leg to a standing position with your feet together.

5. Reverse the movement to come back down to the floor. Repeat all repetitions on one side, and then switch sides.

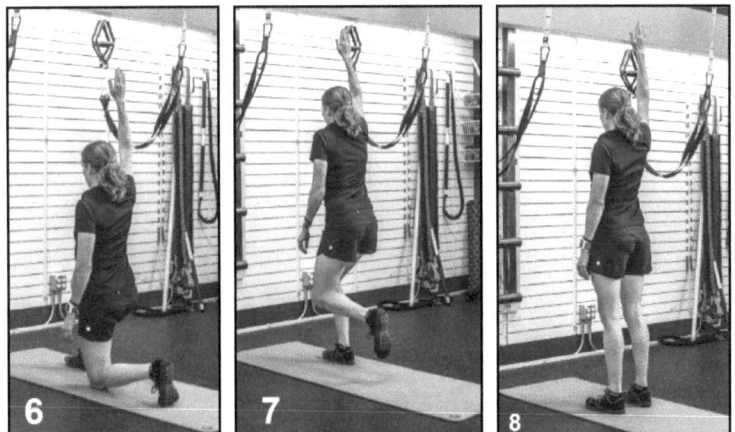

Note: Keep the extended arm straight up and hand pointed at the ceiling throughout the whole movement!

Tips and Progressions:

- You will probably want to reduce repetitions to the 4 to 6 range when doing the full get-up, as the movement involves much more than the half. You can also add weight in the hand of the extended arm to progress the full get-up to a harder level.

Lateral Box Jump Plyometric

This move will build power and control in the hips and legs. The impact will help increase resiliency, and is good for your bone density. The landing part of the movement will train your legs and hips to control and reverse the descent of your body mass. The transition will train your muscles to be able to quickly fire to accelerate your mass forward or upward again.

Primary Focus: Legs and hips.

Secondary Focus: Cardio.

Setup: Straps mid-length to fully extended.

1. Face the anchor, holding the straps. The step should be to the side of your feet.

2. Jump sideways up and onto the step while keeping the toes pointed forward.

3. Jump back down to the starting position.

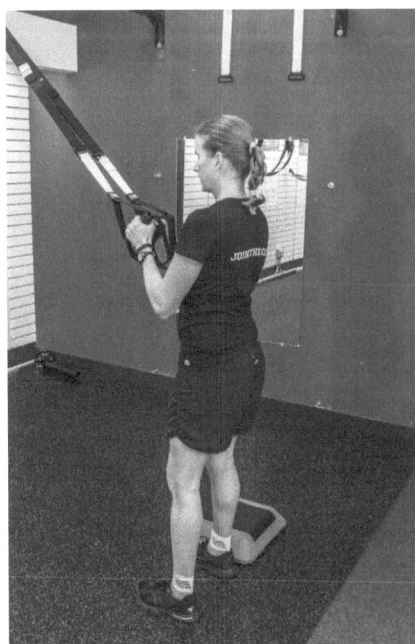

Note: Obtain control of your momentum on the step before jumping back off.

Tips and Progressions:

- The height of the step will determine the level of difficulty. If you have access to multiple levels, start low and progress to higher when ready.

- Make sure the step or box you are using is stable enough to handle your body weight as well as the sideways momentum of the jump.

Starting Position

Finishing Position

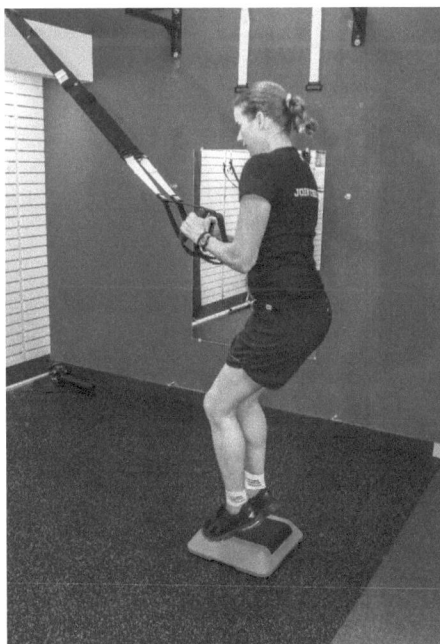

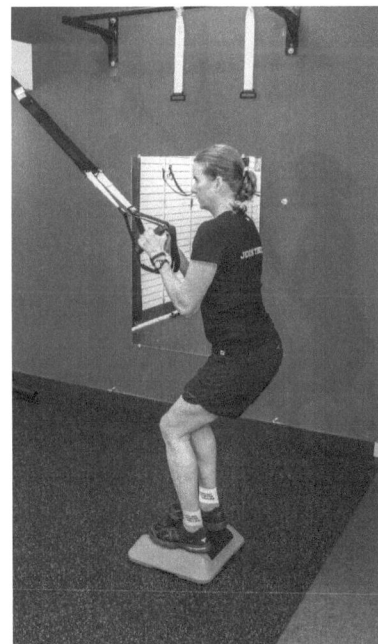

Lateral Cone Hop Intermediate and Advanced, Plyometric

This movement will build power and control in the hips and legs. The impact is great for your bone density. The landing part of the movement will train your legs and hips to control and reverse the descent of your body mass. The heel kick required to clear the cone is relevant to the heel kick in the run stride, if you're a runner.

Primary Focus: Legs and hips.

Secondary Focus: Cardio.

Setup: Straps mid-length to fully extended.

1. Face the anchor, holding the straps. The cone should be to the side of your feet.

2. Jump sideways over the cone. Kick your heels to your butt to help your feet clear the top of the cone.

3. When you land on the other side, quickly jump back over using the same technique.

Tips and Progressions:

- Keep the knees right over the feet during your time on the ground. A common form error is for the knees to cave in.

Starting Position   **Finishing Position**

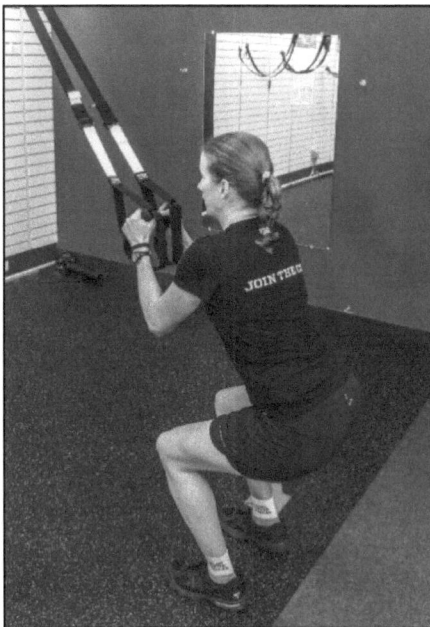

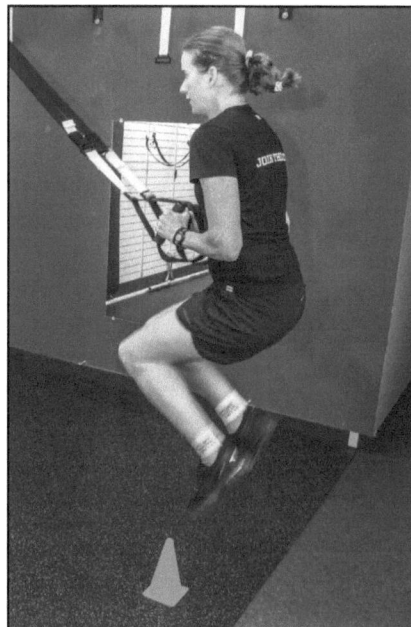

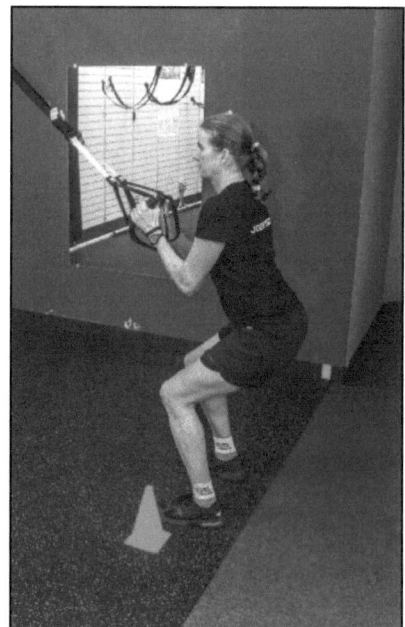

Mogul Plyometric

This will build power and control in the hips and legs. The impact will help increase resiliency and is good for your bone density. The landing part of the movement will train your legs and hips to maintain alignment and regain control against rotational forces.

Primary Focus: Legs and hips.

Secondary Focus: Cardio.

Setup: Straps mid-length to fully extended.

1. Face sideways, holding the straps.

2. Jump and rotate so you land facing in the opposite direction.

3. Reverse the jump back to the starting position. Make sure you obtain control of your rotational momentum before reversing the jump. Jump back down to the starting position.

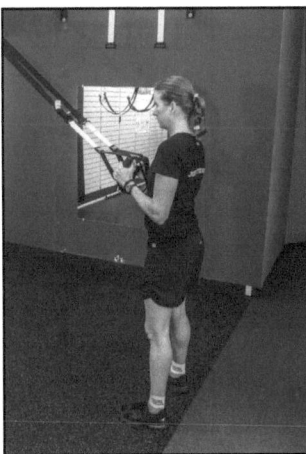

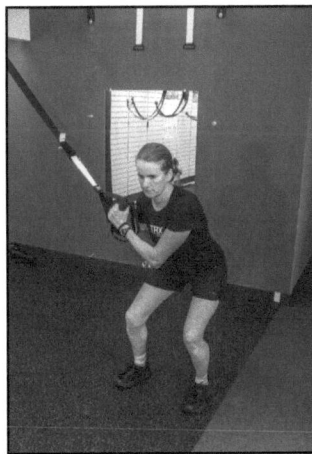

Note: Toes should be pointing 180 degrees from where they were at the start.

Tips and Progressions:

- The rotational forces of the jump may cause your knees and legs to want to torque that direction on landing. The keeps and hips should stay in alignment.

- The depth of the squat and height of the jump can be increased as you improve.

- You can do this one with or without a suspended trainer.

Starting Position   **Finishing Position**

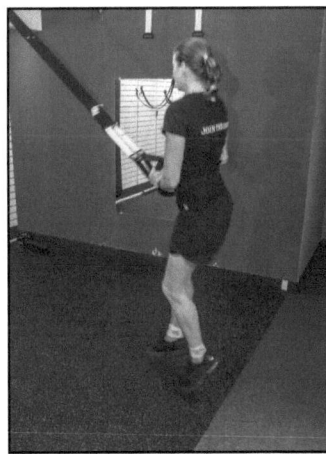

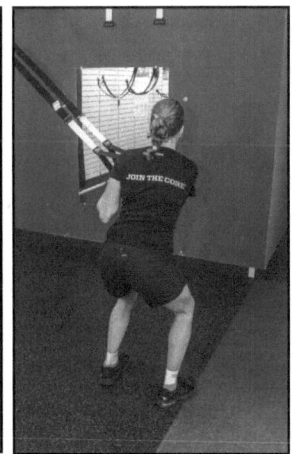

Single-Leg Lateral Box Jump Intermediate and Advanced, Plyometric

This movement will build power and control in the hips and legs. The impact will develop stability and strength when supporting yourself on one leg. Performing this in the single-leg stance will develop the ability to control momentum and maintain alignment in running or hiking, especially on adverse terrain. The impact is also good for your bone density.

Primary Focus: Legs and hips.

Secondary Focus: Cardio.

Setup: Straps mid-length to fully extended.

1. Face the anchor, holding the straps. The step should be to the side of your feet.

2. Get on one leg, and with this leg only, jump sideways up and onto the step while keeping the toes pointed forward.

3. Jump back down to the starting position, landing on the same single leg. Repeat all repetitions on one leg before switching.

Note: Obtain control of your momentum and balance on the step before jumping back off.

Tips and Progressions:

• It's OK to start this one with no height. Just jump to the side.

• The height of the step will determine the level of difficulty. If you have access to multiple levels, start low and progress to higher when ready.

• Make sure the step or box you are using is stable enough to handle your body weight, as well as the sideways momentum of the jump.

Starting Position   **Finishing Position**

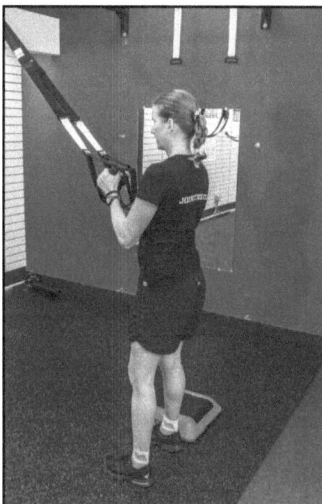

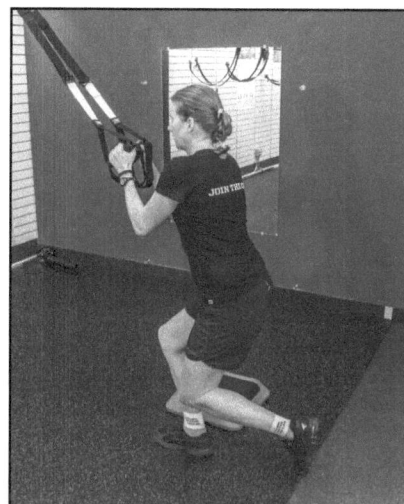

Chapter 15

Sample Workouts

The following section contains some sample workouts. Each workout goes with a corresponding section from earlier in the book. Use them to get started, and progress them when you're ready. Also, use them as templates as your fitness increases, and don't be afraid to replace movements to keep things interesting and challenging. You may do each workout in its entirety, or you may choose parts of any one workout to include in other workouts using other methods of training.

Foundation Workout Level 1

This program will help give you a solid foundation of general strength, stability, and better core engagement. Master this workout and you will become better conditioned to progress to more advanced suspension training workouts.

Frequency: Twice per week, in combination with additional endurance and flexibility training sessions.

Warm-Up

Exercise	Targeted Area	Intensity	Sets	Reps	Rest
Golf Rotation	Upper Torso	Easy to Moderate	2–3	15–20 each side	30 seconds
Squat Row	Legs and Torso	Easy to Moderate	2–3	15–20	30 seconds

Summary of Program

Exercise	Targeted Area	Intensity	Sets	Reps	Rest
Suspended Push-Ups	Chest and Shoulders	Moderate	2–3	15–20	30 seconds
Suspended Row	Back and Biceps	Moderate	2–3	15–20	for all
Split Squat	Legs and Hips	Moderate	2–3	15	or as
Plank	Core	Moderate	2–3	20–60 seconds	needed
Suspended Bicep Curl	Arms	Moderate	2–3	15	
Suspended Tricep Extension	Arms	Moderate	2–3	15	
Hip Hinge	Legs and Hips	Moderate	2–3	15	

Golf Rotation

1. Face the anchor with a shoulder-width stance, and hold the straps.

2. Keep one arm in place, and reach up and slightly behind you with the other arm, rotating your torso and looking in the same direction.

3. Hold for one to three seconds each side. Alternate sides.

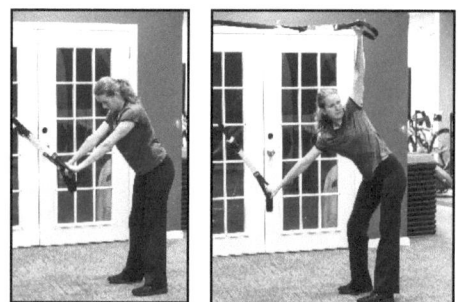

Squat Row

1. Facing the anchor, hold the straps, get into a shoulder-width stance, and lean back slightly on the straps.

2. Sit down into the squat while extending your arms.

3. Push yourself back up with your legs while also simultaneously pulling your upper body toward the straps.

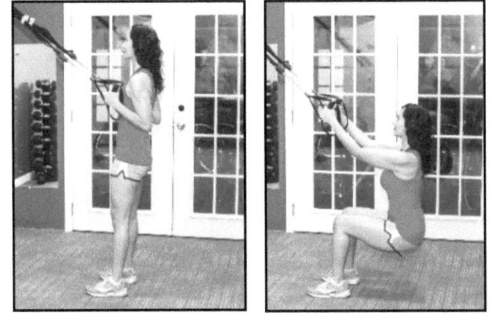

Suspended Push-Up

1. Facing away, hold the end of each strap in each hand, and get into a shoulder-width or slightly wider stance. Keep a straight body position from your head to your feet.

2. Allow your arms to bend, and lower your body until your elbows reach ninety degrees and are aligned with your shoulders.

3. Push yourself back up to the straight-arm position, exhaling as you do so.

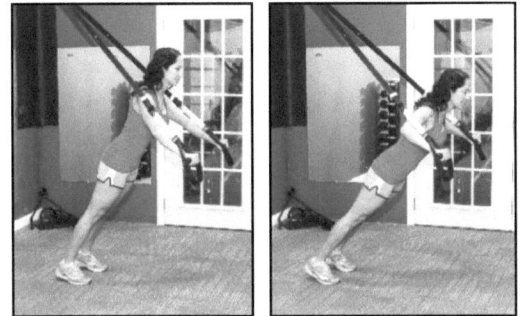

Row

1. Shorten the straps to mid-length, and face toward the anchor point. Straighten your arms and lean back.

2. Pull yourself up until your elbows are bent and at your side. Keep your body straight like a board.

3. Lower yourself back down by allowing the arms to straighten out again until you are back in the starting position.

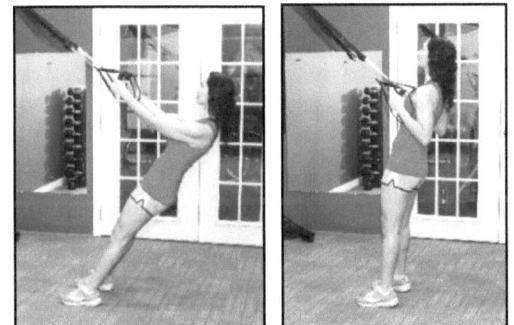

Split Squat

1. Face the anchor and hold the straps in front of you. Take a large step behind you with one leg, while keeping the other leg where it is.

2. Drop the back knee down toward the floor as low as you are comfortable doing. The knee of the front foot should stay directly over that foot.

3. Return to the starting position by pushing through your back toe and the front foot.

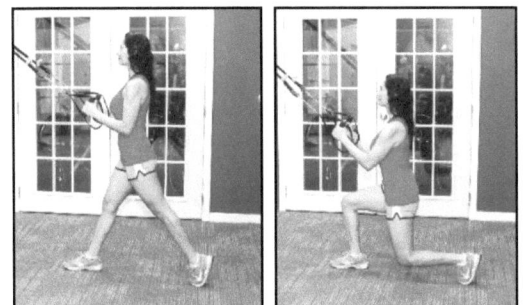

Plank

1. Raise your body up as one unit so you're making contact with the ground with only your forearms and toes. Your body should form a straight line from shoulders to ankles.

2. Engage your core by sucking your belly button into your spine.

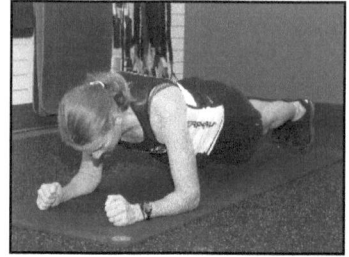

Bicep Curl

1. Face the anchor, holding the straps with your arms fully extended and parallel to the ground.

2. Bring your palms to your forehead, allowing the elbows to bend, and pulling your body up the straps until your elbows are bent to a ninety-degree angle.

3. Allow the arms to extend back to the starting position.

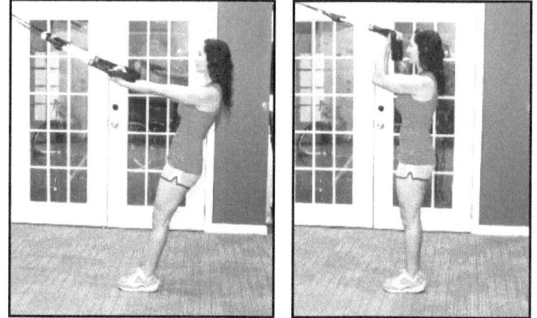

Triceps Extension

1. Facing away, hold the straps with your arms fully extended and parallel to the ground.

2. Start the movement by allowing your elbows to bend and your body to descend toward your hands.

3. Return to the starting position by straightening the arms and pushing the body back up and away from the hands.

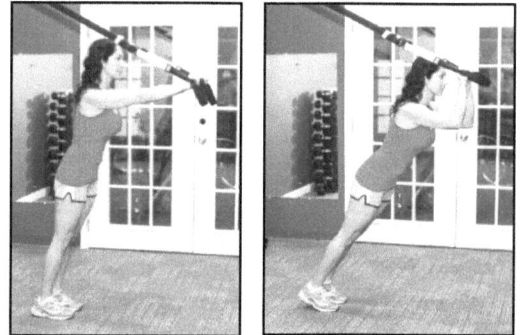

Hip Hinge

1. Facing the anchor, hold the straps with your arms extended in front of you.

2. Lift one leg and extend it behind you while bending forward from the waist (hinging at the hip), and pushing your arms out in front of you.

3. Return to the starting position with both feet on the ground again.

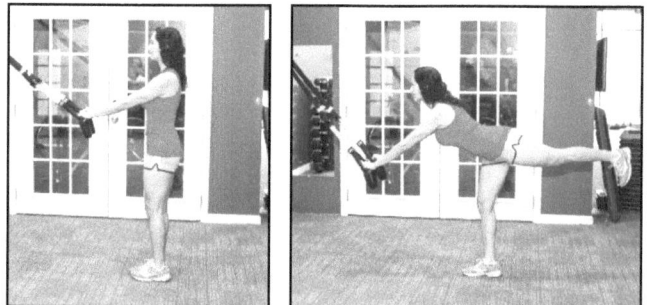

Foundation Workout Level 2

This program consists of more advanced movements than level 1, and movements that can also be progressed. The number of repetitions in some of the sets are lower because the resistance and difficulty of the movement is higher, which emphasizes strength development. If you're unable to perform one of the movements, step back to comparable movements in the level 1 workout, and continue to work on progressing that movement at that level.

Frequency: Twice per week, in combination with additional endurance and flexibility sessions.

Warm-Up

Exercise	Targeted Area	Intensity	Sets	Reps	Rest
Squat Press	Legs and Shoulders	Easy to Moderate	2–3	15 each side	30 seconds
Get-Ups	Total Body	Moderate	2–3	8 each side	30 seconds

Summary of Program

Exercise	Targeted Area	Intensity	Sets	Reps	Rest
Push-Ups (Feet Suspended)	Chest and Shoulders	Hard	2–3	10–15	30 seconds
Suspended Pull-Ups	Back and Biceps	Hard	2–3	10–15	for all
Side Plank	Core	Hard	2–3	15	or as
Sprinter Starts	Legs and Hips	Hard	2–3	20–60 seconds	needed
Reverse Flys	Upper Back	Hard		15	
Pike	Core	Hard		10–15	
Tall Kneeling Rollout	Core	Hard		10–15	

Squat Press

1. Face away from the anchor with a handle in each hand, and the straps on the outside of your arms.

2. Squat down with good form, as low as you are comfortable going.

3. Push back up with your legs and hips as you press your arms overhead.

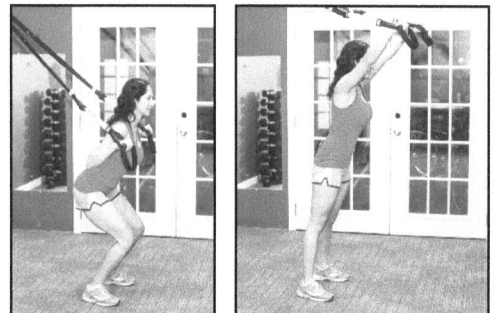

Suspended Get-Up

1. Start the movement by pushing through the hip of the bent leg, while simultaneously pulling yourself with your arms.

2. When you reach the top, immediately continue into a tricep press by pressing and extending the arms until they are straight and at your side, and your feet are together.

3. Descend back to the starting position on the floor by simply performing the movement in reverse.

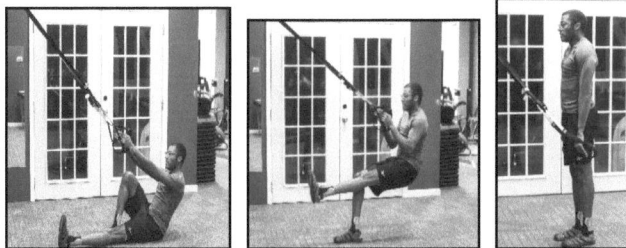

Push-Up (Feet Suspended)

1. Get your toes on the cradles and straighten your legs to get into a suspended straight-arm plank position. Go down until your elbows bend to approximately a ninety-degree angle.

2. At the bottom, push through the floor to raise your body back up to the starting position as one unit.

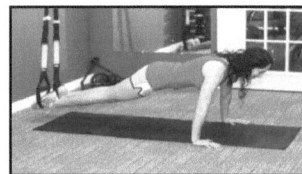

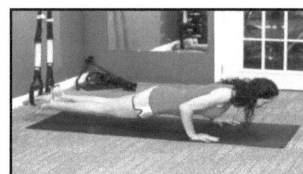

Suspended Pull-Up

1. Start by sitting on the floor with your knees bent directly underneath the suspended trainer. Hold the handles with your palms facing away from you.

2. Pull yourself straight up from the floor and until your chin is level with your hands. Think about pulling yourself over an imaginary bar.

3. Hold your position at the top for a second with good form, and then come back down in a slow, controlled movement.

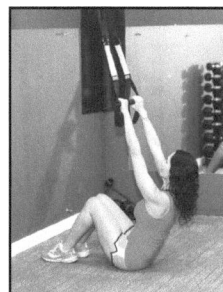

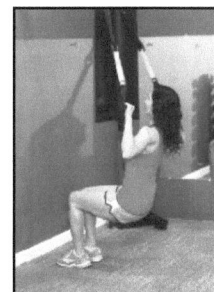

Suspended Side Plank

1. Start with your toes in the cradles and lying sideways this time. Your elbow should be directly underneath the shoulder, and the top leg should be forward.

2. Tighten the core and lift your hips off the floor with your body weight supported by the arm and shoulder and the feet in the cradles.

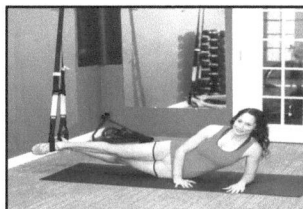

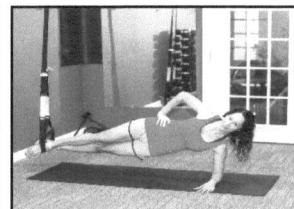

Sprinter Starts

1. Face away from the anchor with the straps underneath your arms, and lean forward into them. Take a large step back with one leg, allowing the front leg to bend.

2. Come back to the starting position by pushing back up through the front leg, and finish the movement by driving the knee of the back leg up and toward your chest. Alternate legs.

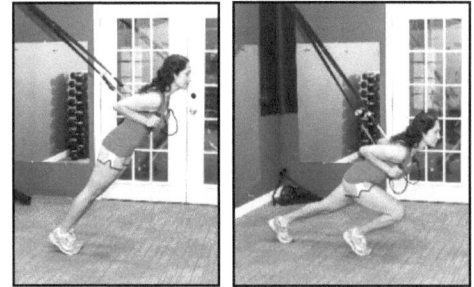

Reverse Fly

1. Face the anchor with your arms extended and a slight backward lean.

2. Keeping the arms straight, open up the arms and bring them back to extend out from your shoulders. This will bring your body forward.

3. Bring the arms back together to the front, maintaining arm extension and a straight body.

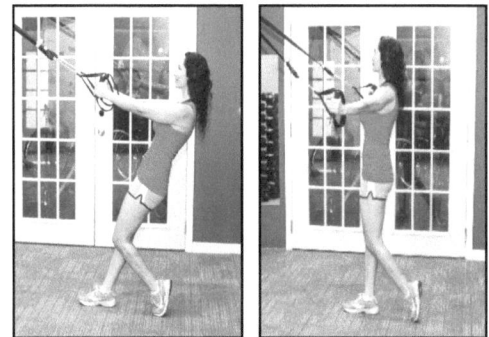

Pike

1. Face away from the suspended trainer on your hands and knees, with your toes in the cradles right underneath the anchor, and your hands underneath your shoulders. To get in starting position, straighten your legs, which is going to lift your knees off the ground.

2. Pull your legs toward your chest by driving your hips upward toward the ceiling.

3. At the top of the movement, pause and slowly go back down to the starting position.

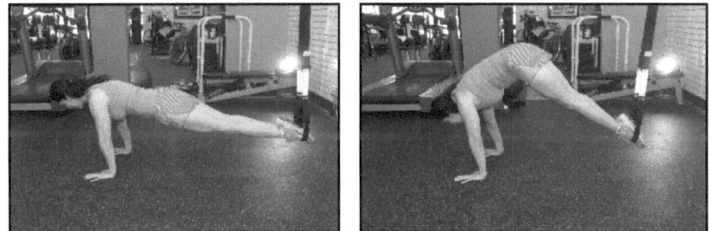

Tall Kneeling Rollout

1. Face the anchor, kneeling on both knees, torso upright, and holding the straps (place a pad, mat, or rolled-up towel under the knees for comfort).

2. Maintain good posture by making yourself tall, keeping shoulders relaxed, putting your chest out, and looking forward. Tighten the core, lean forward, and extend the arms out in front of you.

3. Return to the start by pulling up through both your hips and core and bringing the arms back toward the body.

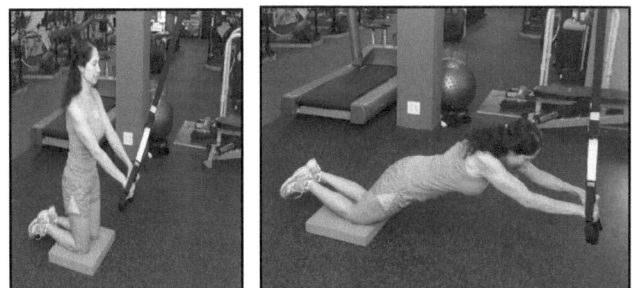

Cardio / Endurance / Fat-Burning Workout Level 1

This workout consists of movements that target the larger muscle groups and multiple muscle groups at the same time. The warm-up movements will loosen you up and get your blood moving, heart rate up, and prepare you for the main sets. Keep the resistances moderate to light to allow for quick transition between movements, with very short recovery times of zero to fifteen seconds. This will keep your heart rate up, and is great for calorie burning and increasing cardiovascular fitness and health.

First time through: It's OK to go a little slower and take a little more rest. As you get comfortable with the movements, increase the intensity. Do this by shortening the rest periods, increasing the resistance, and increasing the speed of the movements during the running, ski jumps, and the cardio sets.

Frequency: Twice per week, in combination with additional endurance and flexibility training sessions.

Warm-Up

Exercise	Targeted Area	Intensity	Sets	Reps	Rest
Mountain Climbers (Hands Suspended)	Full Body	Easy to Moderate	2–3	15–20 each side	30 seconds
Golf Rotation	Upper Torso	Easy to Moderate	2–3	10 each side	30 seconds

Circuit #1: Do the following circuit two to three times. Repeat each movement consecutively to complete one circuit.

Exercise	Targeted Area	Intensity	Sets	Time	Rest
Run in Place	Cardio	Moderate	1	30 seconds	0–15 seconds
Suspended Row	Back and Biceps	Moderate	1	30 seconds	0–15 seconds
Squat Press	All Body	Moderate	1	30 seconds	0–15 seconds
Cardio Activity (see list)	Cardio	Moderate	1	2 minutes	
Rest and Recover		Easy	1	1–2 minutes	

Take a three-to-five-minute rest and water break after the entire first circuit has been completed two to three times.

Circuit #2: Do the following circuit two to three times. Repeat each movement consecutively to complete one circuit.

Exercise	Targeted Area	Intensity	Sets	Reps	Rest
Suspended Push-Ups	Chest and Shoulders	Moderate	1	30 seconds	0–15 seconds
Ski Jumps	Cardio	Moderate	1	30 seconds	0–15 seconds
Squat Row	Legs and Back	Moderate	1	30 seconds	0–15 seconds
Cardio Activity (see list)	Legs and Hips	Moderate	1	3 minutes	
Rest and Recover		Easy	1	1–2 minutes	

Cooldown: Three-to-five-minute walk. Add stretches as needed if you have tight areas.

Mountain Climbers (Hands Suspended)

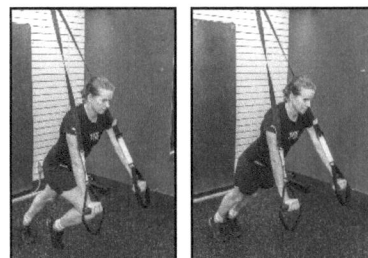

1. Face away from the anchor while leaning forward with your arms fully extended on the straps.

2. Keep a straight body. Drive the knee of one leg toward your chest while maintaining the position of the supporting leg.

3. Bring the leg back down to return to the start position, and switch legs. Alternate legs as if you are marching.

Golf Rotation

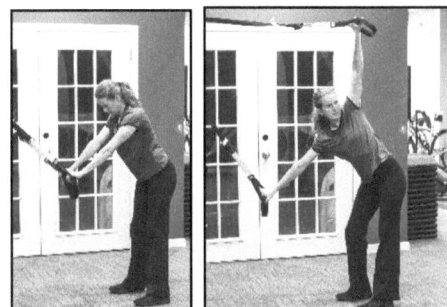

1. Facing the anchor, hold the straps, and get into a shoulder-width stance.

2. Keep one arm in place, and reach up and slightly behind you with the other arm. Look toward the elevated arm.

3. Hold for one second each side. Alternate sides.

Run in Place

1. Face away with the straps underneath your arms this time, and lean forward into the straps.

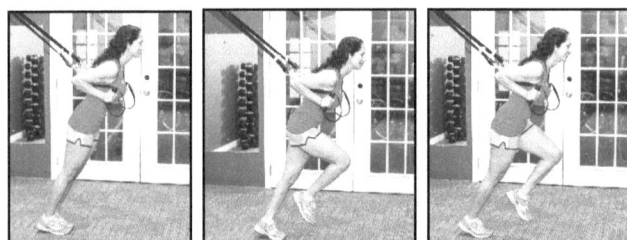

2. Start by jogging in place with small but frequent steps while maintaining forward lean.

3. Increase both the speed of your foot turnover and the height you're lifting your knees as you get comfortable with the movement.

Note: You may do this movement by using the straps or freestanding. Using the straps allows for forward lean, and freestanding allows for more arm movement. Both are good.

Row

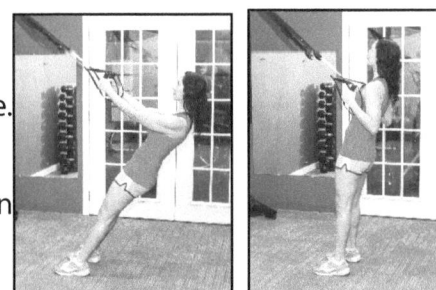

1. Face the anchor, straighten your arms, and lean back.

2. Pull yourself up until your elbows are bent and at your side. Keep your body straight like a board.

3. Lower yourself back down by allowing the arms to straighten out again until you are back in the starting position.

Squat Press

1. Face away from the anchor with a handle in each hand and the straps on the outside of your arms.

2. Drop your hips to the floor behind you while keeping your arms where they are.

3. Push back up with your legs and hips, and press your arms overhead.

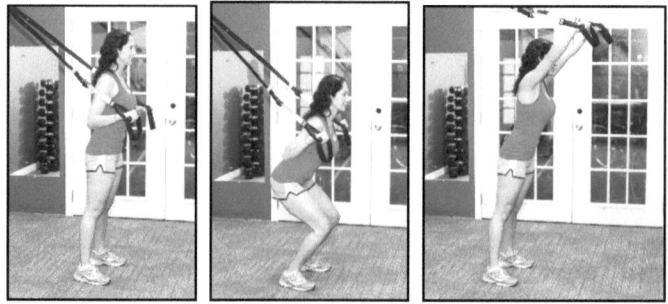

Cardio Activities

Choose from the following based on space and equipment available:

- Walk up stairs

- Power walk

- Jog one minute out and then back

- Jog in place

- Stationary machine such as treadmill, bike, rowing machine, or elliptical

- Side shuffle back and forth

- Jumping jacks

- Knee to elbows

- A dynamic stretch movement that challenges you

- Step aerobics

- Dance or Zumba

- Jump rope

- Kickbox or work on a punching bag

The goal is to challenge your cardiovascular system and get your heart rate up for the time assigned. Pick something you enjoy, and don't be afraid to mix it up!

Suspended Push-Up

1. Face away from the anchor with arms extended, holding the straps.

2. Allow your arms to bend, and lower your body until your elbows reach ninety degrees and are aligned with your shoulders.

3. Push yourself back up to the straight-arm position, exhaling as you do so, and maintain a tight core and straight body from head to ankle.

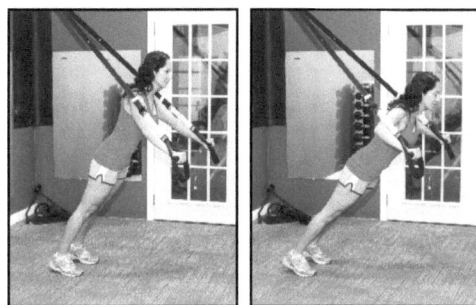

Ski Jumps

1. Face the anchor with a shoulder-width stance, holding one strap one in each hand.

2. Keeping your feet close to each other, perform side-to-side hops over the center line.

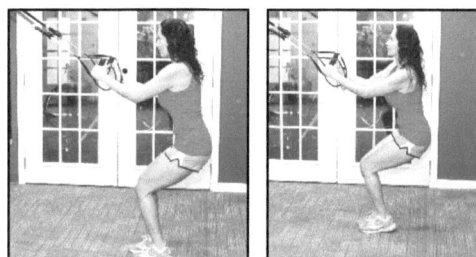

Squat Row

1. Face the anchor, hold the straps with elbows at your side, and lean back slightly.

2. Keeping the arms relaxed and shoulders back, sit down into the squat while extending your arms.

3. Push yourself back up with your legs while simultaneously pulling your upper body toward the straps. Your finish position should be standing tall with your elbows bent at your side.

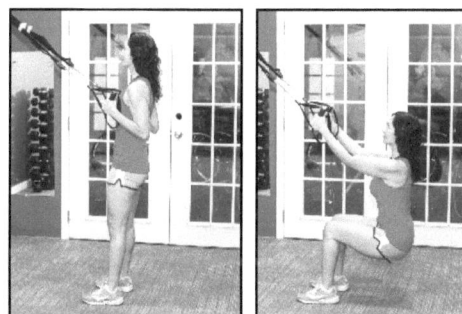

Cardio / Endurance / Fat-Burning Workout Level 2

This workout consists of movements that target multiple muscle groups at the same time as well as large muscle groups. It follows a similar format as the level 1 workout. However, it is assumed you're of an intermediate to advanced fitness level. The movements and cardio suggestions are more advanced and require a higher level of strength and stability. The number of sets is also increased, making it a workout that's both higher intensity and of longer duration. Keep the resistances moderate to allow for quick transition between movements, with very short recovery times of zero to fifteen seconds. This will keep your heart rate up, and is great for calorie burning and increasing cardiovascular fitness and health.

First time through: It's OK to go a little slower and take a little more rest. As you get comfortable with the movements, increase the intensity by shortening the rest periods, increasing the resistance on the suspended movements, and increasing the intensity of the cardio sets.

Warm-Up

Exercise	Targeted Area	Intensity	Sets	Reps	Rest
Streamline Squat	Full Body	Easy to Moderate	2–3	15 each side	30 seconds
Ski Jumps	Legs, Calves, Cardio	Easy to Moderate	2–3	45 seconds	30 seconds

Circuit #1: Do the following circuit three to four times. Repeat each movement consecutively to complete one circuit.

Exercise	Targeted Area	Intensity	Sets	Time	Rest
Push-Ups (Feet Suspended)	Core and Upper Body	Moderate	1	30 seconds	0–15 seconds
Squat to Reverse Fly	Legs and Back	Moderate	1	30 seconds	0–15 seconds
Lunge to Fly	Legs and Chest	Moderate	1	30 seconds	0–15 seconds
Cardio Activity (see list)	Cardio	Moderate	1	3 minutes	
Rest and Recover		Easy	1	1 minute	

Take a three-to-five-minute rest and water break after the entire first circuit has been completed two to three times.

Circuit #2: Do the following circuit three to four times. Repeat each movement consecutively to complete one circuit.

Exercise	Targeted Area	Intensity	Sets	Reps	Rest
Suspended Get-Ups	All Body	Moderate	1	30 seconds	0–15 seconds
Skaters	Cardio	Moderate	1	30 seconds	0–15 seconds
Squat-Press Jumps	Upper Torso and Arms	Moderate	1	30 seconds	0–15 seconds
Cardio Activity (see list)	Cardio	Moderate	1	3 minutes	
Rest and Recover			1	1 minute	

Cooldown: Three-to-five-minute walk. Add stretches if you have tight areas as needed.

Streamline Squat

1. Face the anchor with a shoulder-width stance, holding one handle with both hands and your arms extended overhead.

2. Squeeze the arms together as if you are trying to squeeze your ears with your arms. Go down as low as you are comfortably able into a squat.

3. When you get to the lowest point in your squat, push yourself back up with your legs and hips, exhaling as you do so.

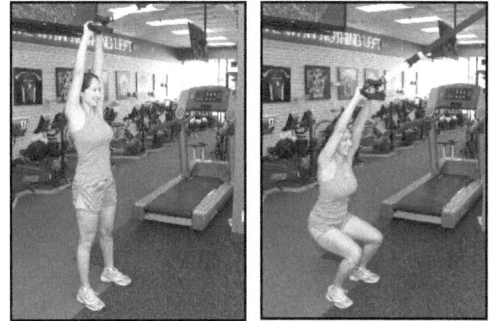

Ski Jumps

1. Face the anchor with a shoulder-width stance, holding one strap in each hand.

2. Keeping your feet close to each other, perform side-to-side hops over the center line.

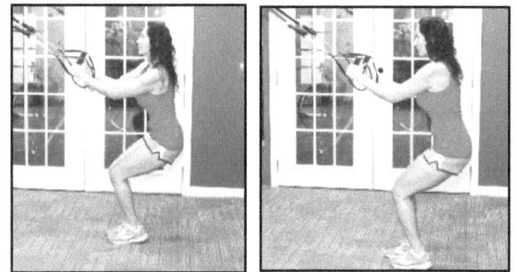

Push-Up (Feet Suspended)

1. Face away from the suspended trainer on your hands and knees, with your toes in the cradles right underneath the anchor. Your hands should be slightly wider than shoulder width, and your thumbs should be aligned with your chest.

2. Start by straightening your legs, which will lift your knees off the ground. Keep your body straight, and go down until your elbows bend to approximately a ninety-degree angle.

3. At the bottom, push through the floor to raise your body back up to the starting position as one unit.

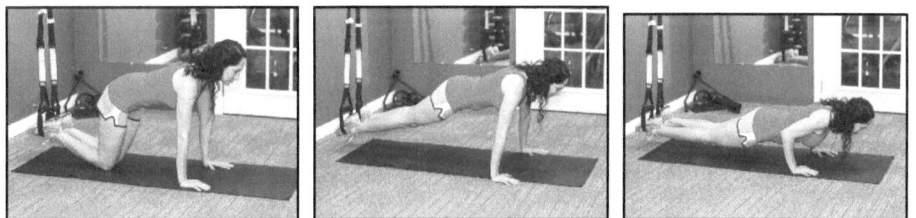

Squat to Reverse Fly

1. Face the anchor and hold the straps with a slightly wider than shoulder-width stance.

2. With straight arms, sit down into the squat as low as you are comfortable with.

3. At the bottom, push back up and extend your arms out to the side until they're in line with your shoulders.

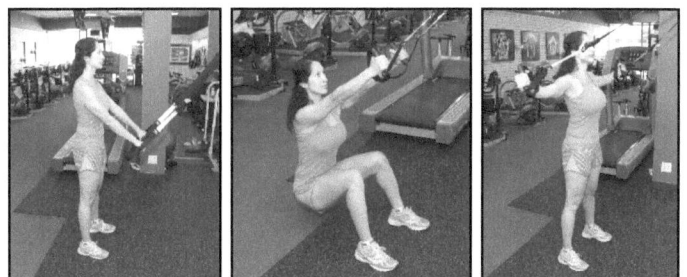

Lunge to Fly

Face away from the anchor and hold the straps out in front of you with your arms extended.

1. Take a big step forward with one foot, and drop the back knee down toward the floor to go down into the lunge. At the same time, allow the arms to open and move from the front to the side.

2. To come back up, push back up through the front leg and squeeze the muscles in your chest to bring your arms back together in front of you.

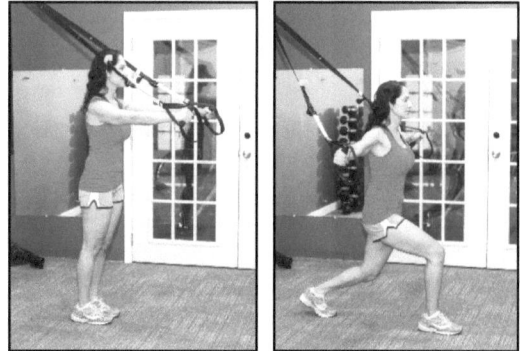

Cardio Activities: Choose from the following based on space and equipment available.

Stairs	Jumping Rope	Jogging	High-Knee Running
Stationary Machine	Jumping Jacks	Side Shuffle	Shuttle Run
Kickboxing	Punching-Bag Work	Dynamic Stretches	Front and Backpedal

The goal is to challenge your cardiovascular system and get your heart rate up for the time assigned. Pick something you enjoy, and don't be afraid to mix it up!

Suspended Get-Ups

1. Begin seated on the floor facing the anchor of the suspension trainer, holding the straps. Extend one leg straight in front of you with the other leg bent at the knee.

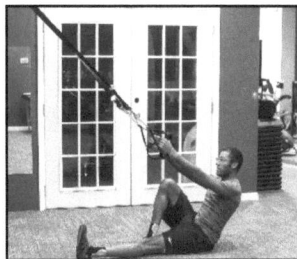

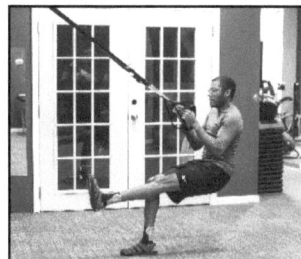

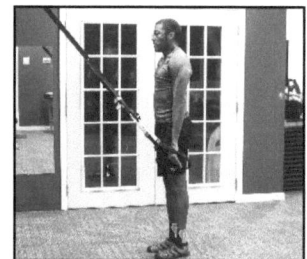

2. Start the movement by pushing through the hip of the bent leg while, simultaneously pulling yourself with your arms. Keep good posture.

3. When you reach the top, your feet will be together. Immediately continue into a tricep extension, straightening the arms until they are fully extended and at your side.

4. To descend back to the starting position on the floor, perform the movement in reverse.

Skaters

1. Face the anchor, holding the straps. Step out to the side with one leg, and drop down into a lateral lunge movement.

2. Push back up through that leg, pushing yourself to the opposite side. Descend toward the floor on other leg and cross the unsupported leg behind you.

3. Push back up through the supported leg and repeat.

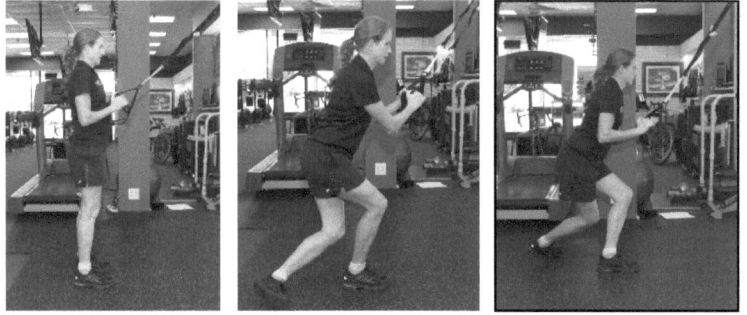

Squat-Press Jump

1. Face away from the anchor, holding the straps at shoulder level.

2. Drop your hips and descend into a squat, keeping your arms in the same position.

3. When you reach the bottom, explode upward while simultaneously pressing your arms up.

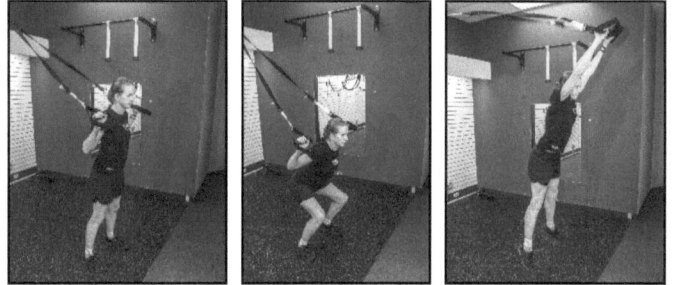

Bone Density Workout Level 1

This is a circuit that can be done by itself as a short workout, or inserted into any other workout to add some impact and high-force work to your routine. Both impact and higher forces generated by the muscles will put strain on the bones to which they are connected. This strain stimulates the bones to increase their strength and density to be able to handle the daily demands placed on them.

I suggest starting with this level 1 circuit. As you improve your fitness, you may be able to progress to the level 2 circuit. Those at a more advanced fitness level may begin with level 2.

Perform a general warm-up of ten minutes, increasing from a moderately easy to moderately hard exertion level.

Level 1 Circuit

Exercise	Targeted Area	Intensity	Sets	Reps	Rest
Suspended Push-Ups	Chest and Shoulders	Heavy	3	8–10	45 seconds
Jump Squat	Legs and Hips	Maximum Power	3	12–15	45 seconds
Suspended Rows	Back and Biceps	Heavy	3	8–10	45 seconds
Jump Rope or Ski Jumps	Full Body	Moderate	3	30 seconds	45 seconds

Suspended Push-Up

1. Facing away, hold the end of each strap in one hand and get into a shoulder-width or slightly wider stance.

2. Allow your arms to bend, and lower your body until your elbows reach ninety degrees and are aligned with your shoulders.

3. Push yourself back up to the straight-arm position, exhaling and maintaining a straight body.

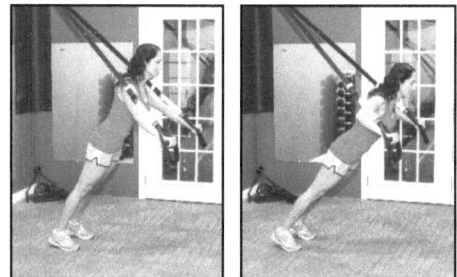

Jump Squat

1. Facing the anchor, hold the straps and stand with your feet a little wider than shoulder width.

2. Keeping the arms relaxed and shoulders back, squat down toward the floor.

3. When you reach the bottom, immediately power back up through the hips and legs and jump as high as you are able.

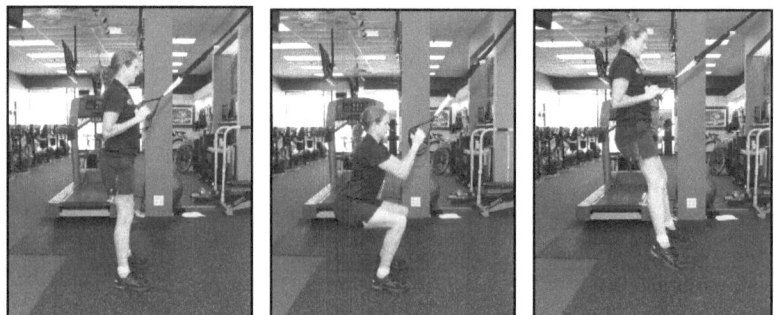

Row

1. Face toward the anchor point, holding the straps. Straighten your arms and lean back.

2. Pull yourself up until your elbows are bent and at your side. Keep your body straight like a board.

3. Lower yourself back down by allowing the arms to straighten out again until you're back in the starting position.

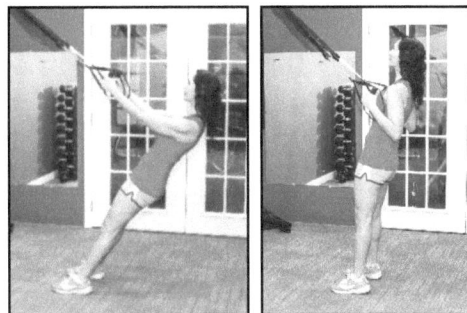

Jump Rope

Jump ropes are inexpensive and easy to transport for use at home, at the gym, or on the road.

Perform this at a moderate pace. If you're not used to jumping rope, start slowly and don't worry about the time as much as getting the feel for the rhythm. If you're comfortable jumping rope, increase your speed and extend the time until you are fatigued.

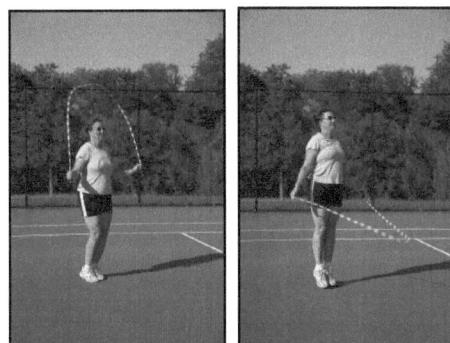

Ski Jumps

1. Face the anchor point with a shoulder-width stance, holding the straps one in each hand.

2. Keeping your feet close to each other, perform side-to-side hops over the center line.

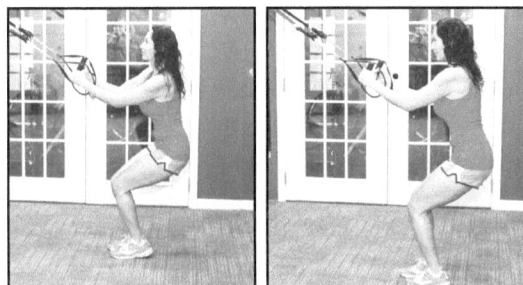

Bone Density Workout Level 2

This is a circuit that can be done by itself as a short workout, or inserted into any other workout to add some impact and high-force work to your routine. Both impact and higher forces generated by the muscles will put strain on the bones to which they're connected. This strain stimulates the bones to increase their strength and density to better handle the daily demands placed on them.

Perform a general warm-up of ten minutes, increasing from a moderately easy to moderately hard exertion level. Include some jump roping if you have one.

Level 1 Circuit

Exercise	Targeted Area	Intensity	Sets	Reps	Rest
Power Push-Ups	Chest and Shoulders	Maximum Power	3	8–10	45 seconds
Split-Squat Jumps	Legs and Hips	Maximum Power	3	12–15	45 seconds
Suspended Pull-Ups	Back and Biceps	Heavy	3	8–10	45 seconds
Squat-Press Jumps	Full Body	Maximum Power	3	30 seconds	45 seconds

Jump Rope

Jump ropes are inexpensive and easy to transport for use at home, at the gym, or on the road. This is part of the warm-up, so do this at a moderate pace if you're not used to jumping rope. If you're comfortable jumping rope, go at a faster speed and extend the time out until you're fatigued. You may also progress to using a weighted rope.

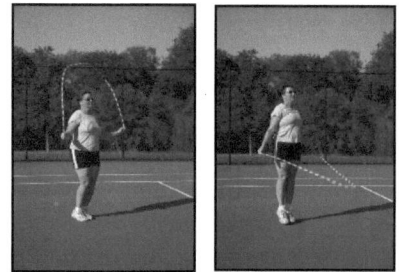

Power Push-Ups

1. Get into your push-up position, and descend until you have a ninety-degree bend in the elbow.

2. Power back up, trying to generate as much force as possible so your hands leave the ground.

3. Catch yourself, control the descent back down, and push up again the same way.

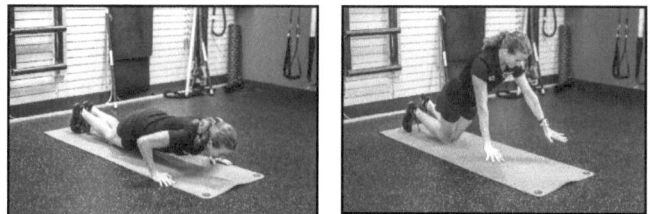

Split-Squat Jump

1. Facing the anchor, hold the straps, and assume a long split-stride position with one leg forward and the other one back behind you.

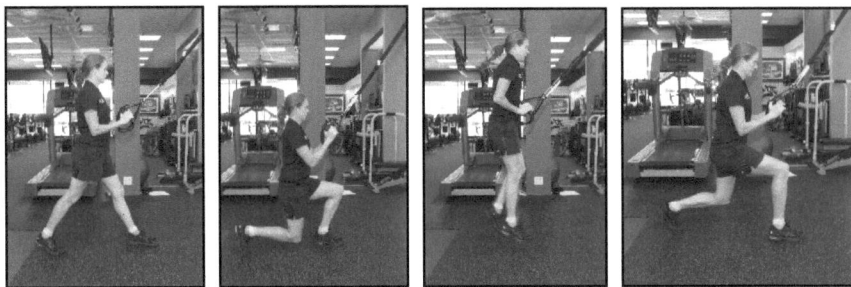

2. Keep the arms relaxed and shoulders back, and drop the back knee down to the floor.

3. When you reach the bottom, immediately power back up through the hips and legs, jump as high as you can, and quickly switch legs while you're in the air. When you land, the leg that was in back is now in front, and vice versa.

Suspended Pull-Up

1. Start by sitting on the floor with your knees bent directly underneath the suspended trainer. Hold the handles with your palms facing away from you.

2. Pull yourself straight up from the floor until your chin is level with your hands. Think about pulling yourself over an imaginary bar.

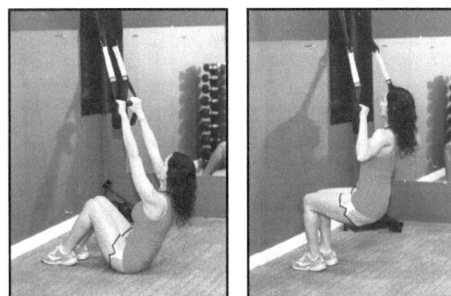

3. Hold your position at the top for a second with good form, and then come back down in a slow, controlled movement.

Squat-Press Jump

1. Face the anchor, holding the straps at shoulder level with a shoulder-width stance.

2. Drop your hips and descend into a squat, keeping your arms in the same position.

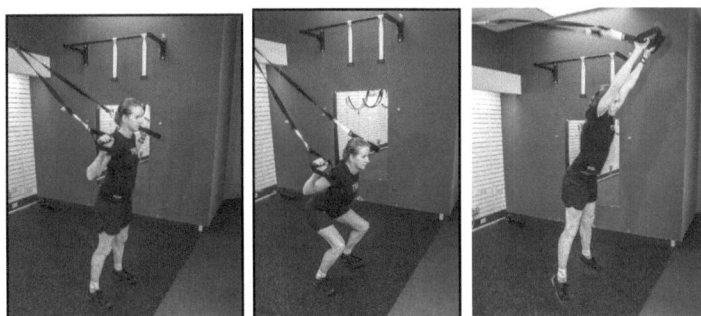

3. When you reach the bottom, explode upward while simultaneously pressing your arms up.

Dynamic Stretch Circuits

Each of these circuits is a balanced selection of three movements targeting different parts of the body. The goal is improvement of both flexibility and stability. They are great as part of a warm-up because they will loosen up your joints, and increase circulation to better prepare you for the workout to come. They're also good to perform between exercises within a workout, or by themselves during active recovery day. Doing some of them after a long day sitting down at the office, or after travel, will help loosen you up and counter the position you may have held for an extended period of time, which will also help prevent detrimental effects on your posture.

Level 1 Circuit

Basic movements that are fundamental to improving the quality of your movement patterns in all endeavors. Master these between progressing to level 2 movements.

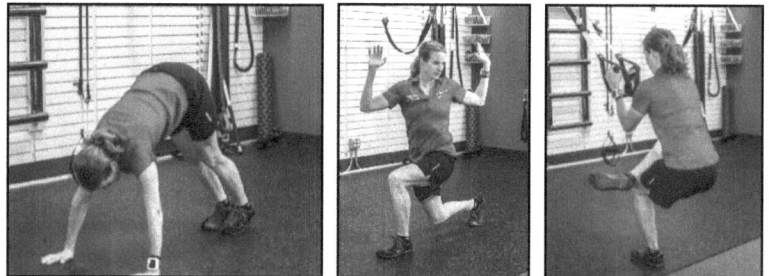

Exercise	Targeted Area	Sets	Reps
Scarecrow Rotation	Upper Torso	1–3	10 each side
Knee Hug	Back of Hips	1–3	10 each side
Quad Stretch Walk	Front of Hips	1–3	10 each side

Level 2 Circuit

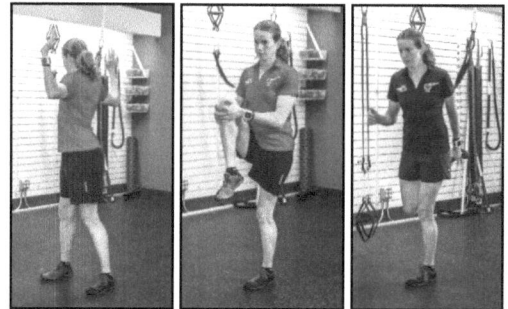

This contains more complex movements requiring greater levels of both stability and mobility that build on the level 1 movements.

Exercise	Targeted Area	Sets	Reps
Inchworms	Hamstrings and Calves	3	6–8
Lunge and Rotate	Torso and Front of Hip Flexors	3	6–8 each side
Hip Drop	Glutes and Hips	3	8–10 each side

CYCLING-SPECIFIC STRENGTH WORKOUT

These circuits are short workouts that can be done alone, in combination with endurance workouts, or extended to longer workouts by adding more movements. Each circuit consists of a pushing, pulling, leg, and core movement. The level 1 circuit is appropriate for all levels. The level 2 circuit contains more advanced movements, and is for intermediate and advanced levels. If you're just starting a strength routine, you will benefit most by mastering the foundation workout first.

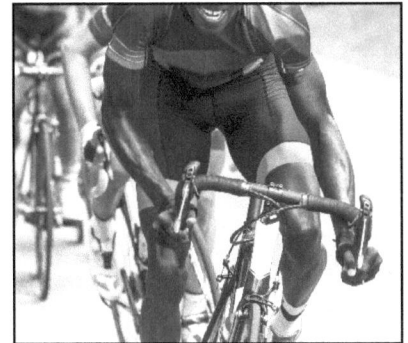

Although these workouts are cycling specific, they're not necessarily specific to where you are in your season, or your cycling discipline. Keep this in mind and adjust as needed to fit your program. See chapter 11 for more information on how to do this. These circuits are merely suggestions. Don't limit yourself to them or be afraid to substitute and progress movements. I chose to base the sets on time. Focus on intensity and quality of repetitions over how many you can get in during the time. You may also choose to base your sets on repetitions.

Frequency: Twice per week, in combination with additional endurance and flexibility training sessions

Warm up with fifteen minutes on a stationary bike or trainer if possible. Include three thirty-second spin-ups of high resistance and high cadence to get the oxygen levels higher in your muscles and your heart rate up.

Level 1

Exercise	Targeted Area	Intensity	Sets	Time	Rest
Suspended Push-Ups	Chest and Shoulders	Moderate/Hard	2–3	20 seconds	30 seconds
Suspended Row	Back and Biceps	Moderate/Hard	2–3	20 seconds	for all
Sprinter Start	Legs and Hips	Moderate/Hard	2–3	20 seconds	or as
Half Get-Ups	Core	Moderate/Hard	2–3	20 seconds	needed

Level 2

Exercise	Targeted Area	Intensity	Sets	Time	Rest
Bear Crawls (Forward and Backward)	Chest, Shoulders, and Core	Hard	2–3	20 seconds	30 seconds
Assisted Pull-Up	Back and Biceps	Hard	2–3	20 seconds	for all
Single-Leg Squats	Legs and Hips	Hard	2–3	20 seconds each	or as
Side Plank	Core	Hard	2–3	20–60 seconds each	needed

*Side plank may be done grounded or suspended.

Cooldown: Easy spin on stationary bike or trainer if possible. Aim for a higher cadence of ninety-plus RPMs for ten to fifteen minutes. This is important to remind the muscles what they're training for! Add stretches if you have tight areas as needed.

RUNNING-SPECIFIC STRENGTH WORKOUT

These circuits are short workouts that can be done alone, in combination with endurance workouts, or extended to longer workouts by adding more movements. Each circuit consists of a pushing, pulling, leg, and core movement. The level 1 circuit is appropriate for all levels. The level 2 circuit contains more advanced movements and is for intermediate and advanced levels. If you're just starting a strength routine, you will benefit most by mastering the foundation workout first.

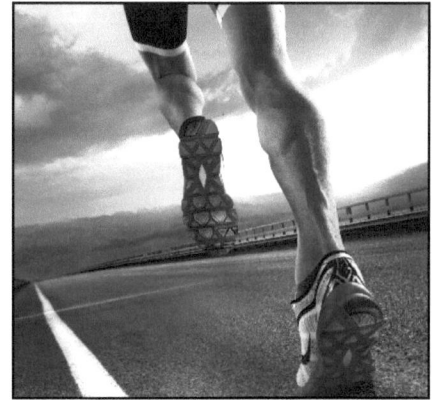

These exercises are selected with the demands of running in mind. They are primarily focused on maintaining strong run mechanics in the upper and lower body, particularly during the single-leg stance. Although these workouts are running specific, they're not necessarily specific to where you are in your season or the exact type of running in which you participate. Keep this in mind and adjust as needed to fit your program. See chapter 12 for more information on how to do this. These circuits are merely suggestions. Don't limit yourself to them or be afraid to substitute and progress movements. I chose to base the sets on time. Focus on intensity and quality of repetitions over how many you can get in during the time. You may also choose to base your sets on repetitions.

Frequency: Twice per week in combination with additional endurance and flexibility training sessions.

Warm up with ten minutes of easy jogging and some dynamic stretches. Include two to three sets of strides or short periods of faster running to get the oxygen levels higher in your muscles and get your heart rate up.

Level 1

Exercise	Targeted Area	Intensity	Sets	Time	Rest
Suspended Push-Ups	Chest and Shoulders	Moderate/Hard	2–3	20	30 seconds
Suspended Row	Back and Biceps	Moderate/Hard	2–3	20	for all
Reverse or Crossover Lunge	Legs and Hips	Moderate/Hard	2–3	20	or as
Plank	Core	Moderate/Hard	2–3	20 seconds	needed

Level 2

Exercise	Targeted Area	Intensity	Sets	Time	Rest
Push-Ups (Feet Suspended)	Chest, Shoulders, and Core	Hard	2–3	20 seconds total	30 seconds
Single-Arm Rows	Back and Biceps	Hard	2–3	20 seconds	for all
Suspended Reverse Lunge or Power Lunge	Legs and Hips	Hard	2–3	20 seconds each	or as
Atomic Crunches	Core	Hard	2–3	20–60 seconds	needed

Cooldown: Perform some additional stretches in areas needed. This workout may be followed up with or preceded by an endurance workout as part of your program.

That's everything!

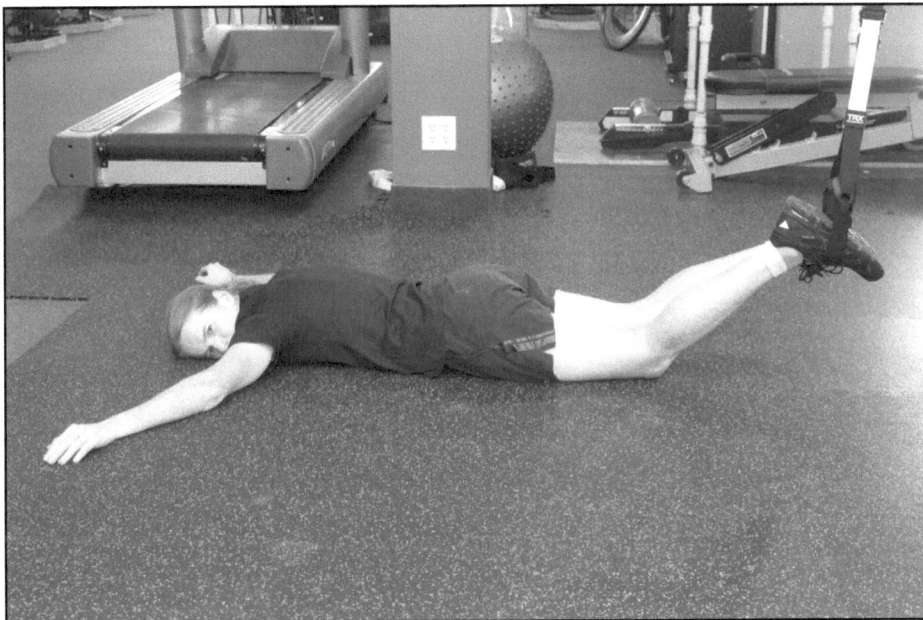

References

Chapter 1

1. Byrne, Jeannette M., Bishop, Nicole S., Caines, Andrew M., Crane, Kalynn A., Feaver, Ashley M. Pearcey, and E. P. Gregory. "Effect of Using a Suspended Training System on Muscle Activation during the Performance of a Front Plank Exercise." *Journal of Strength and Conditioning Research* Vol. 28 (November 2014): 3049–3055.

2. Kibele, Armin, and David G. Behm. "Seven Weeks of Instability and Traditional Resistance Training Effects on Strength, Balance and Functional Performance." *Journal of Strength and Conditioning Research* Vol. 0 (October 2009) 1–8.

3. Snarr, Ronald L., and Michael R. Esco. "Electromyographical Comparison of Plank Variations Performed with and without Instability Devices." *Journal of Strength and Conditioning Research* Vol. 28 (November 2014) 3298–3305.

4. Gillette, Mike. *Rings of Power: The Secrets of Successful Suspended Training.* St Paul, MN: Dragon Door Publications, Inc., 2015.

Chapter 5

1. Fleck, Steven J. "Periodized Strength Training: A Critical Review." *Journal of Strength and Conditioning Research* Vol. 13 (January 1999) 82–89.

Chapter 6

1. Stone, Michael H., and Michael S. Conley. *Essential of Strength Training and Conditioning.* Champaign, IL: Human Kinetics, 1994. Chapter 5.

2. Schoenfeld, Brad, and Jay Dawes. "High-Intensity Interval Training: Applications for General Fitness Training." *Strength and Conditioning Journal* Vol. 41 (December 2009): 44–46.

Chapter 7

1. Mohamad, Nur Ikhwan, Kazunori Nosaka, and John Cronin. "Maximizing Hypertrophy: Possible Contribution of Stretching in the Interset Rest Period." *Strength and Conditioning Journal* Vol. 33 (February 2011): 81–85.

2. Mohamad, Nur Ikhwan, Kazunori Nosaka, and John Cronin. "Brief Review: Maximizing Hypertrophic Adaptation—Possible Contributions of Aerobic Exercise in the Interset Rest Period." *Strength and Conditioning Journal* Vol. 34 (February 2012): 8–15

3. Sooneste, Heiki, Tanimo. "Effects of Training Volume on Strength and Hypertrophy in Young Men." *Journal of Strength and Conditioning Research* Vol. 27 (January 2013): 8–13.

4. Hedrick, Allen. "Training for Hypertrophy." *Strength and Conditioning Journal* Vol. 17 (June 1995): 22–29.

5. Krieger, James W. "Brief Review: Single vs. Multiple Sets of Resistance Exercise for Muscle Hypertrophy: A Meta-Analysis." *Journal of Strength and Conditioning Research* Vol. 24 (April 2010): 1150–1159.

6. Kilen, Anders, Line B. Hjelvang, Niels Dall, Nanna L. Kruse, and Nikolai B. Nordsborg. "Adaptations to Short, Frequent Sessions of Endurance and Strength Training Are Similar to Longer, Less Frequent Exercise Sessions When the Total Volume Is the Same." *Journal of Strength and Conditioning Research* Vol. 20 (November 2015): S46–S51.

7. Willardson, Jeffrey M. "A Brief Review: How Much Rest between Sets?" *Strength and Conditioning Journal* Vol. 30 (June 2008): 44–49.

Chapter 8

1. National Institute of Arthritis and Musculoskeletal and Skin Diseases. "*Osteoporosis*."

http://www.niams.nih.gov/health_info/bone/osteoporosis/.

2. National Osteoporosis Foundation. "*Prevention: Who's at Risk?*"

https://www.nof.org/prevention/general-facts/bone-basics/are-you-at-risk/.

3. Conroy, Brian P., and Roger W. Earle. *Essentials of Strength and Conditioning NSCA*. Champaign, IL: Human Kinetics. Chapter 4.

4. Brentano, Michel A., Eduardo L. Cadore, Eduardo M. Da Silva, Anelise B. Ambrosini, M. Coertjens, Rosemary Petkowicz, Itamara Viero, and Luiz F. M. Kruel. "Physiological Adaptations to Strength and Circuit Training in Postmenopausal Women with Bone Loss." *Journal of Strength and Conditioning Research* Vol. 22 (November 2008): 1816–1825.

5. Donald A. Chu. *Jumping into Plyometrics*. Champaign, IL: Human Kinetics, 1998.

6. Mosti, Mats P., Nils Kaehler, Astrid K. Stunes, Jan Hoff, and Unni Syversen. "Maximal Strength Training in Postmenopausal Women with Osteoporosis or Osteopenia." *Journal of Strength and Conditioning Research* Vol. 27 (October 2013): 2879–2886.

7. Almstedt, Hawley C., Jacqueline A. Canepa, David A. Ramirez, and Todd C. Shoepe. "Changes in Bone Mineral Density in Response to 24 Weeks of Resistance Training in College-Age Men and Women." *Journal of Strength and Conditioning Research* Vol. 25 (April 2011): 1098–1103.

8. Scofield, K. L., and S. Hecht. "Bone Health in Endurance Athletes: Runners, Cyclists, and Swimmers." *Current Sports Medicine Reports* Vol. 11 (November–December 2012): 328–334.

9. Lanye, Jennifer E., and Miriam E. Nelson. "The Effects of Progressive Resistance Training on Bone Density: A Review." *Medicine & Science in Sports & Exercise* Vol. 31 (January 1999): 25–30.

10. Nichols, Jeanne F., and Mitchell J. Rauh. "Longitudinal Changes in Bone Mineral Density in Male Master Cyclists and Nonathletes." *Journal of Strength and Conditioning Research* Vol. 25 (March 2011): 727–734.

11. Olmedillas Hugo, Alejandro González-Agüero Luis A. Moreno, José A. Casajus, and Germán Vicente-Rodríguez. "Cycling and Bone Health: A Systematic Review." *BMC Medicine* (December 2012).

Chapter 9

1. Knudson, Duane. "Program Stretching After Vigorous Physical Training." *Strength and Conditioning Journal* Vol. 32 (December 2010): 55–57.

2. Sands, William A., Jeni R. McNeal, and Steven R. Murray. "Stretching and Its Effects on Recovery: A Review." *Strength and Conditioning Journal* Vol. 35 (October 2013): 30–34.

3. Armiger, P., and M. A. Martyn. *Stretching for Functional Flexibility*. Baltimore, MD: Lippincott Williams and Wilkins, 2010.

4. Mark Kovacs. *Dynamic Stretching*. Berkeley, CA: Ulysses Press, 2010.

Chapter 11

1. Yamamoto, Linda M., Jennifer F. Klau, Douglas J. Casa, William J. Kraemer, Lawrence E. Armstrong, and Carl M. Maresh. "The Effects of Resistance Training on Road Cycling Performance Among Highly Trained Cyclists: A Systematic Review." *Journal of Strength and Conditioning Research* Vol. 24 (February 2010): 560–566.

2. Paton, Carl D., and William G. Hopkins. "Combining Explosive and High Resistance Training Improves Performance in Competitive Cyclists." *Journal of Strength and Conditioning Research* Vol. 19 (April 2005): 826–830.

3. Jackson, Nathaniel P., Matthew S. Hickey, and Raoul F. Reiser. "High Resistance/Low Repetition vs. Low Resistance/High Repetition Training: Effects on Performance of Trained Cyclists." *Journal of Strength and Conditioning Research* Vol. 21 (January 2007): 289–295.

4. Bastiaans, J. J., A. B. van Diemen, T. Veneberg, and A. E. Jeukendrup. "The Effects of Replacing a Portion of Endurance Training by Explosive Strength Training on Performance in Trained Cyclists." *European Journal of Applied Physiology* Vol. 86 (November 2001): 79–84.

5. Bishop, D., D. G. Jenkins, L. T. Mackinnon, M. McEniery, and M. F. Carey. "The Effects of Strength Training on Endurance Performance and Muscle Characteristics." *Medicine & Science in Sports & Exercise* Vol. 31 (June 1999): 886–891.

6. Hickson, R. C., B. A. Dvorak, E. M. Gorostiaga, T. T. Kurowski, and C. Foster. "Potential for Strength and Endurance Training to Amplify Endurance Performance." *Journal of Applied Physiology* Vol. 65 (November 1988): 2285–2290.

7. Rønnestad, B. R., J. Hansen, I. Hollan, and S. Ellefsen. "Strength Training Improves Performance and Pedaling Characteristics in Elite Cyclists." *Scandinavian Journal of Medicine & Science in Sports* Vol. 25 (April 2015): e89–e98.

8. Segerström, Åsa B., Anna M. Holmbäck, Targ Elzyri, Karl-Fredrik Eriksson, Karin Ringsberg, Leif Groop, Ola Thorsson, and Per Wollmer. "Upper Body Muscle Strength and Endurance in Relation to Peak Exercise Capacity during Cycling in Healthy Sedentary Male Subjects." *Journal of Strength and Conditioning Research* Vol. 25 (May 2011): 1413–1417.

9. Maldonado, B. *Preferred Movement Patterns in Cycling*. Minneapolis: Langdon Street Press, 2010.

Chapter 12

1. Piacentini MF, De Ioannon G, Comotto S, Spedicato A, Vernillo G, La Torre A.. "Concurrent Strength and Endurance Training Effects on Running Economy in Master Endurance Runners." *Journal of Strength & Conditioning Research* Vol 27(August 2013): 2295-2303.

2. Støren, O., J. Helgerud, E. M. Støa, and J. Hoff. "Maximal strength training improves running economy in distance runners." *Medicine & Science in Sports & Exercise* (June 2008): 1089-1084.

3. Sato, Kimitake and Moniqu Mokha. "Does Core Strength Training Influence Running Kinetics, Lower-Extremity Stability, and 5000-m Performance in Runners?" *Journal of Strength & Conditioning Research* Vol 23 (January 2009):133-140

4. Esteve-Lanao, Jonathan, Matthew R. Rhea, Steven J. Fleck, Lucia, Alejandro "Running-Specific Periodized Strength Training Attenuates Loss of Stride Length During Intense Endurance Running." *Journal of Strength & Conditioning Research* Vol 22(July 2008): 1176-1183.

5. Berryman, Nicolas, Delphine Maurel, and Laurent Bosquet. "Effect of Plyometric vs. Dynamic Weight Training on the Energy Cost of Running." *Journal of Strength & Conditioning Research* Vol 24(July 2008): 1818-1825.

6. Sedano, Silvia, Pedro J. Marín, Gonzalo Cuadrado, and Juan C. Redondo. "Concurrent Training in Elite Male Runners: The Influence of Strength Versus Muscular Endurance Training on Performance Outcomes." *Journal of Strength & Conditioning Research* Vol 27(September 2013): 2433-2443.

7. Saunders PU, Telford RD, Pyne DB, Peltola EM, Cunningham RB, Gore CJ, Hawley JA. "Short Term Plyometric Training Improves Running Economy in Highly Trained Middle and Long Distance Runners." *Journal of Strength & Conditioning Research* Vol 20(November 2006): 947-954.

8. Taipale, R. S., J. Mikkola, A. Nummela, V. Vesterinen, B. Capostagno, S. Walker, D. Gitonga, W. J. Kraemer, and K. Häkkinen. "Strength training in endurance runners." *International Journal of Sports Medicine* (July 2010).

9. Zouita S,Zouita AB, Kebsi W, Dupont G, Ben Abderrahman A, Ben Salah FZ, Zouhal H. "Strength Training Reduces Injury Rate in Elite Young Soccer Players During One Season." *Journal of Strength & Conditioning Research* Vol 30(May 2016): 1295-1307

Index

ABOUT THE AUTHOR

Tracy holds a B.S. in Biology and an M.S. in Human Performance from the University of Wisconsin at La Crosse, and is a certified strength and conditioning specialist (CSCS) through the NSCA. Tracy is a Level 2 USA Cycling coach and a Level 1 USA Triathlon coach. She holds a Level 2 Functional Movement Systems screening certification, which enables her to examine and assess basic movement patterns for dysfunction and make corrections. She also holds a TRX® Suspension Training Advanced Group certification.

In her spare time, Tracy's personal passion is training and competing in triathlons, road races, and criteriums. She has several age-group wins and podiums in triathlons, and podiums in the Texas Racing Cup series for cycling. She currently lives in Dallas with her husband, who runs Cycling Center Dallas, a wattage-based training facility for cyclists and triathletes. They share their house with many bikes, two crazy dogs, and one plant.

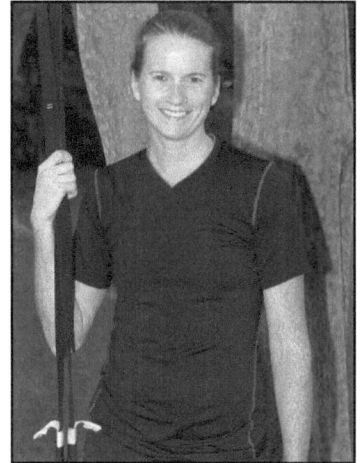

www.ingramcontent.com/pod-product-compliance
Lightning Source LLC
Chambersburg PA
CBHW041419290326
41932CB00042B/17